Advances in Clinical Dentistry

Advances in Clinical Dentistry

Editor: Dave Clark

FOSTER ACADEMICS

www.fosteracademics.com

www.fosteracademics.com

FOSTER ACADEMICS

Cataloging-in-Publication Data

Advances in clinical dentistry / edited by Dave Clark.
p. cm.
Includes bibliographical references and index.
ISBN 978-1-63242-500-3
1. Dentistry. 2. Dental therapeutics. 3. Dental care. 4. Teeth--Diseases. I. Clark, Dave.
RK61 .A38 2017
617.6--dc23

Foster Academics,
118-35 Queens Blvd., Suite 400,
Forest Hills, NY 11375, USA

ISBN 978-1-63242-500-3 (Hardback)

Printed and bound in China.

Contents

Preface

Dentistry refers to practice of diagnosing, preventing and treating the various disorders related to oral cavity, dentition and oral mucosa. The varied branches of dentistry include forensic odontology, dental public health, oral implantology, periodontology, orthodontics, etc. This book unfolds the innovative aspects of oral healthcare and dentistry which will be crucial for the progress of this field in the future. The various advancements in this area are glanced at and their applications as well as ramifications are looked at in detail in the text. With state-of-the-art inputs by acclaimed experts of this field, the book targets students and professionals. It will help new researchers by foregrounding their knowledge in this branch.

After months of intensive research and writing, this book is the end result of all who devoted their time and efforts in the initiation and progress of this book. It will surely be a source of reference in enhancing the required knowledge of the new developments in the area. During the course of developing this book, certain measures such as accuracy, authenticity and research focused analytical studies were given preference in order to produce a comprehensive book in the area of study.

This book would not have been possible without the efforts of the authors and the publisher. I extend my sincere thanks to them. Secondly, I express my gratitude to my family and well-wishers. And most importantly, I thank my students for constantly expressing their willingness and curiosity in enhancing their knowledge in the field, which encourages me to take up further research projects for the advancement of the area.

Editor

1

Amelogenesis Imperfecta and Generalized Gingival Overgrowth Resembling Hereditary Gingival Fibromatosis in Siblings: A Case Report

Emre Yaprak,[1] Meryem Gülce Subaşı,[2] Mustafa Avunduk,[3] and Filiz Aykent[4]

[1] *Department of Periodontology, Faculty of Dentistry, Kocaeli University, Kocaeli, Turkey*
[2] *Department of Prosthodontics, Faculty of Dentistry, Aydın University, İzzettin Çalışlar Cad., No. 31/A, Bahçelievler, İstanbul, Turkey*
[3] *Department of Pathology, Meram Faculty of Medicine, Necmettin Erbakan University, Konya, Turkey*
[4] *Department of Prosthodontics, Faculty of Dentistry, Selcuk University, Konya, Turkey*

Correspondence should be addressed to Meryem Gülce Subaşı, gulce2subasi@yahoo.co.uk

Academic Editors: D. Ram and J. J. Segura-Egea

Amelogenesis imperfecta (AI) is a group of hereditary disorders primarily characterized by developmental abnormalities in the quantity and/or quality of enamel. There are some reports suggesting an association between AI and generalized gingival enlargement. This paper describes the clinical findings and oral management of two siblings presenting both AI and hereditary gingival fibromatosis (HGF) like generalized gingival enlargements. The treatment of gingival enlargements by periodontal flap surgery was successful in the management of the physiologic gingival form for both patients in the 3-year follow-up period. Prosthetic treatment was also satisfactory for the older patient both aesthetically and functionally.

1. Introduction

Amelogenesis imperfecta (AI) is a group of hereditary disorders primarily characterized by developmental abnormalities in the quantity and/or quality of enamel, such as hypoplasia, hypomaturation, and/or hypocalcification [1, 2]. Dental anomalies such as multiple impacted teeth, failed tooth eruption, congenitally missing teeth, open occlusal relationship, taurodontism [3–8], pulpal calcification, hypercementosis, root or crown resorption, and root malformations [9–13] can be detected in AI patients.

Teeth attrition can be observed as a result of AI [14, 15]. Dentin hypersensitivity and decreased occlusal vertical dimension due to attrition causes a restrictive effect on teeth function and individual oral hygiene applications. Unaesthetic appearance is also disturbing factor for the AI patients, because of both color defects and shape abnormalities [16, 17]. Witkop's classification which, based on clinical and hereditary conditions, is the most frequently used among various classifications of AI [18–24].

Hereditary gingival fibromatosis (HGF) is a rare disorder characterized by the proliferate fibrous overgrowth of the gingival tissue that can occur as an isolated disease or as part of a syndrome or chromosomal abnormality [25, 26]. There are some reports suggesting an association between AI and gingival enlargement [12, 27–31]. However, the certain mechanism of the association of AI and gingival overgrowth remains in suspense.

This paper describes the rehabilitations of two female siblings presenting AI and HGF like generalized gingival enlargement.

2. Case Presentation

Systemically healthy 12 and 19 years old female siblings, complaining of insufficient chewing functions due to hypersensitivity of the teeth and esthetic problems because of both gingival enlargement and the color of the teeth were admitted to the Periodontology Clinics at the Faculty of Dentistry,

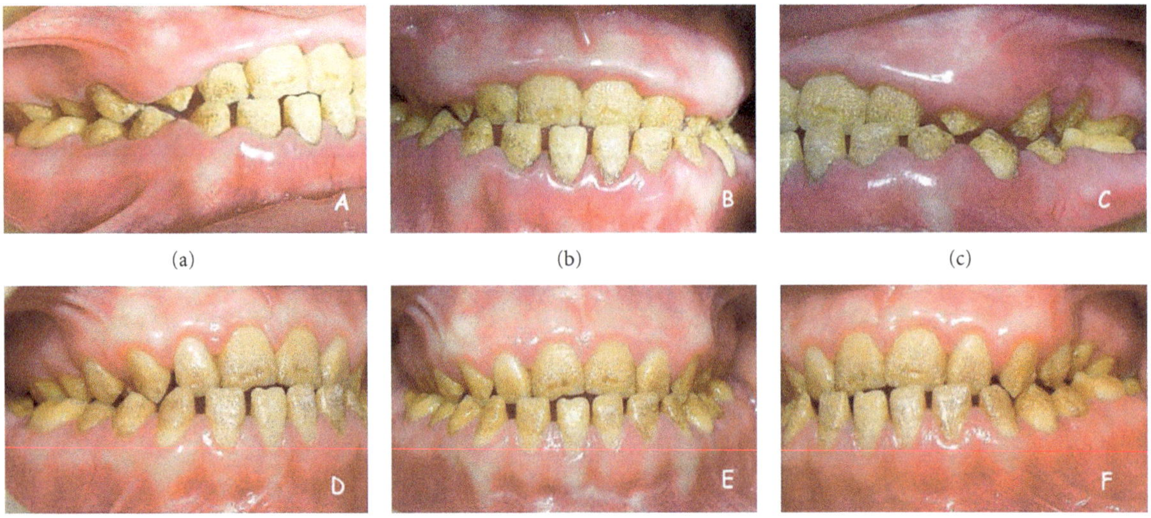

(a) (b) (c)

(d) (e) (f)

Figure 1: Initial aspect of the 12-year-old patient displays diffuse gingival enlargements covering almost all teeth ((a), (b), and (c)). Appropriate gingival form is established by periodontal flap surgery and maintained for 3 years ((d), (e), and (f)).

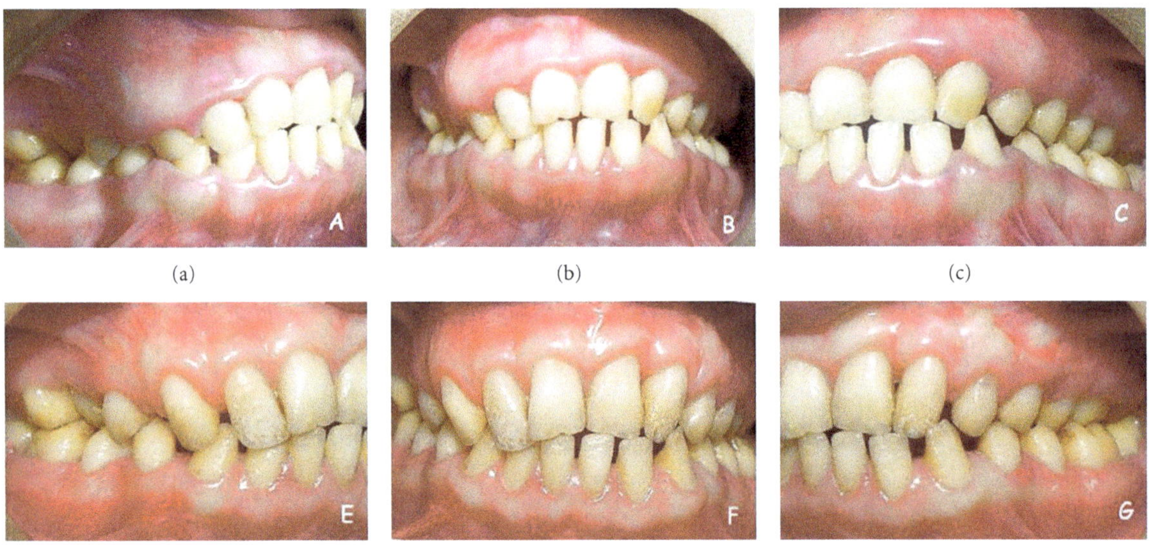

(a) (b) (c)

(d) (e) (f)

Figure 2: Initial appearance of 19-year-old patient presents more mild gingival enlargements comparing with her younger sibling ((a), (b), and (c)). Appropriate gingival form is constituted by periodontal flap surgery at the 3rd month before prosthetic treatment ((d), (e), and (f)).

Selcuk University. Medical conditions of the patients were normal and there were no signs of any syndrome. Intraoral examination of both patients revealed yellowish-brown, rough, and atypical enamel formation. Generalized fibrotic gingival enlargements with secondary inflammation covering almost all teeth were also seen. Clinical crown lengths were short because of AI and diffuse gingival enlargement in both patients (Figures 1(a), 1(b), and 1(c)) and Figures 2(a), 2(b), and 2(c). However, these findings were more severe in the younger sister. O'Leary plaque index [32] was found 83% in younger and 71% in older patient. Radiographic examination showed normal dentin formation and pulp chamber, but enamel appeared to be thin in each patient (Figure 3). The other family members were examined except grand-parents and no familial occurrence of AI or gingival hyperplasia was observed.

Clinical findings determined the diagnosis as a pitted hypoplastic type of amelogenesis imperfecta in younger and a rough hypoplastic type of amelogenesis imperfecta in older patient. Histological investigations showed

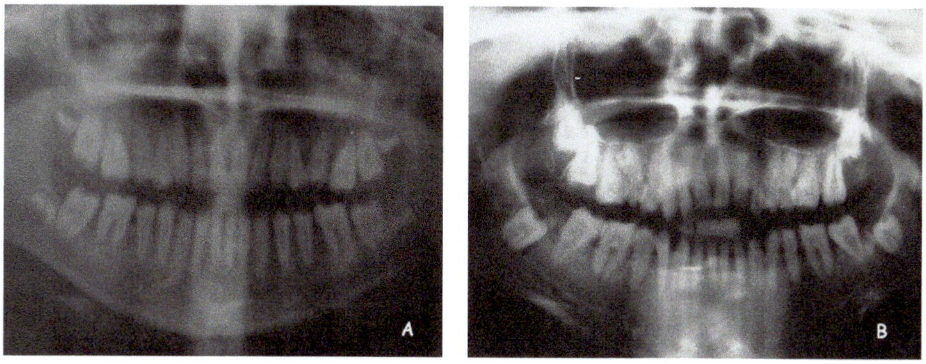

(a) (b)

FIGURE 3: Panoramic radiography shows reduction of enamel thickness for younger (a) and older (b) patients.

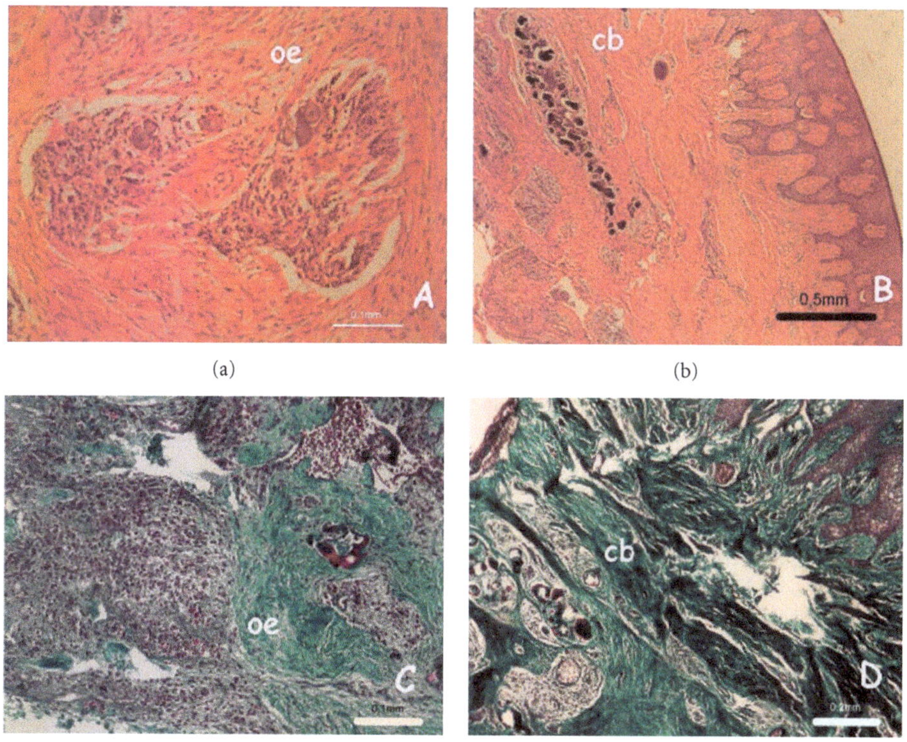

(c) (d)

FIGURE 4: Odontogenic epithelium (oe), and calcified bodies (cb) were seen in hematoxylin and eosin ((a) and (b)) and Masson's trichrome ((c) and (d)) stainings of younger ((a) and (c)) and older ((b) and (d)) patients.

mononuclear inflammatory infiltrate, calcified bodies, and odontogenic epithelium in a dens-fibrovascular-connective tissue (Figure 4). Because of fibrotic appearance, hereditary pattern, and histological character, the lesions were described as HGF like gingival enlargements with secondary inflammatory involvement for both patients.

The reduction of the gingival inflammation which was the main objective of the initial periodontal therapy was realized by oral hygiene motivation, scaling and root planning. Dental hypersensitivity limiting the plaque control was removed by fluoride gel applications and fluoride mouth washes. After obtaining an adequate hygiene and reduction of inflammation, excessive gingival tissues were excised by internal bevel incision with full-thickness flap elevation under local anesthesia. Maxillary and mandibular labial frenectomy and vestibuloplasty applications were done also during the surgery. In addition, some alveolar bone resection was applied to the right upper quadrant of the older patient. Thus, physiological gingival form and sufficient crown lengthening were constituted before the prosthetic treatment. In the follow-up period, at 3rd year, there was no sign for recurrence of gingival enlargement in both patients (Figures 1(d), 1(e), and 1(f) and Figure 5(b)).

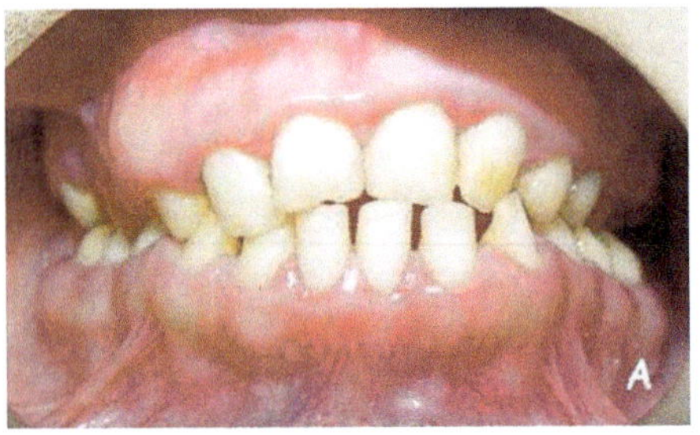

(a)

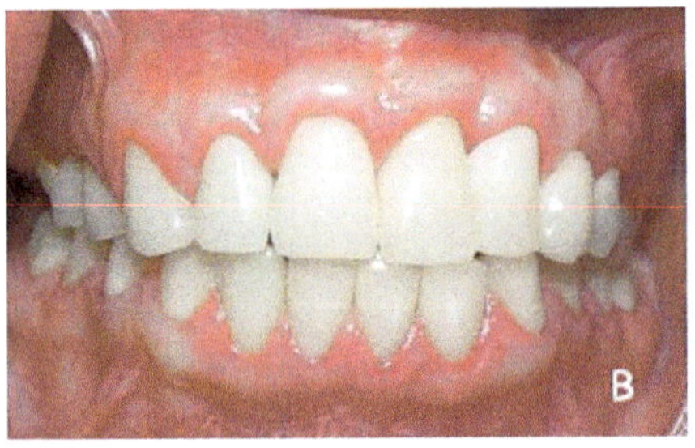

(b)

Figure 5: Preoperative (a) and the final (b) intra oral appearances of 19-year-old patient at the 3rd year.

After the periodontal therapy, two siblings were oriented to the department of prosthodontics. Clinical examination of younger patient revealed Angle Class III dental relationship, posterior cross-bite, pitted enamel defect, teeth attrition, and low vertical dimension. The older patient had Angle Class I dental relationship, posterior cross-bite, yellowish-brown teeth, rough enamel surface, teeth hypersensitivity, multiple diastema and normal occlusal vertical dimension. Radiographic examination of each patient, showed reduction of enamel. In the older patient as well as enamel wear maxillary right canine was congenitally missing. Both patients were diagnosed hypoplastic amelogenesis imperfecta. Since the younger patient did not complete developmental period, prosthodontic treatment was delayed.

For the older patient, residual maxillary right primary canine was extracted, maxillary right lateral, mandibular left, and right first molar teeth received endodontic treatment. Full mouth all-ceramic fixed partial dentures (Zirconia FPDs) were planned to maintain more effective chewing function and also to obtain a better aesthetic appearance. Maxillary and mandibular anterior and posterior teeth were prepared for full ceramic restorations. To prevent the exposition of the pulp mandibular, four incisors were prepared creating a chamfer cervical finish line and the others were prepared with a rounded shoulder finish line. After completion of the preparations, gingival retraction was made and definitive impressions were made using a vinyl polysiloxane impression material (Elite H-D; Zhermack, Rovigo, Italy). Laboratory processed provisional restorations were cemented with noneugenol temporary cement (Temp Bond NE; Kerr, Salerno, Italy). The maxillary and mandibular casts with trimmed dies of prepared teeth were obtained from the type 4 dental stone (Elite Rock; Zhermack, Rovigo, Italy). Then the casts were mounted onto an articulator (Stratos 100; Ivoclar Vivadent, Schaan, Liechtenstein) using interocclusal records. Maxillary anterior right 4-unit zirconia FPD and 23 zirconia crowns were fabricated. The patient's natural occlusal scheme (right side group functional occlusion, left side canine protected occlusion) and anterior guidance were preserved in the definitive restorations. The crowns evaluated intraorally, adjusted, and cemented with a resin cement (Multilink; Ivoclar-Vivadent, Schaan, Liechtenstein). Postoperative care instructions were given to the patient on home care and periodic call visits. After the prosthetic treatment, the patient was satisfied both functionally and aesthetically (Figure 5(b)). Recall evaluations at 6-month intervals were performed for a period of 3 years. In the follow-up period, at 3rd year there was no sign for recurrence of gingival enlargement in both patients.

3. Discussion

This paper described two female siblings presenting both AI and HGF like generalized gingival enlargements. The treatment of gingival overgrowth by periodontal flap surgery was successful in the management of the physiologic gingival form and the constitution of crown lengthening before prosthetic treatment.

In the literature, there are case reports presenting an association between AI and gingival enlargement and most of these [12, 27–31, 33] reported a gingival enlargement accompanied with AI as an inflammatory gingival hyperplasia due to rough surface of the enamel increasing bacterial plaque accumulation. Histological findings similar to these reports such as mononuclear inflammatory infiltrate, calcified-bodies and odontogenic epithelium in a dens-fibrovascular-connective tissue, and ulceration of mucosa were also seen in current paper. Although Macedo et al. [33] considered these findings as occasional, these histological findings can be seen in HGF [34, 35].

This paper suggests an association between AI and HGF like overgrowth based on histological, clinical findings, and also hereditary pattern of siblings. A former report had a hypothesis that rough enamel surface due to AI increases bacterial plaque accumulation and this accumulation causes inflammatory gingival hyperplasia [33]. This consideration is fairly reasonable, but, however, there are many cases [16, 36, 37] of AI not presenting any gingival enlargements even inflammatory hyperplasia. So, whether there is another possible mechanism in the etiology of such generalized overgrowths in AI patients remains as a question. Beyond the separate histopathologic examinations, some case-control studies evaluating the role of fibroblastic activities, growth factors, are needed to determine the certain mechanisms of such gingival overgrowths with AI, and whether such enlargements resemble HGF or not.

AI has a large group of hereditary patterns such as autosomal dominant, autosomal recessive, sex-linked, and spodadic AI [1, 38–40]. HGF is also usually identified as an autosomal dominant condition although recessive forms are described in the literature [25, 35, 41, 42]. Some genetic linkage studies are needed to evaluate whether there is a genetic transition between AI and such gingival overgrowths or not.

Prosthetic rehabilitation is another important issue for the management of the aesthetical and functional complaints of AI patients. There are several prosthetic treatment alternatives for these patients. Porcelain fused to metal crowns, all ceramic crowns, laminate veneers, and overdentures can be used for the prosthetic treatment of AI patients [11, 17, 43]. The treatment plan is related to many factors such as number of permanent teeth, intraoral situation at the time of the treatment was planned, type and severity of disorder, patient's occlusion, occlusal vertical dimension, age, socioeconomic status of the patient, and patients expectation.

In this paper, considering these factors fixed full-mouth all ceramic prosthetic restorations were planned for the older patient. With the help of the prostheses adequate crown form, shape, and smooth crown surfaces were constituted and poor chewing functions were improved. Insufficient esthetic was also recovered by color management.

4. Conclusion

This paper describes clinical findings and oral rehabilitation of two female siblings presenting AI and HGF like generalized gingival enlargements. Periodontal flap surgery was successful in the treatment of gingival overgrowth of both patients. After the periodontal treatment of the older patient, full ceramic fixed restorations were effective to eliminate tooth hypersensitivity, improve esthetics, and restore function. The 3-year recall examination revealed no signs of deterioration in the restorations. The patient did not experience tooth sensitivity or any other complication associated with the oral rehabilitation. The patient's esthetic and functional expectations were also satisfied.

References

[1] P. J. M. Crawford, M. Aldred, and A. Bloch-Zupan, "Amelogenesis imperfecta," *Orphanet Journal of Rare Diseases*, vol. 2, no. 1, article 17, 2007.

[2] P. S. Hart, T. C. Hart, J. P. Simmer, and J. T. Wright, "A nomenclature for X-linked Amelogenesis imperfecta," *Archives of Oral Biology*, vol. 47, no. 4, pp. 255–260, 2002.

[3] M. J. Aldred and P. J. Crawford, "Variable expression in Amelogenesis imperfecta with taurodontism," *Journal of Oral Pathology*, vol. 17, no. 7, pp. 327–333, 1988.

[4] K. M. S. Ayers, B. K. Drummond, W. J. Harding, S. G. Salis, and P. N. Liston, "Amelogenesis imperfecta—multidisciplinary management from eruption to adulthood. Review and case report," *New Zealand Dental Journal*, vol. 100, no. 4, pp. 101–104, 2004.

[5] J. Congleton and E. J. Burkes, "Amelogenesis imperfecta with taurodontism," *Oral Surgery Oral Medicine and Oral Pathology*, vol. 48, no. 6, pp. 540–544, 1979.

[6] T. Lykogeorgos, K. Duncan, P. J. M. Crawford, and M. J. Aldred, "Unusual manifestations in X-linked Amelogenesis imperfecta," *International Journal of Paediatric Dentistry*, vol. 13, no. 5, pp. 356–361, 2003.

[7] K. Ooya, J. Nalbandian, and T. Noikura, "Autosomal recessive rough hypoplastic Amelogenesis imperfecta. A case report with clinical, light microscopic, radiographic, and electron microscopic observations," *Oral Surgery Oral Medicine and Oral Pathology*, vol. 65, no. 4, pp. 449–458, 1988.

[8] G. B. Winter, "Amelogenesis imperfecta with enamel opacities and taurodontism: an alternative diagnosis for 'idiopathic dental fluorosis'," *British Dental Journal*, vol. 181, no. 5, pp. 167–172, 1996.

[9] M. A. Collins, S. M. Mauriello, D. A. Tyndall, and J. T. Wright, "Dental anomalies associated with Amelogenesis imperfecta: a radiographic assessment," *Oral Surgery, Oral Medicine, Oral Pathology, Oral Radiology, and Endodontics*, vol. 88, no. 3, pp. 358–364, 1999.

[10] R. Greenfield, V. Iacono, S. Zove, and P. Baer, "Periodontal and prosthodontic treatment of Amelogenesis imperfecta: a clinical report," *The Journal of Prosthetic Dentistry*, vol. 68, no. 4, pp. 572–574, 1992.

[11] J. C. Nel, J. A. Pretorius, A. Weber, and J. T. Marais, "Restoring function and esthetics in a patient with Amelogenesis imperfecta," *International Journal of Periodontics and Restorative Dentistry*, vol. 17, no. 5, pp. 479–483, 1997.

[12] E. Peters, M. Cohen, and M. Altini, "Rough hypoplastic Amelogenesis imperfecta with follicular hyperplasia," *Oral Surgery Oral Medicine and Oral Pathology*, vol. 74, no. 1, pp. 87–92, 1992.

[13] H. K. Yip and R. J. Smales, "Oral rehabilitation of young adults with Amelogenesis imperfecta," *International Journal of Prosthodontics*, vol. 16, no. 4, pp. 345–349, 2003.

[14] I. C. Mackie and A. S. Blinkhorn, "Amelogenesis imperfecta: early interception to prevent attrition," *Dental Update*, vol. 18, no. 2, pp. 79–80, 1991.

[15] S. Sundell, "Hereditary Amelogenesis imperfecta. I. Oral health in children," *Swedish Dental Journal*, vol. 10, no. 4, pp. 151–163, 1986.

[16] K. Gokce, C. Canpolat, and E. Ozel, "Restoring function and esthetics in a patient with Amelogenesis imperfecta: a case report," *Journal of Contemporary Dental Practice*, vol. 8, no. 4, pp. 95–101, 2007.

[17] W. P. Williams and L. H. Becker, "Amelogenesis imperfecta: functional and esthetic restoration of a severely compromised dentition," *Quintessence International*, vol. 31, no. 6, pp. 397–403, 2000.

[18] M. J. Aldred and P. J. Crawford, "Amelogenesis imperfecta—towards a new classification," *Oral Diseases*, vol. 1, no. 1, pp. 2–5, 1995.

[19] M. J. Aldred, R. Savarirayan, and P. J. M. Crawford, "Amelogenesis imperfecta: a classification and catalogue for the 21st century," *Oral Diseases*, vol. 9, no. 1, pp. 19–23, 2003.

[20] A. I. DARLING, "Some observations on Amelogenesis imperfecta and calcification of the dental enamel," *Proceedings of the Royal Society of Medicine*, vol. 49, no. 10, pp. 759–765, 1956.

[21] S. Hart, T. Hart, C. Gibson, and J. T. Wright, "Mutational analysis of X-linked Amelogenesis imperfecta in multiple families," *Archives of Oral Biology*, vol. 45, no. 1, pp. 79–86, 2000.

[22] G. B. Winter and A. H. Brook, "Enamel hypoplasia and anomalies of the enamel," *Dental Clinics of North America*, vol. 19, no. 1, pp. 3–24, 1975.

[23] C. J. Witkop, "Amelogenesis imperfecta, dentinogenesis imperfecta and dentin dysplasia revisited: problems in classification," *Journal of Oral Pathology*, vol. 17, no. 9-10, pp. 547–553, 1988.

[24] C. J. WITKOP, "Hereditary defects in enamel and dentin," *Acta Genetica et Statistica Medica*, vol. 7, no. 1, pp. 236–239, 1957.

[25] I. P. Baptista, "Hereditary gingival fibromatosis: a case report," *Journal of Clinical Periodontology*, vol. 29, no. 9, pp. 871–874, 2002.

[26] L. Häkkinen and A. Csiszar, "Hereditary gingival fibromatosis: characteristics and novel putative pathogenic mechanisms," *Journal of Dental Research*, vol. 86, no. 1, pp. 25–34, 2007.

[27] M. Atasu, S. Biren, and G. Mumcu, "Hypocalcification type Amelogenesis imperfecta in permanent dentition in association with heavily worn primary teeth, gingival hyperplasia, hypodontia and impacted teeth," *Journal of Clinical Pediatric Dentistry*, vol. 23, no. 2, pp. 117–122, 1999.

[28] M. T. Brennan, B. C. O'Connell, T. E. Rams, and A. C. O'Connell, "Management of gingival overgrowth associated with generalized enamel defects in a child," *Journal of Clinical Pediatric Dentistry*, vol. 23, no. 2, pp. 97–102, 1999.

[29] L. Feller, Y. Jadwat, M. Bouckaert, A. Buskin, and E. J. Raubenheimer, "Enamel dysplasia with odontogenic fibroma-like hamartomas: review of the literature and report of a case," *Oral Surgery, Oral Medicine, Oral Pathology, Oral Radiology and Endodontology*, vol. 101, no. 5, pp. 620–624, 2006.

[30] A. Hirshberg, A. Buchner, and D. Dayan, "The central odontogenic fibroma and the hyperplastic dental follicle: study with Picrosirius red and polarizing microscopy," *Journal of Oral Pathology and Medicine*, vol. 25, no. 3, pp. 125–127, 1996.

[31] W. F. van Heerden, E. J. Raubenheimer, A. F. Dreyer, and A. M. Benn, "Amelogenesis imperfecta: multiple impactions associated with odontogenic fibromas (WHO) type," *The Journal of the Dental Association of South Africa*, vol. 45, no. 11, pp. 467–471, 1990.

[32] T. O'Leary, "The periodontal screening examination," *Journal of Periodontology*, vol. 38, no. 6, pp. 617–624, 1967.

[33] G. O. Macedo, R. S. Tunes, A. C. F. Motta et al., "Amelogenesis imperfecta and unusual gingival hyperplasia," *Journal of Periodontology*, vol. 76, no. 9, pp. 1563–1566, 2005.

[34] G. Farrer-Brown, R. B. Lucas, and D. Winstock, "Familial gingival fibromatosis: an unusual pathology," *Journal of Oral Pathology*, vol. 1, no. 2, pp. 76–83, 1972.

[35] O. Günhan, D. G. Gardner, H. Bostanci, and M. Günhan, "Familial gingival fibromatosis with unusual histologic findings," *Journal of Periodontology*, vol. 66, no. 11, pp. 1008–1011, 1995.

[36] H. Akin, S. Tasveren, and D. Y. Yeler, "Interdisciplinary approach to treating a patient with Amelogenesis imperfecta: a clinical report," *Journal of Esthetic and Restorative Dentistry*, vol. 19, no. 3, pp. 131–135, 2007.

[37] G. A. Thompson and J. M. Schwartz, "Oral rehabilitation of a patient with Amelogenesis imperfecta," *Journal of Prosthodontics*, vol. 6, no. 4, pp. 257–264, 1997.

[38] P. J. M. Crawford and M. J. Aldred, "X-linked Amelogenesis imperfecta: presentation of two kindreds and a review of the literature," *Oral Surgery Oral Medicine and Oral Pathology*, vol. 73, no. 4, pp. 449–455, 1992.

[39] C. Kärrman, B. Bäckman, M. Dixon, G. Holmgren, and K. Forsman, "Mapping of the locus for autosomal dominant Amelogenesis imperfecta (AIH2) to a 4-Mb YAC contig on chromosome 4q11-q21," *Genomics*, vol. 39, no. 2, pp. 164–170, 1997.

[40] M. Michaelides, A. Bloch-Zupan, G. E. Holder, D. M. Hunt, and A. T. Moore, "An autosomal recessive cone-rod dystrophy associated with Amelogenesis imperfecta," *Journal of Medical Genetics*, vol. 41, no. 6, pp. 468–473, 2004.

[41] L. Bozzo, O. P. de Almeida, C. Scully, and M. J. Aldred, "Hereditary gingival fibromatosis. Report of an extensive four-generation pedigree," *Oral Surgery, Oral Medicine, Oral Pathology*, vol. 78, no. 4, pp. 452–454, 1994.

[42] R. D. Coletta, O. P. Almeida, E. Graner, R. C. Page, and L. Bozzo, "Differential proliferation of fibroblasts cultured from hereditary gingival fibromatosis and normal gingiva," *Journal of Periodontal Research*, vol. 33, no. 8, pp. 469–475, 1998.

[43] R. W. Li, "Adhesive solutions: report of a case using multiple adhesive techniques in the management of enamel hypoplasia," *Dental Update*, vol. 26, no. 7, pp. 277–287, 1999.

2

Inflammatory Myofibroblastic Tumor of the Lung and the Maxillary Region: A Benign Lesion with Aggressive Behavior

Lorena Gallego,[1] Tania R. Santamarta,[2] Verónica Blanco,[3] Luis García-Consuegra,[2] Tommaso Cutilli,[4] and Luis Junquera[2,5]

[1] *Department of Oral and Maxillofacial Surgery, Cabueñes Hospital, 33394 Gijón, Spain*
[2] *Department of Oral and Maxillofacial Surgery, Central University Hospital, 33306 Oviedo, Spain*
[3] *Department of Pathology, Central University Hospital, 33306 Oviedo, Spain*
[4] *Italy Health Sciences Department, Maxillofacial Surgery Unit, University of L'Aquila, 67100, Italy*
[5] *Oral and Maxillofacial Surgery, Dental School, University of Oviedo, Catedrático José Serrano Street, 33009 Oviedo, Spain*

Correspondence should be addressed to Luis Junquera; junquera@uniovi.es

Academic Editors: M. A. Qudeimat and S. R. Watt-Smith

Inflammatory myofibroblastic tumor (IMT) is a rare mass-forming lesion characterized by fibroblastic or myofibroblastic spindle cell proliferation with varying degrees of inflammatory cell infiltration. Although it has been reported in virtually every organ in the body, the lung is the most common site of involvement. Extrapulmonary IMTs, although rare, have been reported and are characterized by different, more aggressive behavior. We report an extremely rare case of maxillary metastases of pulmonary IMT. Lung IMT was initially misdiagnosed, and oral lesion mimicked clinically and radiologically a radicular cyst. On histologic examination, cells exhibited diffuse and intense immunoreactivity for α-smooth muscle actin and vimentin whereas both pulmonary and oral IMTs presented absence of cellular atypia and lack of expressivity of oncogenic determinants. Distant metastases of lung IMT are extremely unusual, and this is the first report to our knowledge with this particular clinical course. Despite the possibility that the present case could also represent a metachronous multifocal IMT, with pulmonary and extrapulmonary lesions, similar histopathological and immunohistochemical patterns in lung and maxillary region suggest a metastatic course.

1. Introduction

Inflammatory myofibroblastic tumor (IMT) is a rare mass-forming lesion characterized by fibroblastic or myofibroblastic spindle cell proliferation with varying degrees of inflammatory cell infiltration. Because of these unknown factors, IMT was referred to by several different terms until the World Health Organization (WHO) classified IMT as a distinct entity in 1994 [1]. IMTs belong to the group of soft tissue tumours and have also been named plasma cell granuloma, inflammatory pseudotumour, xanthoma xanthomous pseudotumour, fibrous histiocytoma or histiocytoma, mast cell tumour or mast cell granuloma. The majority of IMT lesions are present in the lungs. Extrapulmonary IMTs, although rare, have also been reported and are characterized by different, more aggressive behavior. The frequency of upper respiratory tract accounts for 11% of extrapulmonary cases and the remainder of the head and neck sites, less than 5% [2].

We report an extremely rare case of maxillary metastases of pulmonary IMT. Distant metastases of lung IMT are extremely unusual, and this is the first report to our knowledge with this particular clinical course. Histological and immunohistological findings are analyzed.

2. Case Report

In February 2011, a 53-year-old female patient was referred to our Department of Oral and Maxillofacial Surgery with a chief complaint of swelling and pain of the left upper maxillary region. The symptoms were noticed 2 months previously, after root canal treatment of upper left canine.

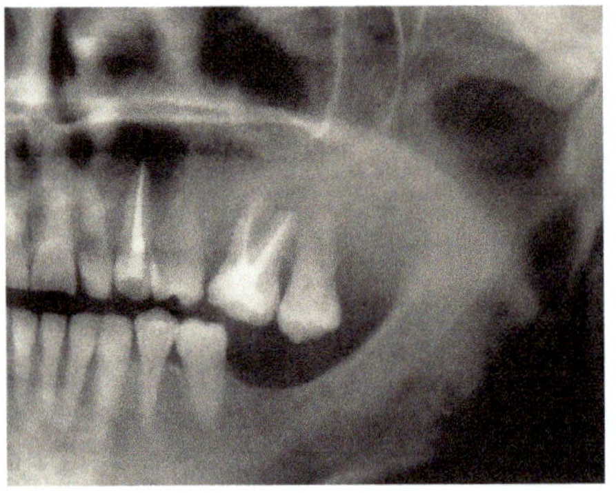

Figure 1: Panoramic radiograph revealing a radiolucency of about 2 cm of diameter in the periapical region of the endodontically treated left canine.

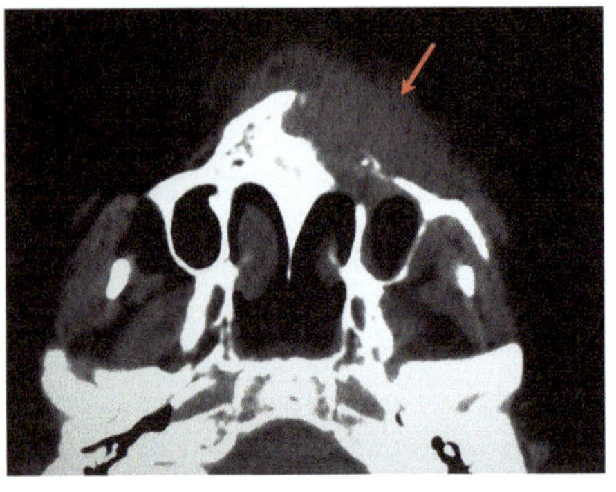

Figure 2: Axial CT image showing an infiltrative mass in the left maxillary region with destruction of the maxillary bone anteriorly wall, invading skin.

There was no medical history of note but a remarkable history of pneumonia surgically treated two years ago.

Extraorally, the swelling was diffuse, nontender, with increased local surface temperature and redness in the left infraorbital region. Intraorally, no lesions were observed. There was noted pain on percussion of the endodontically treated canine and adjacent premolar teeth. Radiograph showed root canal filling extending 1 mm beyond the canine root apex and imprecise periapical radiolucency with a diameter of about 2 cm (Figure 1). No root resorption was detected. Previous radiographs nine months before root canal treatment showed no clear radiolucency. Then, a provisional diagnosis of radicular cyst was considered, and a decision was made to perform periapical surgery under local anaesthesia.

Intraoperatively, a cyst-like lesion with unclear margins occupied with globular soft tissue was discovered. All surgical material was sent for histopathologic examination. A postoperative CT showed an infiltrative lesion in the left maxillary sinus with destruction of the maxillary bone anteriorly and minimal destruction of the infraorbital wall, invading skin (Figure 2).

Although the histopathologic examination was consistent with an active and chronic inflammation without atypical mitosis, a lymphoproliferative or malignant tumor was suspected due to the CT images. A skin and subcutaneous tissue biopsy was performed. Histopathology examination revealed again inflammatory changes without a definitive diagnosis of the lesion.

Then, the patient underwent a total excision of the mass under general anaesthesia in April 2011. Postoperative histopathology of the surgically excised material revealed a solid, nonencapsulated mass, which is composed of compact spindle cells sprinkled with inflammatory cells, with a predominance of plasma cells and lymphocytes (Figure 3(a)). Special stains for microorganisms, including mycobacteria, fungi, and virus, were negative. The neoplastic cells showed myofibroblastic phenotype and reacted immunologically with vimentin and alpha-smooth muscle actin (Figures 3(b) and 3(c)), while a smaller number was positive for CD5, CD20, and Ki67 (Figure 3(d)). Staining for desmin, CD117, p53, and S100 was negative. With these findings, the diagnosis of IMT was made.

As referred, the patient had a remarkable history of pneumonia surgically treated in January 2009. Histology of lung demonstrated intra-alveolar inflammatory cell infiltration and prominent lymphoid infiltrate with obliteration of bronchiolar space. At that time, the diagnosis based on computed tomography (CT) and histopathology study of surgical specimen was cryptogenic organizing pneumonia (Figure 4). Corticosteroid and calcifediol therapy was prescribed for ten-month duration. During the steroid therapy, the symptoms disappeared and a marked shrinkage of the mass and radiographic improvement was achieved. Prednisolone was gradually tapered and finally discontinued in February 2010, and no regrowth of the tumor was observed. After treatment, CT scans of the chest showed no significant changes in lesion size. The patient was still controlled by Respiratory Care Department.

In view of such findings in maxillary region, histopathological results of the previous lung lesion, initially suggesting a cryptogenic organizing pneumonia, were carefully revised. A complete immunohistochemical staining was performed to rule out a possible metastases of previous misdiagnosed lung IMF. In fact, inflammatory cells, with a predominance of plasma cells and lymphocytes (Figure 5(a)), reacted immunologically exactly the same as maxillary IMT. Lung tumor cells reacted positive with vimentin and alpha-smooth muscle actin (Figures 5(b) and 3(c)), smaller number was positive for Ki67 (Figure 5(d)), and staining for desmin, CD117, p53 and S100 was negative. Thus, considering these findings, the specimen was diagnosed as lung IMT with metastasis to the maxillary region.

The patient's recovery was uneventful. At her most recent followup, 20 months after maxillary resection, there was no sign of oral recurrence. The pulmonary IMT is carefully reviewed with no regrowth or chest symptoms observed to date.

3. Discussion

IMT was first reported in 1905 by Birch-Hirschfield, but its etiology remains unknown. In 1994, the World Health

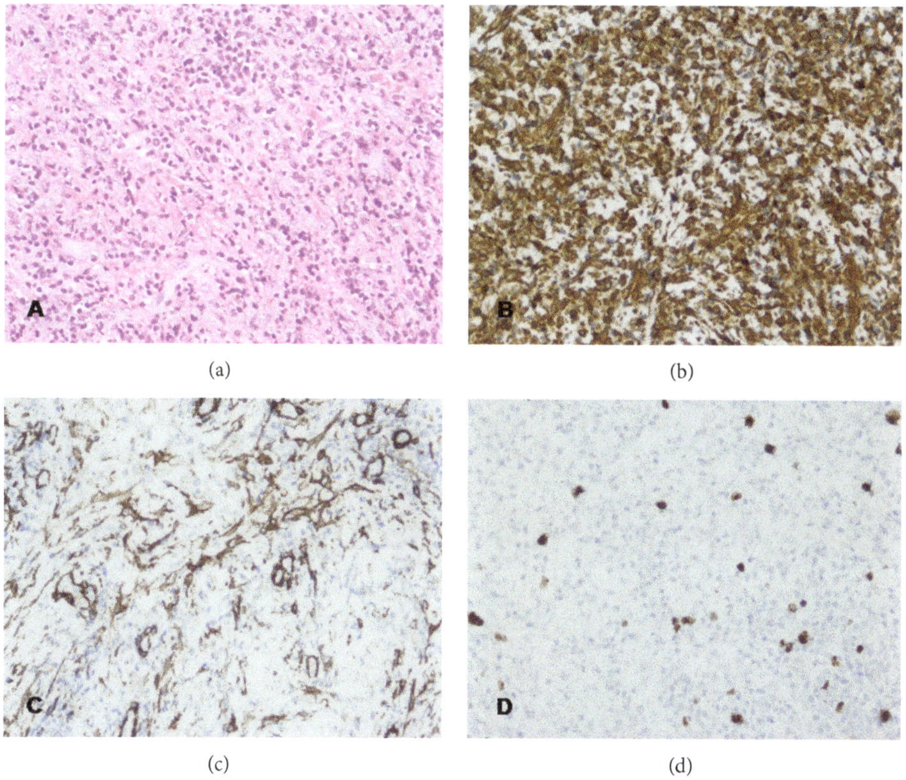

FIGURE 3: Histological and immunohistochemical examination of the maxillary mass. (a) Hematoxylin-eosin staining demonstrating spindle cells sprinkled with inflammatory cells, with a predominance of plasma cells and lymphocytes (original magnification ×200). (b) immunohistochemical staining showing strong reactivity for vimentin (original magnification ×200). (c) Immunohistochemical staining showing moderate reactivity for α-smooth muscle actin (original magnification ×200). (d) Immunohistochemical staining showing focal and weak immunoreactivity of the tumor cells for Ki-67 (original magnification ×200).

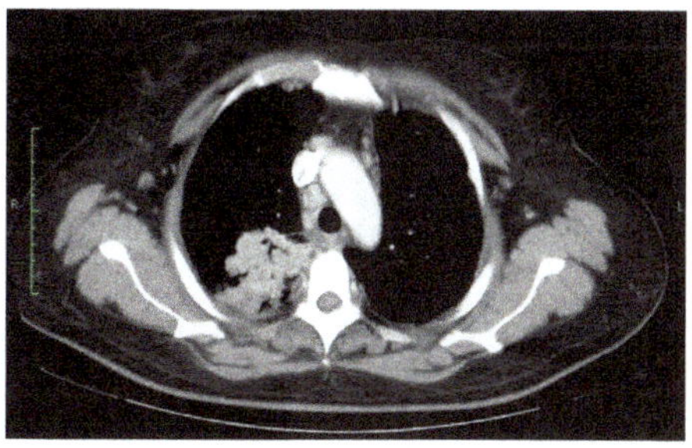

FIGURE 4: Computed tomography (CT) scan showing an irregular mass in the right lung field. This lesion was initially diagnosed as a cryptogenic organizing pneumonia.

Organization defined IMT as an intermediate soft tissue tumor that is composed of myofibroblast-differentiated spindle cells and accompanied by numerous inflammatory cells, plasma cells, and/or lymphocytes [1]. The term pseudotumor was coined because these lesions mimic expansive, invasive malignant tumors, both clinically and radiologically. Recently, the concept of IMT being a benign reactive lesion has been challenged owing to the clinical demonstration of recurrences as high as 37%, cytogenetic evidence of acquired clonal chromosomal abnormality, and the presence of regional metastases [3–5]. The term inflammatory fibrosarcoma (IFS) is used to describe the most aggressive varieties with documented metastasis [6].

Although it has been reported in virtually every organ and site in the body, the lung is the most common site of involvement. When the tumor arises in the lungs it appears as a nodular lesion, usually with completely benign behavior. However, the occurrence of the tumor at extrapulmonary sites, histologically the same, may be accompanied with some special aggressive characteristics and then classified as IFS [7]. It is worth mentioning that the WHO does not classify IFS as a single entity; however, based on the study by Meis and Enzinger [4], several authors share the opinion that there is a difference between these 2 tumors (focused on the metastatic potential of each).

Pseudotumours are relatively rare in the head and neck, excluding the orbit and cerebrum. IMT has been reported to occur in the larynx, orbit, maxillary sinus, mandible, mouth, parapharyngeal space, tonsils, thyroid, parotid, and lacrimal glands [8]. Associated clinical findings include fever, tenderness, and erythema over the affected region. The imaging findings of IMT are a mildly enhancing soft-tissue mass without any internal calcification or bone destruction

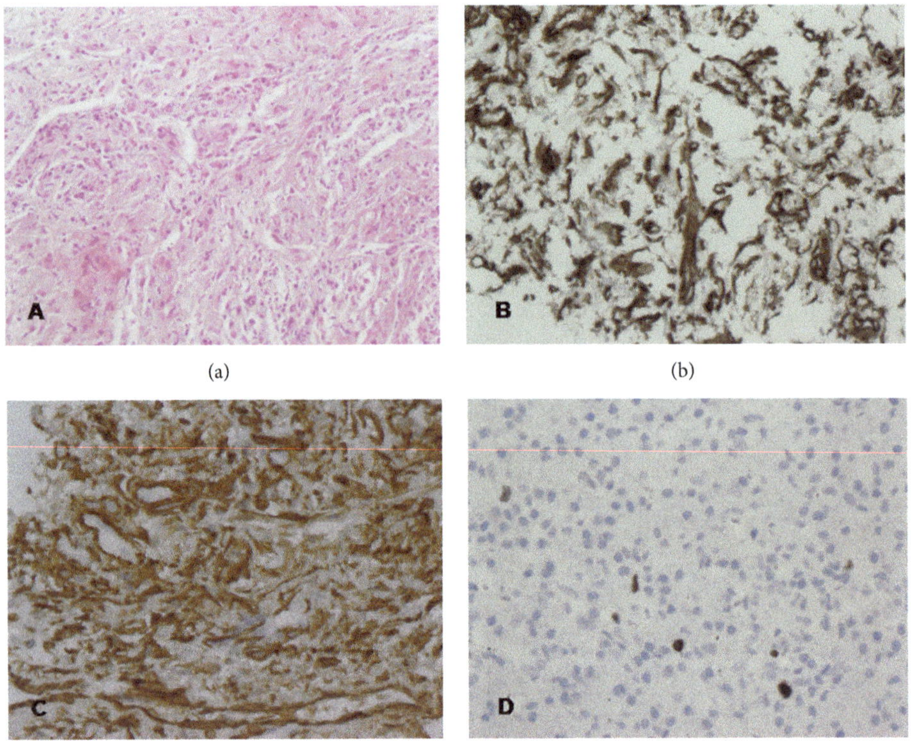

(a) (b) (c) (d)

Figure 5: Histological and immunohistochemical examination of the pulmonary mass. (a) Hematoxylin-eosin staining demonstrating spindle cells sprinkled, with a predominance of plasma cells and lymphocytes (original magnification ×200). (b) immunohistochemical staining showing strong reactivity for vimentin (original magnification ×400). (c) Immunohistochemical staining showing strong reactivity for α-smooth muscle actin (original magnification ×400). (d) Immunohistochemical staining showing weak immunoreactivity of the tumor cells for Ki-67 (original magnification ×400).

revealed by contrast-enhanced CT, although in our case, the tumor had infiltrated all the bony walls of the involved sinus, indicating an aggressive variety of IMT.

Histologically, IMT is composed of inflammatory cells, histiocytes, and fibroblasts. The specific components of IMT can vary and range from those that are dominated by plasma cells to those primarily comprised of myofibroblasts and fibroblasts [9]. The recent WHO classification of soft tissue tumors recognizes 3 basic variants of IMT: (1) loosely organized myofibroblasts in an edematous myxoid background with plasma cells, lymphocytes, eosinophils, and blood vessels, resembling nodular fasciitis; (2) dense aggregates of spindle cells arrayed in a variable myxoid and collagenized background and admixed with a distinctive inflammatory infiltrate, diffuse clusters of plasma cells, and lymphoid nodules, resembling fibrous histiocytoma or fibromatosis; and (3) collagen sheets with scattered plasma cells and eosinophils resembling a scar or desmoid tumor [10]. Cytologic atypia with nuclear pleomorphism and increased mitotic activity are uncommon features and may be associated with malignant transformation.

We report a case of lung IMT with distant maxillary metastases. This is, to the best of our knowledge, the first report of diagnosis of a maxillary IMT after pulmonary manifestation. Despite the possibility that the present case could also represent a metachronous multifocal IMT, with pulmonary and extrapulmonary lesions, similar histopathological and immunohistochemical patterns in lung and maxillary region suggest a metastatic course. With regard to the present case, the supporting histology was more congruent with a diagnosis of IMT than IFS, as evidenced by the absence of frequent mitotic figures, unapparent cellular atypia, and lack of expressivity of several oncogenic determinants, such as p53 and Ki-67. Otherwise, the clinical course of our report suggests biologic aggressiveness, due to the presence of metastases. Those findings disagree with studies that associated potential for aggressive growth, recurrence, and malignant transformation with a high degree of atypia, presence of ganglion-like cells, increased mitotic figures, multinodularity, DNA aneuploidy, elevated Ki-67 proliferative index, and oncogenic protein overexpression, such as ALK, p53, and bcl-2 [11].

A simple excision is the proposed and mainly applied treatment, including postoperative reassessment for at least 10 years. Local recurrence could be related with inadequate resection of the lesion or tumors. The difficulty of completely excising the tumor in most of the cases is related to its location and its vicinity to valuable structures, which by definition are numerous in the head and neck area [12]. Although the number of oral IMTs is limited, seems to exhibit a more favourable clinical course and is distinguished, to date, by the lack of recurrence, malignant transformation, metastasis, and mortality. Metastasis is seen in less than 5% of the cases of IMT [7, 13]. However, bearing in mind the fact that IMT could be multifocal, it is difficult to distinguish between a real metastasis and a synchronous or metachronous primary lesion, as the case reported. Adjuvant radiotherapy has also been reported for the treatment of IMT but because of the small number of reports, it is difficult to adopt safe conclusions.

4. Conclusion

In summary, a case of maxillary metastases of pulmonary IMT is described. Lung IMT was initially misdiagnosed, and oral lesion mimicked clinically and radiologically a radicular cyst. On histologic examination, cells exhibited diffuse and intense immunoreactivity for α-smooth muscle actin and vimentin whereas both pulmonary and oral IMTs presented absence of cellular atypia and lack of expressivity of oncogenic determinants. This is the first report to our knowledge of an IMT of the lung with oral metastasis.

References

[1] J. M. Coindre, "Histologic classification of soft tissue tumors (WHO, 1994)," *Annales de Pathologie*, vol. 14, no. 6, pp. 426–427, 1994.

[2] A. W. H. Shek, P. C. Wu, and N. Samman, "Inflammatory pseudotumour of the mouth and maxilla," *Journal of Clinical Pathology*, vol. 49, no. 2, pp. 164–167, 1996.

[3] R. Biselli, C. Ferlini, A. Fattorossi et al., "Inflammatory myofibroblastic tumor (inflammatory pseudotumor). DNA flow cytometric analysis of nine pediatric cases," *Cancer*, vol. 77, pp. 778-784, 1996.

[4] J. M. Meis and F. M. Enzinger, "Inflammatory fibrosarcoma of the mesentery and retroperitoneum: a tumor closely simulating inflammatory pseudotumor," *American Journal of Surgical Pathology*, vol. 15, no. 12, pp. 1146–1156, 1991.

[5] C. F. Poh, R. W. Priddy, and D. M. Dahlman, "Intramandibular inflammatory myofibroblastic tumor—a true neoplasm or reactive lesion?" *Oral Surgery, Oral Medicine, Oral Pathology, Oral Radiology and Endodontology*, vol. 100, no. 4, pp. 460–466, 2005.

[6] I. Dimitrakopoulos, K. Psomaderis, F. Iordanidis, and D. Karakasis, "Inflammatory myofibroblastic tumor of the maxillary sinus: a case report," *Journal of Oral and Maxillofacial Surgery*, vol. 65, no. 2, pp. 323-326, 2007.

[7] K. Watanabe, T. Tajino, M. Sekiguchi, and T. Suzuki, "Inflammatory myofibroblastic tumor (inflammatory fibrosarcoma) of the bone," *Archives of Pathology and Laboratory Medicine*, vol. 124, no. 10, pp. 1514–1517, 2000.

[8] K. A. Eley and S. R. Watt-Smith, "Intraoral presentation of inflammatory myofibroblastic tumor (pseudotumor) at the site of dental extraction: report of a case and review of the literature," *Journal of Oral and Maxillofacial Surgery*, vol. 68, no. 8, pp. 2016–2020, 2010.

[9] J. K. Brooks, N. G. Nikitakis, B. F. Frankel, J. C. Papadimitriou, and J. J. Sauk, "Oral inflammatory myofibroblastic tumor demonstrating ALK, p53, MDM2, CDK4, pRb, and Ki-67 immunoreactivity in an elderly patient," *Oral Surgery, Oral Medicine, Oral Pathology, Oral Radiology and Endodontology*, vol. 99, no. 6, pp. 716–726, 2005.

[10] C. M. Coffin and J. A. Fletcher, "Inflammatory myofibroblastic tumour: World Health Organization classification of tumours," in *Pathology and Genetics of Tumours of Soft Tissue and Bone*, C. D. M. Fletcher, K. K. Unni, and F. Mertens, Eds., IARC Press, Lyon, France, 2002.

[11] J. W. Hussong, M. Brown, S. L. Perkins, L. P. Dehner, and C. M. Coffin, "Comparison of DNA ploidy, histologic, and immunohistochemical findings with clinical outcome in inflammatory myofibroblastic tumors," *Modern Pathology*, vol. 12, no. 3, pp. 279–286, 1999.

[12] C. J. Wales, L. M. Carter, and P. H. Whitfield, "Facial pseudotumours. A case report and review of their management," *British Journal of Oral and Maxillofacial Surgery*, vol. 46, no. 1, pp. 57–58, 2008.

[13] A. K. Petridis, R. G. Hempelmann, H. H. Hugo, T. Eichmann, and H. M. Mehdorn, "Metastatic low-grade inflammatory myofibroblastic tumor (IMT) in the central nervous system of a 29-year-old male patient," *Clinical Neuropathology*, vol. 23, no. 4, pp. 158–166, 2004.

3

Prosthodontic Rehabilitation of Hereditary Ectodermal Dysplasia in an 11-Year-Old Patient with Flexible Denture: A Case Report

Neha Jain,[1] Dinesh Naitam,[2] Arti Wadkar,[3] Anuradha Nemane,[4] Shiva Katoch,[5] and Ashish Dewangan[2]

[1] *Department of Prosthodontics, Manav Rachna Dental College, Faridabad 121004, India*
[2] *Department of Prosthodontics, Rungta College of Dental Sciences and Research, Kohka-Kurud Road, Kurud, Bhilai 490024, India*
[3] *Department of Prosthodontics, Nair Hospital Dental College, Mumbai 400008, India*
[4] *Department of Prosthodontics, YMT Dental College, Navi Mumbai 410210, India*
[5] *Department of Prosthodontics, D.A.V. Dental College, Solan 173212, India*

Correspondence should be addressed to Jain Neha, nejamaverick@gmail.com

Academic Editors: D. Cogulu, J. C. de la Macorra, A. Milosevic, and A. Scribante

Hereditary ectodermal dysplasia is a rare group of inherited disorders characterized by aplasia or dysplasia of two or more tissues of ectodermal origin such as hair, nails, teeth, and skin. The dental characteristics of this syndrome include anodontia or hypodontia of the primary and/or permanent teeth, hypoplastic conical teeth, and underdevelopment of the alveolar ridges. The options for a definitive treatment plan include fixed, removable or implant-supported prostheses, singly or in combination. This clinical report describes the prosthetic rehabilitation of an 11-year-old boy with hereditary ectodermal dysplasia. Maxillary flexible removable partial denture and mandibular conventional complete denture were fabricated to establish an acceptable masticatory function, speech, and esthetics for the patient.

1. Introduction

Ectodermal dysplasia (ED) is a large, heterogeneous group of inherited disorders that are characterized by primary defects in the development of two or more tissues derived from the embryonic ectoderm. The syndrome involves overlapping features, thereby complicating a definitive classification. The two main categories of ED are the Hidrotic (Clouston's syndrome) and Hypohidrotic (Christ-Siemens-Touraine syndrome) forms [1]. The difference between the two is in terms of sweat gland manifestations. Hidrotic ectodermal dysplasia has an autosomal dominant inheritance where sweat glands are normal which are absent in Hypohidrotic ectodermal dysplasia. The latter (HED) has an X-linked recessive inheritance and is the most common form of ED syndrome affecting men more severely and frequently [1]. The incidence of HED is about 1/100,000 [2].

Patients with HED have absent or decreased sweating because of lack of sweat glands producing extremely high fevers because their skin cannot control temperature properly. The skin is thin with light coloring. Hair may be absent or very thin. After puberty hair growth improves in some patients. The eyebrows, eyelashes, and other body hair may also be absent or sparse. Fingernails and toenails may show faulty development and be small, thick or thin, brittle, discolored, cracked, and/or ridged.

Extraoral manifestations include frontal bossing, depressed nasal bridge, protuberant lips, and hypotrichosis. The dental characteristics include anodontia or hypodontia of the primary and/or permanent teeth, hypoplastic conical teeth, and underdevelopment of the alveolar ridges [3, 4]. When teeth are missing the alveolar bone in which they are ordinarily embedded does not develop well, leading to a reduced vertical dimension and a typical aged appearance in the face [5, 6]. The deviation from normal facial growth of HED subjects tends to lessen with age when rehabilitated with functional and prosthetic appliances [7].

Factors such as patient's age, stage of growth in conjunction with the missing teeth, soft tissue defects, existence of malformed dentition, and psychological status must be considered in the treatment planning [8]. Since patients with ED have psychosocial issues due to the orofacial manifestations presenting at such young age therefore restoring appearance and function is more challenging than usual. There are multiple treatment options for this condition, but the most frequent prosthetic treatment of ED in young patients is removable prosthodontics [9]. There is enough literature on complete dentures being quite commonly fabricated for anodontia patients till a more definitive prosthesis is fabricated [10].

This clinical report explores the use of flexible denture base material for the fabrication of maxillary removable partial denture (RPD) and conventional acrylic resin for fabrication of mandibular complete denture for a paediatric patient with hypohydrotic ectodermal dysplasia.

2. Case Report

An 11-year-old boy reported with chief complaint of inability to masticate and unesthetic appearance. He desired replacement of his missing teeth. The patient gave history of lack of sweating, dryness of skin, and raised body temperature. Extraoral examination revealed sparse hair, frontal bossing, depressed nasal bridge, prominent supra orbital ridges, sunken cheeks, hyperpigmented skin around the eyes, protuberant lips, and decreased lower facial height (Figure 1). Nails appeared normal.

Intraoral examination revealed absence of saliva and dry oral mucosa. Cone-shaped teeth were present in 11, 12, and 23 region with underdeveloped edentulous mandibular alveolar ridge (Figure 2).

Panoramic radiograph showed presence of 11, 12, and 23 with complete root formation and there was no evidence of any impacted tooth (Figure 3).

Family history revealed similar findings in his 18-year old brother. Clinical findings and family history suggested a diagnosis of hypohydrotic ectodermal dysplasia [11].

Hand wrist radiograph (Figure 4) was taken and evaluated to assess the skeletal development of the patient.

After studying the skeletal maturation indicators as given by Fishman [12], it was found that no definitive prosthesis could be planned for another 6 years as the skeletal maturation was incomplete. Maxillary flexible RPD and mandibular complete denture were planned to provide immediate aesthetic results, reestablish the occlusion by replacing missing teeth and allow the patient to become familiar with removable prosthesis before delivery of the definitive prostheses [13]. Valplast flexible partial denture was planned for maxillary arch due to its favourable properties like esthetics, strength, biocompatibility, and comfort to the patient [14]. Valplast flexible denture base material uses the RetentoGrip

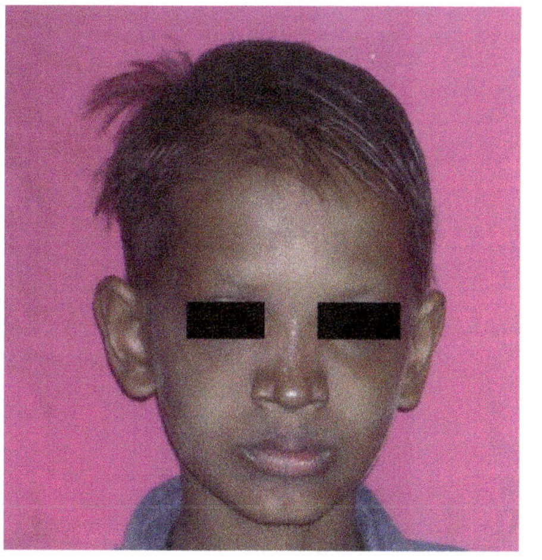

FIGURE 1: Pretreatment extraoral view.

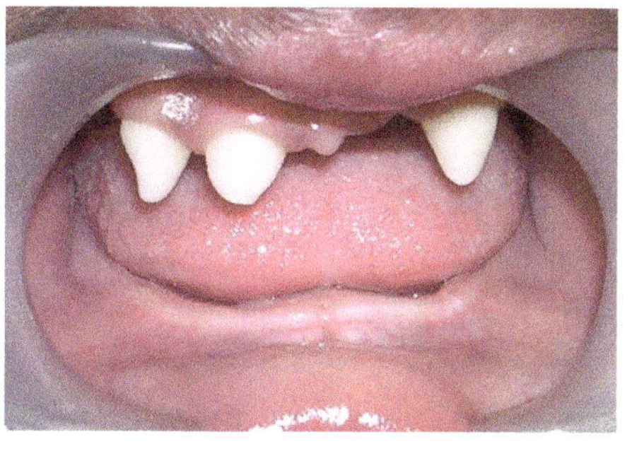

FIGURE 2: Pretreatment intraoral view.

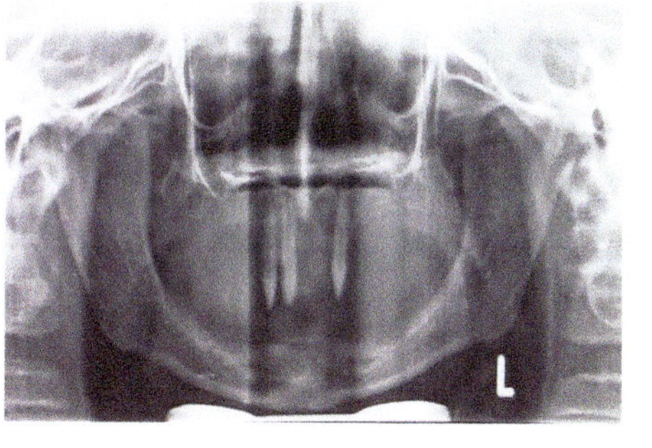

FIGURE 3: Orthopantograph-showing presence of 11, 12, and 23.

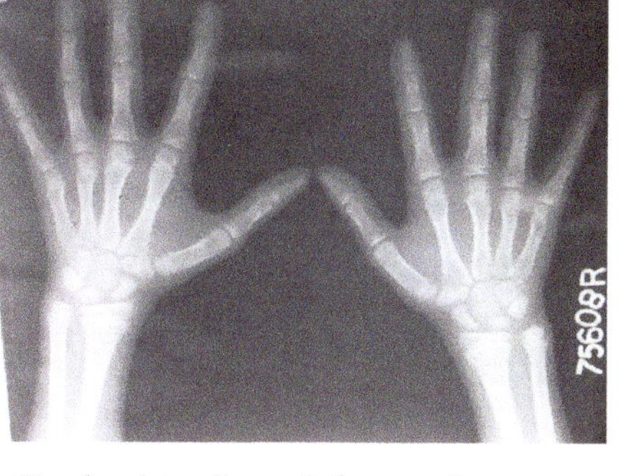

FIGURE 4: Hand-wrist radiograph for growth-spurt assessment.

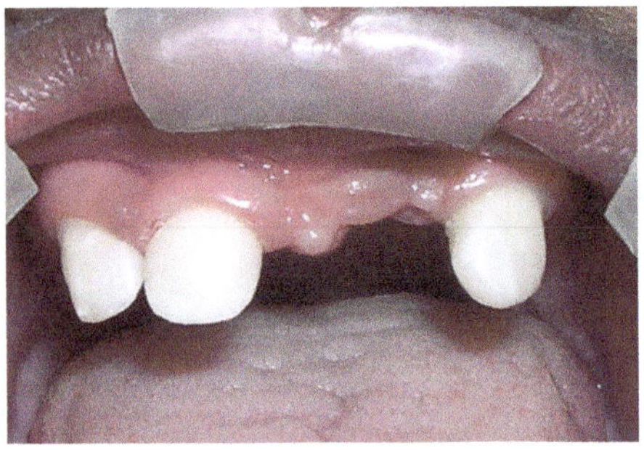

FIGURE 5: Composite restorations of 11, 12, and 23.

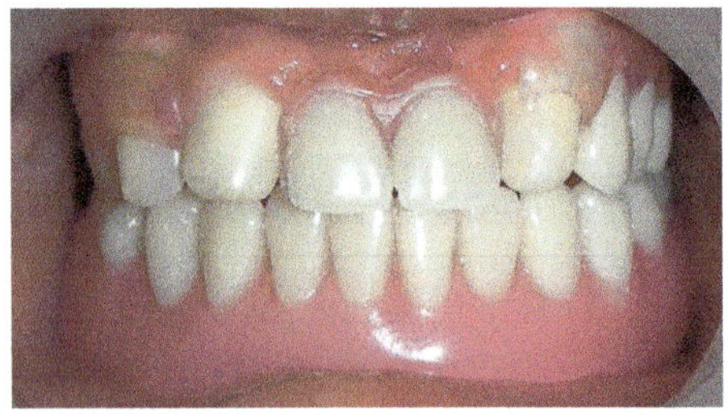

FIGURE 6: Post insertion Intraoral view.

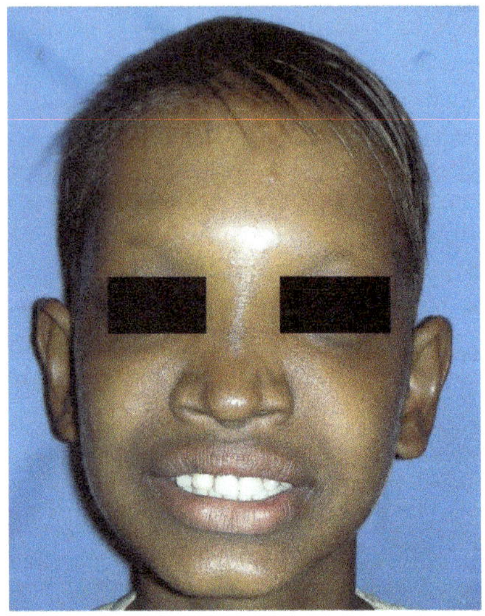

FIGURE 7: Post insertion Extraoral view.

tissue bearing technique for retention, and hence no tooth or tissue, preparation is needed [15].

Maxillary right central and lateral incisors and maxillary left canine were morphologically restored with composite resin to produce 0.25-mm undercuts [16] (Figure 5).

Primary impressions were made with irreversible hydrocolloid impression material as it is comfortable and can be easily removed from undercut area. Casts were prepared with type III dental stone. Custom trays were prepared, and border moulding was done with heavy body polyvinyl siloxane material. The final impressions of the maxillary and mandibular arches were made with medium and light body type of rubber base impression material, respectively. Maxillo-mandibular relation was recorded, and the master casts were mounted on a semiadjustable articulator. The teeth were arranged according to a balanced occlusal scheme [17]. Try-in was done and after careful evaluation the maxillary prostheses were fabricated in Valplast resin by injection moulding technique, and the mandibular prosthesis was fabricated in the conventional heat cure acrylic resin. The dentures were then inserted in the patient's mouth (Figures 6 and 7).

Prior to insertion the valplast partial was immersed for a minute in warm water. The heat exposure will assure a very smooth initial insertion and allows the denture to adapt to the underlying tissue. The patient was educated about proper insertion and the removal of the prostheses and instructed about maintaining denture hygiene. Recall was done after 24 hrs to make necessary adjustments. Future visits were scheduled for 6 months to monitor bone growth and for denture relining.

3. Discussion

An early age prosthodontic intervention helps the child to adjust with the prosthesis and develop normal appearance, speech, mastication, and swallowing as well as temporomandibular joint function. The intraoral prosthesis can be modified during growth spurts or rapid growth periods. Apart from dental benefits, an early age intervention also provides psychosocial benefits [18].

Reduced alveolar bone height with "knife-edge" morphology and limited remaining tooth structure make prosthodontic rehabilitation a challenging task. The replacement of teeth by implants is usually restricted to patients with completed craniofacial growth and is probably best to hold off until adolescence. Implants placed in ED patients younger than 18 years have a higher risk of failure [19]. Implant insertion in children or adolescents can have several unfavourable potential effects including trauma to tooth germs and multidimensional restrictions of skeletal craniofacial growth. In this case implant therapy was not the treatment choice due to ongoing growth and development and insufficient alveolar bone support.

For young patients the use of removable partial denture (RPD) is a reversible treatment that can significantly improve functions and esthetics without jeopardizing compromised dentitions [20]. The use of metal clasps on anterior teeth may cause esthetic problems with the use of cast partial denture [21]. Recently, acetal resins have been used as an alternative tooth-coloured denture clasp material to improve esthetics [22]. The therapeutic use of thermoplastic materials like valplast has increased drastically in the late decade. This new procedure, during which a fully polymerized basic material is softened by heat (without chemical changes) and injected afterwards, has opened up a new chapter in making dentures.

Flexible dentures have got various advantages over the traditional rigid denture bases [23]. Translucency of the material picks up underlying tissue tones, making it almost impossible to detect in the mouth. No clasping is visible on tooth surfaces (when used in manufacturing of clear clasps), improving aesthetics. The material is exceptionally strong and flexible. Good biocompatibility is achieved because the material is free of monomer and metal, these being the principle causes of allergic reactions in conventional denture materials. Flexible dentures will not cause sore spots due to negative reaction to acrylic resins and will absorb small amounts of water to make the denture more soft tissue compatible. There is no requirement of tooth preparation as in case of cast partial denture.

Although dentures are poor alternatives to healthy dentition, they create conditions for the maintenance of a normal, satisfactory daily diet for the child. This is very important, considering that the establishment of lifelong dietary patterns occurs during childhood [24]. When planning dentures in these patients, care should be taken to obtain a wide distribution of occlusal load fully extending the denture base hence balanced occlusion should be the preferred occlusal scheme.

In this case the patient was very comfortable with the valplast partial denture due to its light weight and was quite satisfied with the esthetics because of absence of the metallic part usually seen in other cast partial dentures. Good retention was observed, and the parents reported a significant improvement in terms of speech and mastication.

4. Clinical Significance

The present clinical report demonstrated that maxillary flexible RPDs associated with direct composite restorations and mandibular complete denture are a reversible, relatively inexpensive method of treatment for ectodermal dysplasia patients especially during their growth years. The esthetic, light weight, and good retentive and fracture properties of the flexible denture base materials make them a good alternative to the conventional cast partial dentures.

5. Manufacturers' Details

Irreversible Hydrocolloid-Tropicalgin, Zhermack, Italy.

Type III dental stone-Kalabhai, Mumbai, India.

Semiadjustable Articulator-Teledyne Hanau, Buffalo, New York, USA.

Composite Resin-Filtek Z350, 3 M ESPE, Seefeld, Germany

Rubber Base impression material-AFFINIS Heavy body, Medium body, Light body; Coltene Whaledent.

Autopolymerising resin for custom trays-Pyrex; Pyrex polymer, Roorkee, India.

Valplast Resin-Valplast Int.Corp, Long Island City, New York, U.S.A.

References

[1] I. Tarjan, K. Gabris, and N. Rozsa, "Early prosthetic treatment of patients with ectodermal dysplasia: a clinical report," *Journal of Prosthetic Dentistry*, vol. 93, no. 5, pp. 419–424, 2005.

[2] S. A. Wiśniewski, A. Kobielak, W. H. Trzeciak, and K. Kobielak, "Recent advances in understanding of the molecular basis of anhidrotic ectodermal dysplasia: discovery of a ligand, ectodysplasin A and its two receptors," *Journal of Applied Genetics*, vol. 43, no. 1, pp. 97–107, 2002.

[3] A. Itthagarun and N. M. King, "Ectodermal dysplasia: a review and case report," *Quintessence International*, vol. 28, no. 9, pp. 595–602, 1997.

[4] M. A. Pigno, R. B. Blackman, R. J. Cronin Jr., and E. Cavazos, "Prosthodontic management of ectodermal dysplasia: a review of the literature," *Journal of Prosthetic Dentistry*, vol. 76, no. 5, pp. 541–545, 1996.

[5] T. J. Vergo, "Prosthodontics for pediatric patients with congenital/developmental orofacial anomalies: a long-term follow-up," *Journal of Prosthetic Dentistry*, vol. 86, no. 4, pp. 342–347, 2001.

[6] A. J. Hickey and M. Salter, "Prosthodontic and psychological factors in treating patients with congenital and craniofacial defects," *Journal of Prosthetic Dentistry*, vol. 95, no. 5, pp. 392–396, 2006.

[7] C. Dellavia, F. Catti, C. Sforza, D. G. Tommasi, and V. F. Ferrario, "Craniofacial growth in ectodermal dysplasia: an 8 year longitudinal evaluation of Italian subjects," *Angle Orthodontist*, vol. 80, no. 4, pp. 733–739, 2010.

[8] J. A. Hobkirk, F. Nohl, B. Bergendal, K. Storhaug, and M. K. Richter, "The management of ectodermal dysplasia and severe hypodontia. International conference statements," *Journal of Oral Rehabilitation*, vol. 33, no. 9, pp. 634–637, 2006.

[9] K. A. Vieira, M. S. Teixeira, C. G. Guirado, and M. B. D. Gavião, "Prosthodontic treatment of hypohidrotic ectodermal dysplasia with complete anodontia: case report," *Quintessence International*, vol. 38, no. 1, pp. 75–80, 2007.

[10] A. S. Bidra, J. W. Martin, and E. Feldman, "Complete denture prosthodontics in children with ectodermal dysplasia: review of principles and techniques," *Compendium of Continuing Education in Dentistry*, vol. 31, no. 6, pp. 426–433, 2010.

[11] A. A. Weech, "Hereditary ectodermal dysplasia (congenital ectodermal defect)," *American Journal of Diseases of Children*, vol. 37, pp. 766–790, 1929.

[12] L. S. Fishman, "Radiographic evaluation of skeletal maturation. A clinically oriented method based on hand-wirst films," *Angle Orthodontist*, vol. 52, no. 2, pp. 88–112, 1982.

[13] M. S. Chen, W. A. Eichhold, W. A. Welker, and C. C. Chien, "Simplicity in interim tooth-supported removable partial denture construction," *The Journal of Prosthetic Dentistry*, vol. 54, no. 5, pp. 740–744, 1985.

[14] A. Bhargava, A. Nagpal, M. Kumar, and R. Bhargav, "Flexible dentures demystified," *Dental Technician*, vol. 2, pp. 18–21, 2010.

[15] D. M. Eid, "A new material for partial dentures. An unbreakable thermoplastic resin paraformaldehyde and its Co-polymers," *Egyptian Dental Journal*, vol. 17, no. 1, pp. 1–22, 1971.

[16] C. B. Jenkins and D. C. Berry, "Modification of tooth contour by acid-etch retained resins for prosthetic purposes," *British Dental Journal*, vol. 141, no. 3, pp. 89–90, 1976.

[17] D. P. NaBadalung, "Prosthodontic rehabilitation of an anhidrotic ectodermal dysplasia patient: a clinical report," *The Journal of Prosthetic Dentistry*, vol. 81, no. 5, pp. 499–502, 1999.

[18] A. J. Hickey and T. J. Vergo, "Prosthetic treatments for patients with ectodermal dysplasia," *Journal of Prosthetic Dentistry*, vol. 86, no. 4, pp. 364–368, 2001.
[19] A. K. Yap and I. Klineberg, "Dental implants in patients with ectodermal dysplasia and tooth agenesis: a critical review of the literature," *The International Journal of Prosthodontics*, vol. 22, no. 3, pp. 268–276, 2009.
[20] G. N. Graser and G. S. Rogoff, "Removable partial overdentures for special patients," *Dental clinics of North America*, vol. 34, no. 4, pp. 741–758, 1990.
[21] T. E. Donovan and G. C. Cho, "Esthetic considerations with removable partial dentures," *Journal of the California Dental Association*, vol. 31, no. 7, pp. 551–557, 2003.
[22] A. J. Beaumont, "An overview of esthetics with removable partial dentures," *Quintessence International*, vol. 33, no. 10, pp. 747–755, 2002.
[23] N. S. Sunitha, K. N. Jagadeesh, S. D. Kalavathi, and K. R. Kashinath, "'Flexible dentures'—an alternate for rigid dentures?" *Journal of Dental Sciences & Research*, vol. 1, pp. 74–79, 2010.
[24] E. Kravitz, R. L. Pollack, and D. H. Mueller, "Nutrition during pregnancy, infancy, childhood, and adolescence," *Journal of Pedodontics*, vol. 7, no. 3, pp. 182–195, 1983.

Multifocal Epithelial Hyperplasia of Oral Cavity Expressing HPV 16 Gene: A Rare Entity

M. P. V. Prabhat,[1] Chintamaneni Raja Lakshmi,[1] N. Sai Madhavi,[1] Sujana Mulk Bhavana,[1] Gummadapu Sarat,[1] and Kodali Ramamohan[2]

[1] *Department of Oral Medicine and Radiology, Drs. Sudha and Nageswara Rao Siddhartha Institute of Dental Sciences, Gannavaram Mandal, Krishna District, Andhra Pradesh 521286, India*
[2] *Department of Oral and Maxillofacial Surgery, Drs. Sudha and Nageswara Rao Siddhartha Institute of Dental Sciences, Gannavaram Mandal, Krishna District, Andhra Pradesh 521286, India*

Correspondence should be addressed to Chintamaneni Raja Lakshmi; lakshmi.chintamaneni@yahoo.com

Academic Editors: J. H. Jeng and P. I. Varela-Centelles

Focal epithelial hyperplasia is a rare contagious disease caused by human papilloma virus. Usually HPV involves either cutaneous or mucosal surfaces, whereas concomitant mucocutaneous involvement is extremely rare. We report such a unique case of multifocal epithelial hyperplasia involving multiple sites of oral cavity along with skin lesions in a 65-year-old female. We also discuss the probable multifactorial etiology and variable clinical presentations of the lesions, including evidence of HPV 16 expression, as detected by polymerase chain reaction. The present report illustrates the need for careful examination and prompt diagnosis of the disease, as it might be associated with high risk genotypes such as HPV 16 and 18.

1. Introduction

Human papilloma virus (HPV) infection is known to induce proliferative lesions on the skin and mucosa which may be benign or malignant. Over 120 genotypes have been identified in the HPV family, among which HPV 16 and 18 are considered to be high risk genotypes owing to their malignant potential. Benign oral lesions associated with HPV include squamous papilloma, verruca vulgaris, condyloma acuminatum, focal epithelial hyperplasia, and malignant variants like verrucous carcinoma and squamous cell carcinoma [1].

Focal epithelial hyperplasia of the oral cavity is a benign infectious disease caused by HPV, clinically presenting as multiple, well circumscribed papules on the oral mucosa, primarily involving gingiva, buccal, or labial mucosa [2]. The lack of sufficient literature and the asymptomatic nature of the condition make the clinical diagnosis difficult.

We hereby report a unique case that presented clinically as multifocal epithelial hyperplasia of the oral mucosa in concurrence with the skin lesions.

2. Case Report

A 65-year-old female patient presented with complaint of sensitivity of teeth since 2 months. Her past medical, dental, and personal histories were noncontributory. On extra oral examination multiple warts were seen involving face, scalp (Figures 1 and 2), and trunk. Intraoral examination showed multiple coalescent papillary projections, involving oral mucosa. The lesion was seen involving the labial gingiva of anterior teeth encroaching through the interdental papilla and involving palate (Figures 3 and 4). Predominant lesion was seen on palate extending bilaterally involving marginal gingiva of all the maxillary teeth and mid-palatine raphe and posteriorly till maxillary tuberosity region (Figure 4). Similar papillary lesions were seen involving labial gingiva of lower anterior teeth (Figure 3), dorsum of the tongue (Figure 5), and commissural areas of both right and left buccal mucosa (Figure 6). Lateral border of tongue appeared fissured with loss of papilla and melanin pigmentation. The patient observed these lesions for the past 6-7 months which were gradually spreading and were asymptomatic.

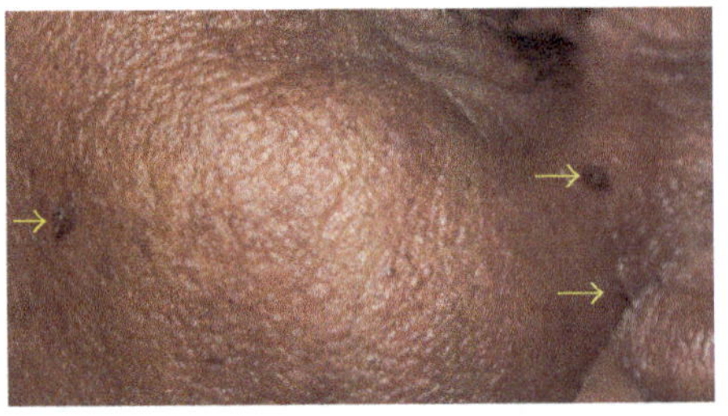

FIGURE 1: Multiple warts were seen involving face.

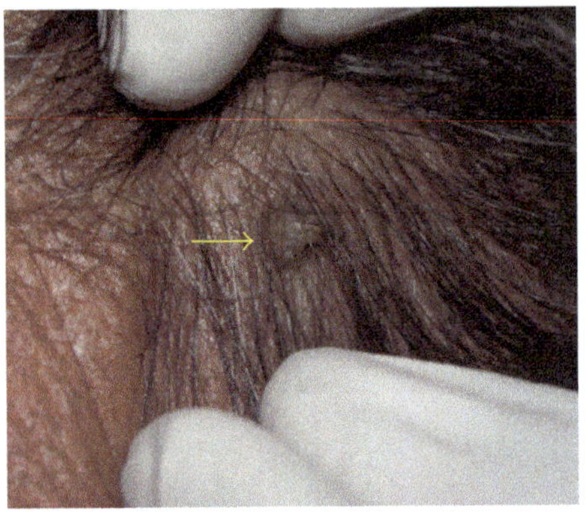

FIGURE 2: Wart seen on the scalp.

Based upon the clinical features, a provisional diagnosis of HPV associated multifocal papillomatosis was established although verrucous leukoplakia, Cowden's syndrome, and verrucous carcinoma were included in the differential diagnosis. Radiological investigations revealed no underlying bony invasion. Routine blood investigations revealed no abnormality. As the present case is a disseminated form of HPV, human immunodeficiency virus (HIV) testing was done and was reported as negative. Biopsy procedures included excision of facial wart and incisional biopsy from the palate. Microscopic picture of the biopsy specimen from skin wart revealed papillomatous epidermis, evident koilocytes with shrunken nucleus surrounded by perinuclear halo in upper epidermis. Specimen from palate revealed presence of multiple papillary epithelial projections with fibrovascular connective tissue cores. The spinous layer of the epithelium demonstrated koilocytes, suggestive of papillary epithelial hyperplasia (Figures 7, 8, and 9). The palatal specimen was further subjected to molecular diagnostics using polymerase chain reaction (PCR), which revealed the presence of HPV 16 genotype using VIC HPV 16 type specific probe.

3. Discussion

Focal epithelial hyperplasia of the oral cavity was first reported among Navajo Indians as multiple nodular elevations, similar to those described in South American Indians and Eskimos of Greenland and Alaska [3]. The first case report was published by Dr. Heck and his team in 1965, following which it came to be known as Heck's disease.

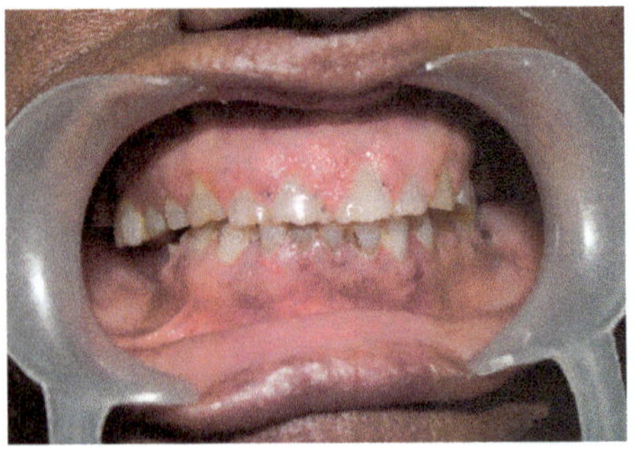

FIGURE 3: Multiple coalescent papillary projections involving upper and lower anterior gingiva.

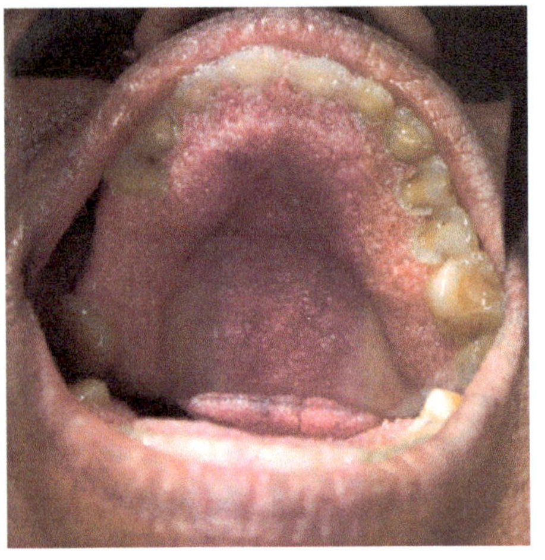

FIGURE 4: Extensive lesion seen involving palate.

So far the literature reported less than 20 cases in humans [4]; hereby we present a rare case of multifocal epithelial hyperplasia expressing HPV 16 genotype.

Over the past few years HPV 13, 32, 1, 6, 11, and 16 were the common subtypes studied in association with the disease. Although HPV is known to be the etiological agent, possibility of genetic predisposition, nutritional deficiencies and environmental factors like poverty and lack of hygiene, role of immunosuppression have been suggested as the other risk factors [4, 5]. In the present case, genetic association was ruled out and no positive history was revealed when enquired about other risk factors; however, factors like low socioeconomic profile and poor maintenance of hygiene can possibly be attributed to the disease manifestation.

Focal epithelial hyperplasia predominantly affects patients between the 1st and 2nd decades of life with a female predilection. The most frequent site was the lower lip [4]. In this case the lesion presented at an unusual age of 65 years involving multiple sites like gingiva, palate, tongue, and commissural areas of both right and left buccal mucosa. Based upon the clinical findings, provisional diagnosis of multifocal epithelial hyperplasia was given, whereas differential diagnosis included verrucous leukoplakia and verrucous carcinoma.

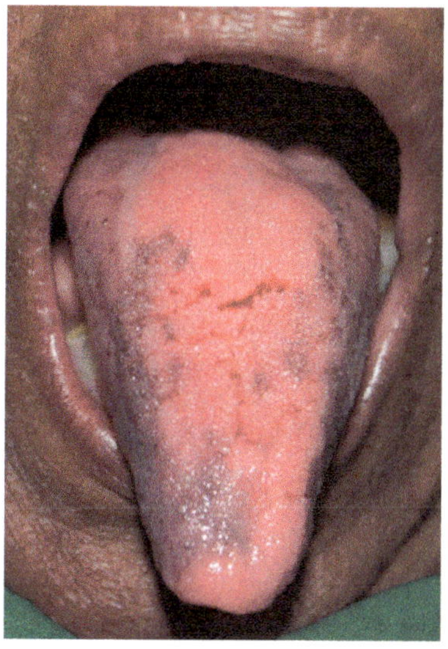

FIGURE 5: Papillary lesions with fissuring seen on the dorsum of tongue.

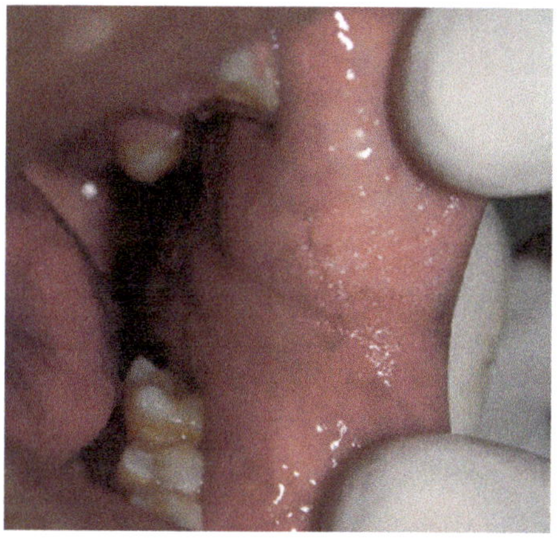

FIGURE 6: Papillary lesion at the left commissural area.

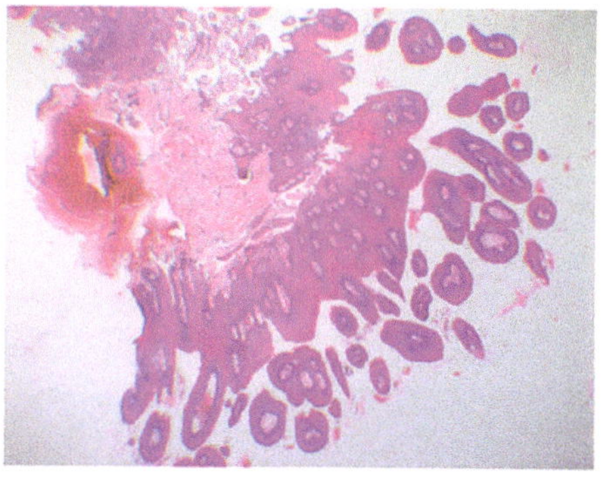

FIGURE 7: Photomicrograph of the lesion showing multiple papillary epithelial projections with fibrovascular connective tissue cores (H&E, 4x).

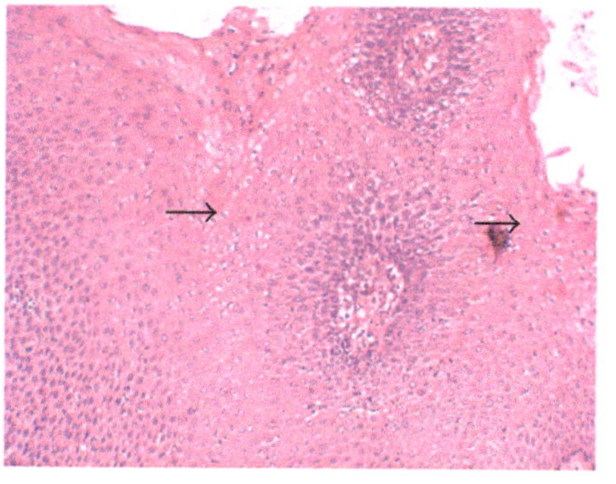

FIGURE 8: Photomicrograph of the lesion showing koilocytes (arrows) in the epithelium. Koilocytes display a hyperchromatic shrunken nucleus with clear cytoplasm (perinuclear halo) (H&E, 10x).

The diagnosis of Heck's disease is mainly based on the clinical picture and histopathological findings. The prominent microscopic features consist of parakeratin layering, extensive acanthosis, epithelial cells of the spinous layer with enlarged nucleus, degeneration of koilocytes, and mitosoid cells [6]. Our case demonstrated multiple papillary epithelial projections with fibrovascular connective tissue cores and presence of koilocytes in the spinous layer of the epithelium favouring the diagnosis. Differential diagnosis includes condyloma acuminatum, verruca vulgaris, papilloma, irritation fibroma, and Cowden syndrome as they are known to have some clinical similarities like lesion type, color, and location.

Recent advancements in molecular biology techniques for HPV testing include light microscopy; electron microscopy; nonamplified molecular techniques like in situ hybridization, southern blot, and dot blot hybridization; target amplification using PCR; signal amplified techniques like hybrid capture technology; and gene expression using DNA microarrays [1]. In the present case the specific histopathologic features in conjunction with the clinical picture drove us towards molecular analysis, so as to rule out the possible association of human papilloma virus. The PCR analysis of the biopsy sample isolated the HPV 16 genotype; however, other common strains associated with oral lesions were ruled out using type specific probes. Studies have clearly established HPV as a definitive risk for oropharyngeal cancer and oral potentially malignant disorders [7–11]. In recent reports, HPV type 16 has been identified in 90% of HPV-associated head and neck tumours and has been found in 50% of oropharyngeal head and neck squamous cell carcinoma [1]. So far, the literature reported HPV 1, 6, 11, 13, and 32 to be commonly associated with Heck's disease and are known to be benign in nature; association of HPV 16 in our case may indicate a malignant potential of the lesion.

Lesions that do not remit or cause functional and/or aesthetic problems can be removed by various modalities like surgery, cryotherapy, electrocoagulation, laser, chemical agents (e.g., retinoic acid), or immunostimulants (e.g., interferon) [4]. Harris Ricardo et al. treated 4 cases of focal epithelial hyperplasia using 80% of trichloroacetic acid and observed resolution of the lesions within 45 days [6]. The prognosis of the disease is good, as most of the lesions remit spontaneously, although periodical clinical followups

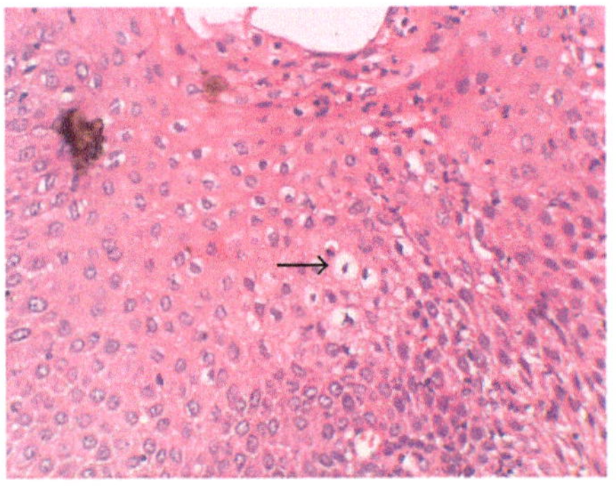

FIGURE 9: High power photomicrograph of the lesion demonstrating koilocytes (arrows) in the spinous layer (H&E, 20x).

are crucial [4]. Considering the multifocal presentation of the case, we advised laser ablation of the entire lesion. Inspite of explaining about high malignant potential of the lesion, sadly the patient was not willing to receive treatment due to the asymptomatic nature of the disease. Hence, we advised periodic long-term followups to monitor the status of the lesion.

4. Conclusion

The present case highlighted a rare presentation of HPV 16 infection as multifocal epithelial hyperplasia of the oral cavity with associated skin lesions. Clinicians need to be aware of such rare presentations to facilitate a prompt diagnosis and better treatment outcome, as certain strains like HPV 16 and 18 are known to have high malignant potential.

Conflict of Interests

The authors would like to declare that there is no conflict of interest or financial support regarding this case report.

References

[1] K. L. Kumaraswamy and M. Vidhya, "Human papilloma virus and oral infections: an update," *Journal of Cancer Research and Therapeutics*, vol. 7, no. 2, pp. 120–127, 2011.

[2] H. Al-Azmi and H. Hanafy, "Human papillomavirus: manifestations, prevention and treatment: an overview," *The Gulf Journal of Dermatology and Venereology*, vol. 19, no. 1, pp. 1–28, 2012.

[3] L. dos Santos-Pinto, E. M. A. Giro, C. A. Pansani, J. Ferrari, E. M. S. Massucato, and L. C. S. Luis Carlos Spolidório, "An uncommon focal epithelial hyperplasia manifestation," *Journal of Dentistry for Children*, vol. 76, no. 3, pp. 233–236, 2009.

[4] A. Bascones-Martínez, S. Cok, C. Bascones-Ilundáin, S. Arias-Herrera, R. Gomez-Font, and J. Bascones-Ilundáin, "Multifocal epithelial hyperplasia: a potentially precancerous disease?" *Oncology Letters*, vol. 3, no. 2, pp. 255–258, 2012.

[5] S. Beaudenon, F. Praetorius, and D. Kremsdorf, "A new type of human papillomavirus associated with oral focal epithelial hyperplasia," *Journal of Investigative Dermatology*, vol. 88, no. 2, pp. 130–135, 1987.

[6] J. Harris Ricardo, M. Carmona Lorduy, and A. Díaz Caballero, "Treatment of focal epithelial hyperplasia with trichloroacetic acid," *Revista Clínica de Periodoncia, Implantología y Rehabilitación Oral*, vol. 5, no. 3, pp. 140–143, 2012.

[7] A. Y. Babiker, F. M. Eltom, M. S. Abdalaziz, A. Rahmani, S. Abusail, and H. G. Ahmed, "Screening for high risk human papilloma virus (HR-HPV) subtypes, among Sudanese patients with oral lesions," *International Journal of Clinical and Experimental Medicine*, vol. 6, no. 4, pp. 275–281, 2013.

[8] S. Syrjänen, G. Lodi, I. von Bültzingslöwen et al., "Human papillomaviruses in oral carcinoma and oral potentially malignant disorders: a systematic review," *Oral Diseases*, vol. 17, no. 1, pp. 58–72, 2011.

[9] J. V. Gonzalez, R. A. Gutierrez, A. Keszler et al., "Human papillomavirus in oral lesions," *Medicina*, vol. 67, no. 4, pp. 363–368, 2007.

[10] C. Simionescu, C. L. . Mărgăritescu, C. Valentina Georgescu, and M. Surpăţeanu, "HPV and p53 expression in dysplastic lesions and squamous carcinomas of the oral mucosa," *Romanian Journal of Morphology and Embryology*, vol. 46, no. 2, pp. 155–159, 2005.

[11] A. Al-Osman, J. B. Perry, and C. Birek, "Extensive papillomatosis of the palate exhibiting epithelial dysplasia and HPV 16 gene expression in a renal transplant recipient," *Journal of the Canadian Dental Association*, vol. 72, no. 4, pp. 331–334, 2006.

5

Ulcerative Lichen Planus in Childhood

Chiyadu Padmini,[1] K. Yellamma Bai,[2] Vinil Chaitanya,[3] and M. Shilpa Reddy[4]

[1] *Department of Pedodontics and Preventive Dentistry, Malla Reddy Institute of Dental Sciences, Suraram, Zediametla, Hyderabad 500055, Andhra Pradesh, India*
[2] *Department of Pedodontics and Preventive Dentistry, Malla Reddy College of Dental Sciences for Women, India*
[3] *Department of Oral Medicine and Radiology, Malla Reddy Institute of Dental Sciences, Suraram, Zediametla, Hyderabad 500055, Andhra Pradesh, India*
[4] *Department of Conservative Dentistry and Endodontics, Malla Reddy Institute of Dental Sciences, Suraram, Zediametla, Hyderabad 500055, Andhra Pradesh, India*

Correspondence should be addressed to Chiyadu Padmini; abcdentalhospital@gmail.com

Academic Editors: V. Brailo, Y.-K. Chen, and Y.-C. Hung

Lichen planus (LP) is a chronic inflammatory mucocutaneous condition which is relatively common in adults but rarely affects children. The present study is a report on an unusual case of ulcerative oral LP involving the dorsum of tongue in a 12-year-old boy. Patient complained of painful oral lesion on the tongue which was burning in nature and obstructing talking and eating spicy foods. On intraoral examination, a white ulcerative lesion on the dorsum of tongue was observed. Diagnosis was made based on clinical examination and histopathological features. We instituted local treatment and patient responded well to the treatment. Although rarely reported in childhood, lichen planus should be considered in a differential diagnosis of hyperkeratotic, reticular, and ulcerative lesions of the oral mucosa in children.

1. Introduction

Lichen planus (LP) is an autoimmune, chronic, inflammatory disease that affects mucosal and cutaneous tissues. The exact etiology of LP is unknown, but it is believed to result from an abnormal T cell-mediated immune response in which basal epithelial cells are recognized as foreign because of changes in the antigenicity of their cell surface [1]. Oral lichen planus (OLP) is a common disease in the middle aged and elderly population and has a prevalence of about 0.5% to 2%. By contrast, oral lichen planus in childhood (OLP) is rare and it was first reported in the 1920s. Oral mucosal involvement in adults itself accounts for 0.5% to 19%, while in children, it is very uncommon [2].

The oral lesions are more pleomorphic than those of their cutaneous forms and subtypes are categorized as reticular, papular, plaque-like, atrophic, erosive, and bullous [3]. The erosive form is extremely rare in children and few reports on this subject have been published in the literature.

Herewith, we are presenting a case of a 12-year-old boy having erosive lichen planus without cutaneous involvement, who responded very well to the treatment. This paper also reviews ulcerative oral lichen planus in children and emphasizes its diagnosis from other oral white and red lesions in children.

2. Case Report

A 12-year-old boy reported to the Department of Pedodontics and Preventive Dentistry, with the chief complaint of ulcer on his dorsum of the tongue which is causing burning sensation on consuming spicy foods from past 1 year (Figure 5).

There is no significant medical history observed. On extra oral examination, patient was normal. On intraoral examination, a single irregular red and white ulcerative lesion measuring approximately 2.5×1.0 cm in size with granulation tissue at the centre surrounded by an inflammatory red border on the dorsum of the tongue was noticed. There was a depapillation of filiform papillae in and around the lesion (Figure 1). Oral hygiene of the patient was good without any dental restorations.

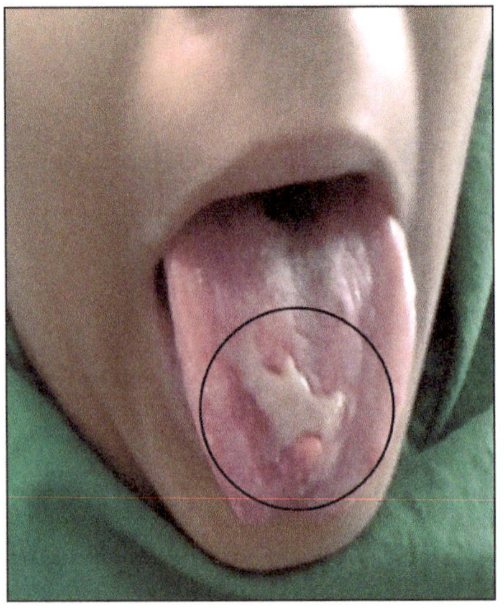

Figure 1: Dorsum of tongue showing ulcerative lesion.

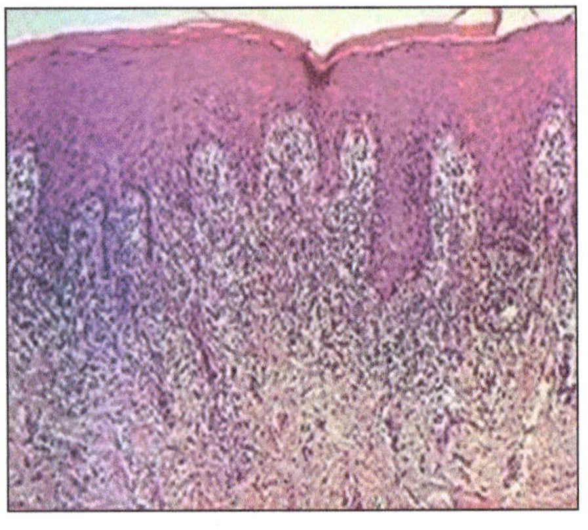

Figure 2: Photomicrograph (5x magnification) of the lesion.

The differential diagnosis was lichen planus and lichenoid lesions. To exclude lichenoid reaction, we investigated his medical status and there was no history of any drug intake. The patient and his parents also denied any habits that may potentially cause oral mucosal ulcerations.

Histopathological examination showed hyperparakeratosis of stratified squamous epithelium and basal cell degeneration with dense band-linked lymphocytic infiltration at the epithelial-connective tissue interface (Figure 2). Both clinical and histopathological features were consistent with ulcerative oral lichen planus.

Specific treatment for ulcerative OLP was topical 0.1% triamcinolone acetonide combined with 1% clotrimazole 3–5 times per day for a duration of one week. Topical anesthetic was given for the pain relief. First review of the patient after 15 days showed significant reduction in both symptoms and signs of the oral lesions (Figure 3). After 15 days, there was good prognosis in the recovery of ulcerative lichen planus (Figure 6). Erosive oral ulcerative oral lichen planus had completely healed at the end of 30 days (Figures 4 and 7). Patient was observed on periodic recall followup.

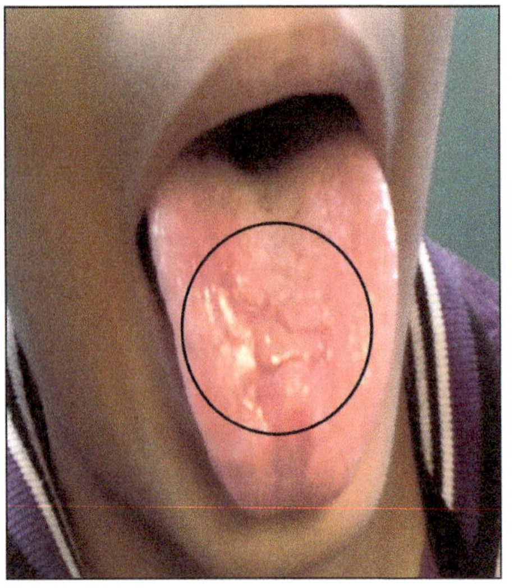

Figure 3: Mid treatment (15th day of treatment) showing reduction in size & healing of the ulceration.

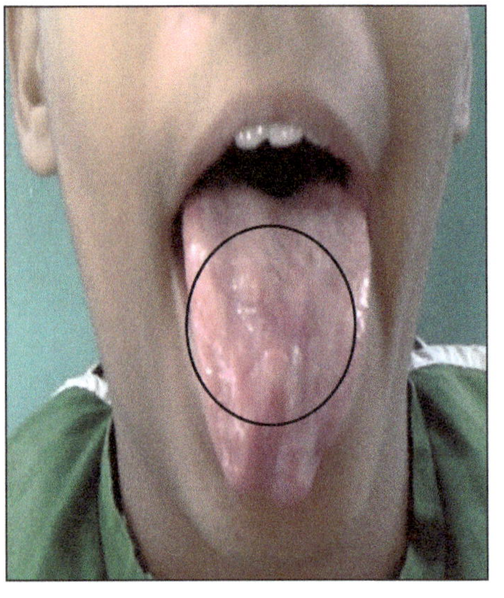

Figure 4: Complete healing of ulcer on tongue (after 30 days of treatment).

3. Discussion

Oral lichen planus in childhood (OLPc) is rare and only a few reports are available in the literature [4]. Oral lichen planus can be divided into a hyperkeratotic (white) variant, commonly without symptoms, a reticular type with Wickham striae (often symmetrical), and papular and plaque-like types.

The atrophic/erythematous (red) variant and the erosive/ulcerative (yellow) variant often have persistent symptoms of pain or stinging aggravated during talking and eating spicy foods. These variants may occur together in one patient or may transform from one to another. The lesions were found more commonly on the buccal mucosa (often symmetrical), lateral margins of the tongue, gingiva, and lips.

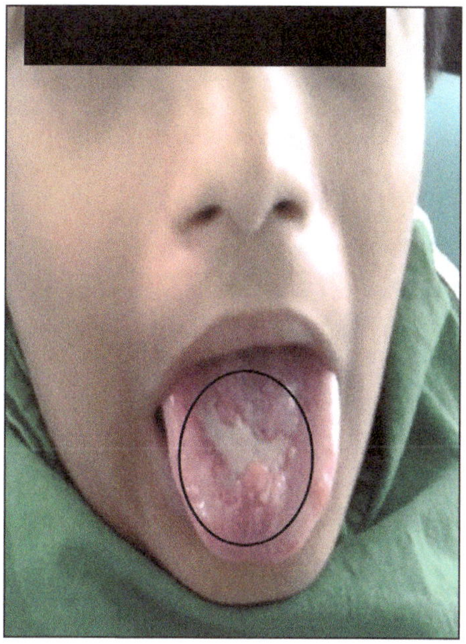

FIGURE 5: Pretreatment photograph showing ulcer on dorsum of tongue.

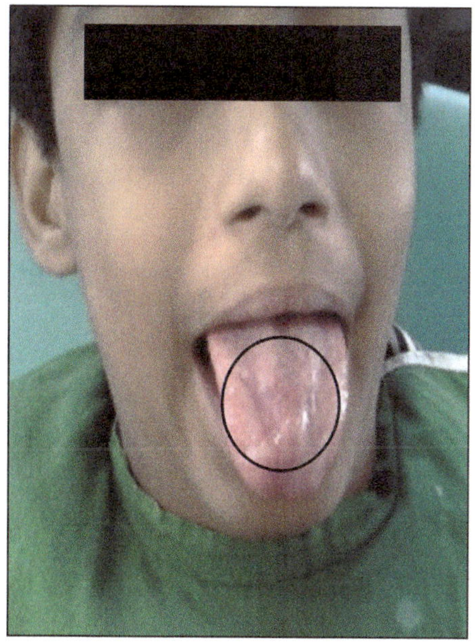

FIGURE 7: Posttreatment photograph showing complete healing of ulceration.

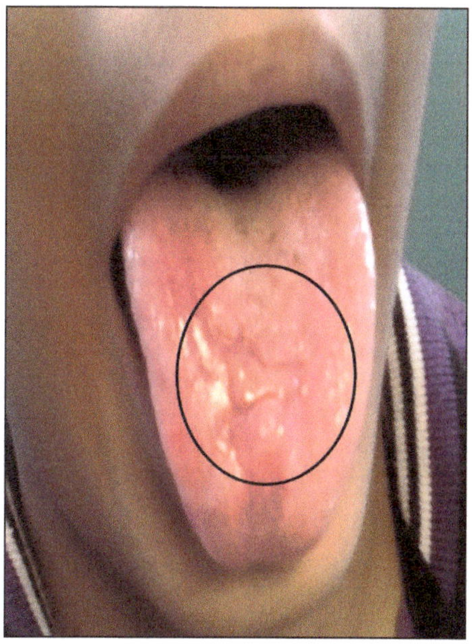

FIGURE 6: Mid treatment photograph showing resolution size of the lesion.

Whereas cutaneous LP is self-limiting, ulcerative OLP is chronic, and rarely undergoes spontaneous remission. The family history of LP is more commonly positive in patients with LP in childhood than in adulthood. The exact cause of ulcerative OLP remains unknown, but an immune-mediated (T cell dependant) pathogenesis has been reported.

OLP in childhood was first described in 1920 and since then only few articles have been published and most of the studies have suggested that childhood LP is more common in tropical countries like India [5]. Sharma and Maheshwari reported 50 children with LP and with concomitant oral lesions in 15 of them and they stated that the oral mucosa seems to be less commonly involved in children with LP than in adults [6].

Predisposing conditions such as graft-versus-host disease, active hepatitis, and hepatitis B immunization are rather frequently mentioned in these reports. Kanwar and Kumar reported only one case having oral ulcerative lichen planus out of 25 patients with cutaneous lichen planus [7].

The mean interval between vaccination and LP onset was three years, ranging between three months and 11 years. Handa and Sahoo reported 87 patients with childhood LP in India. Seven patients showed involvement of the oral mucosa and only one patient had oral ulcerative lichen planus without skin involvement [8].

A 10-year retrospective study was done by Ronald Laeijendecker et al., which was comprised of 10,000 patients below 18 years, with a boy to girl ratio of 1 : 1, and which has shown that the only 3 patients (0.03%) were diagnosed with oral lichen palnus [9]. A study done in the United Kingdom by Alam and Hamburger on boys aged between 6 and 14 years over a period of 20 years has proved that only 6 boys have been diagnosed with OLP and interestingly among 6 patients, 4 were Asians [10]. In 1994, Scully et al. reported 3 girls with OLP, one of whom was from Asian origin [11].

The difference in the prevalence of OLP in children (0.03%) versus that of OLP in adults (0.5%–2%) is understood by less number of associated systemic diseases in children, autoimmune diseases, infections, drug usage, and dental restorations in childhood; this may reduce the risk for developing OLP in childhood [12]. Moreover, the diagnosis of OLP may be missed due to irregular dental checkups, lack of symptoms, and ignorance by clinicians in diagnosing the condition.

The prognosis and the effect of treatment in OLP in children seem to be more favorable than in OLP in adults, which usually persists for many years in spite of intensive treatment and thorough investigation of associated factors. Malignant transformation of ulcerative OLP in adults is 0.07% to 5%; however, malignant transformation of OLP in children is not documented in the literature till now [13].

4. Conclusion

Oral lichen planus in childhood is rare, especially erosive form; diagnosis should be based on children presenting with ulcerative white lesion in oral cavity. The schedule of followup of OLP in children should be 7 days, 15 days, and 30 days after diagnosis to assess healing. Patient should be reviewed twice a year for regular followups after complete progress of the present condition. However, generally, the prognosis of oral lichen planus in childhood seems to be more favorable compared to adults.

References

[1] S. Patel, C. M. Yeoman, and R. Murphy, "Oral lichen planus in childhood: a report of three cases," *International Journal of Paediatric Dentistry*, vol. 15, no. 2, pp. 118–122, 2005.

[2] D. Eisen, "The clinical features, malignant potential, and systemic associations of oral lichen planus: a study of 723 patients," *Journal of the American Academy of Dermatology*, vol. 46, no. 2, pp. 207–214, 2002.

[3] J. M. Aguirre, J. V. Bagán, C. Rodriguez et al., "Efficacy of mometasone furoate microemulsion in the treatment of erosive-ulcerative oral lichen planus: pilot study," *Journal of Oral Pathology and Medicine*, vol. 33, no. 7, pp. 381–385, 2004.

[4] F. Cottoni, P. Ena, G. Tedde, and M. A. Montesu, "Lichen planus in children: a case report," *Pediatric Dermatology*, vol. 10, no. 2, pp. 132–135, 1993.

[5] A. J. Kanwar and D. De, "Lichen planus in childhood: report of 100 cases," *Clinical and Experimental Dermatology*, vol. 33, pp. 423–427, 2008.

[6] R. Sharma and V. Maheshwari, "Childhood lichen planus: a report of fifty cases," *Pediatric Dermatology*, vol. 16, no. 5, pp. 345–348, 1999.

[7] A. J. Kanwar and D. De, "Lichen planus in childhood: report of 100 cases," *Clinical and Experimental Dermatology*, vol. 35, no. 3, pp. 257–262, 2010.

[8] S. Handa and B. Sahoo, "Childhood lichen planus: a study of 87 cases," *International Journal of Dermatology*, vol. 41, no. 7, pp. 423–427, 2002.

[9] R. Laeijendecker, T. Van Joost, B. Tank, A. P. Oranje, and H. A. M. Neumann, "Oral lichen planus in childhood," *Pediatric Dermatology*, vol. 22, no. 4, pp. 299–304, 2005.

[10] F. Alam and J. Hamburger, "Oral mucosal lichen planus in children," *International Journal of Paediatric Dentistry*, vol. 11, no. 3, pp. 209–214, 2001.

[11] C. Scully, O. P. de Almeida, and R. Welbury, "Oral lichen planus in childhood," *British Journal of Dermatology*, vol. 130, no. 1, pp. 131–133, 1994.

[12] M. Rybojad, I. Moraillon, S. Laglenne et al., "Lichen plan del'enfant," *Annales de Dermatologie et de Venereologie*, vol. 125, no. 10, pp. 679–681, 1998.

[13] A. Pakfetrat, A. Javadzadeh-Bolouri, S. Basir-Shabestari, and F. Falaki, "Oral lichen planus: a retrospective study of 420 Iranian patients," *Medicina Oral, Patologia Oral y Cirugia Bucal*, vol. 14, no. 7, pp. E315–E318, 2009.

6

Pathophysiology of Barodontalgia: A Case Report and Review of the Literature

Marcus Stoetzer,[1] Christoph Kuehlhorn,[2] Martin Ruecker,[1] Dirk Ziebolz,[3] Nils Claudius Gellrich,[1] and Constantin von See[1,2]

[1] *Department of Oral and Maxillofacial Surgery, Hanover Medical School, Carl-Neuberg-Straße 1, 30625 Hanover, Germany*
[2] *Munster Military Medical Center, Munster, Germany*
[3] *Department of Preventive Dentistry, Periodontology and Cariology, University of Goettingen Medical Centre, Goettingen, Germany*

Correspondence should be addressed to Marcus Stoetzer, marcus_stoetzer@web.de

Academic Editors: M. Darling, C. Farah, A. Kasaj, L. N. De. Souza, and P. I. Varela-Centelles

Changes in ambient pressure occur during flying, diving, or hyperbaric oxygen therapy and can cause different types of pathophysiological conditions and pain including toothache (barodontalgia). We report the case of a patient with severe pain in the region of his mandibular left first molar, which had been satisfactorily restored with a conservative restoration. Pain occurred during an airplane flight and persisted after landing. Radiology revealed a periapical radiolucency in the region of the distal root apex. Pain relief was achieved only after endodontic treatment. On the basis of this paper, we investigated the aetiology and management of barodontalgia. Dentists should advise patients to avoid exposure to pressure changes until all necessary surgical, conservative, and prosthetic procedures have been completed. The influence of pressure divergences should be noted at any time. Under changed environment pressures may be the changing perception of pathologies.

1. Introduction

Changes in ambient pressure, for example, during flying, diving or hyperbaric oxygen therapy, can lead to barotrauma. Flying and diving are usually associated with different types of pressure changes. During commercial flights, for example, aircraft personnel are exposed to only minor pressure differences but exposure lasts for a relatively long period of time. By contrast, military and aerobatic pilots are subjected to rapid pressure changes and strong acceleration forces. As a result of the higher density of the surrounding medium, divers are exposed to very high ambient pressures. Compared with aircraft personnel, however, the duration of exposure is usually short. Depending on diving depth and technique, there are considerable differences in the breathing gases used. In addition to changes in ambient pressure, this causes further physiological and metabolic changes in the human body. Barodontalgia was reported to occur during flying at altitudes of 600–1500 m and during diving at depths of 10–25 m [1].

A generally accepted classification of barodontalgia was developed by Ferjentsik and Aker [2] and is primarily based on the underlying causes and clinical symptoms (Table 1).

In general, barotrauma is defined as pressure-induced damage that can occur both at high and low pressures. The pathology of barotrauma is directly related to Boyle's law, which states that, if temperature remains constant, the volume of a fixed mass of an ideal gas is inversely proportional to the pressure of the gas. As pressure increases, the volume of a confined gas decreases. Vice versa, volume increases as pressure decreases. Pain during ascent can indicate the presence of a disease of vital pulp tissue (pulpitis). Pain during descent can be indicative of pulp necrosis or facial barotraumas [1].

Pressure differences occur in the human body when a gas-filled cavity cannot communicate with the exterior and pressure cannot be equalized. Clinically, the resulting pressure difference between the gas-filled cavity and the exterior environment can lead to pain, oedema, or vascular gas embolism [3]. This type of pain often occurs in the

Table 1: Classification of barodontalgia.

Class	Cause	Symptoms
Class I	Irreversible pulpitis	Sharp pain on ascent
Class II	Reversible pulpitis	Dull pain on ascent
Class III	Necrotic pulp	Dull pain on descent
Class IV	Periapical pathology	Severe persistent pain on ascent or descent

lungs, the middle ear, or the maxillary sinus (barosinusitis) [4, 5]. In the majority of cases, barosinusitis develops in the presence of acute or chronic maxillary sinusitis. Headaches, numbness, or dental pain in the region of the maxillary posterior teeth occurs as a result of a difference in pressure. A problem in clinical diagnosis is that it is difficult to differentiate between barosinusitis and barodontalgia on the basis of maxillary pain [6, 7].

In general, barodontalgia is defined as pain that occurs in the region of the teeth after pressure changes [8]. This phenomenon was first observed in air crews during World War II and was given the name "aerodontalgia." Later it was also detected in divers. The incidence of this type of tooth pain is 0.26–2.8% in aircraft personnel, air passengers, and divers [6, 9, 10]. A statistical difference between diving and flying personnel has not been reported.

2. Diagnosis and Treatment

A 26-year-old male patient presented with pain in the left mandibular region which had persisted for five days. He reported that the pain had occurred when he had been flying in an airplane and had appeared suddenly at the end of the climb. When asked to describe the intensity of pain using a 0 (no pain) to 10 (worst pain) numerical rating scale (NRS), he rated his pain as 8. At ground level, the patient had been free of pain for approximately five hours. His dental pain had then increased again to a score of 6 to 7 and was described as a dull throbbing local ache. The patient had taken a daily dose of 1600–2400 mg of ibuprofen over a period of four days to relieve his pain since immediate dental care had been unavailable.

Upon clinical examination, the mandibular left first molar (tooth 36) (Figure 1), which had been satisfactorily restored with a conservative restoration, was tender to percussion. A periodontal examination of the left mandible was unremarkable. A vitality test of the mandibular left first molar indicated that the tooth was nonvital.

A radiographic examination showed a well-restored dentition in the left mandible. A single-tooth radiograph of tooth 36 revealed an enlarged periodontal space and a periapical radiolucency in the region of the distal root of tooth 36 (Figure 2).

Following the administration of local anaesthesia and the application of a dental rubber dam, endodontic treatment of tooth 36 was instituted. After access cavity preparation, pulp was removed and three root canals were exposed (Figure 3). During the procedure, no pus was present. Severe

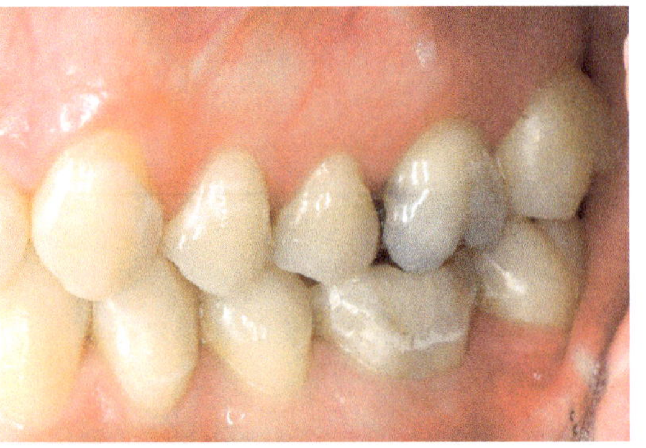

Figure 1: An intraoral clinical examination of the mandible did not reveal macroscopically detectable pathologies.

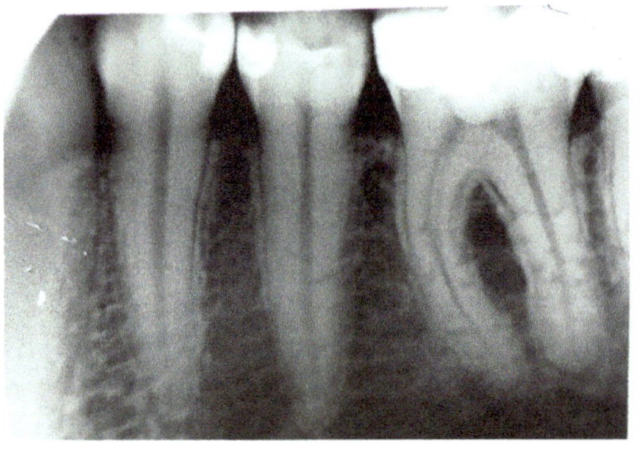

Figure 2: Radiolucency image of tooth 36 showing a periapical radiolucency in the region of the mesial and distal root apices.

bleeding from both mesial root canal orifices, however, was noted. The distal root canal showed in particular gangrenous decomposition of pulp tissue.

The root canals were enlarged using Gates Glidden drills (Dentsply, USA) and prepared with nickel-titanium (Ni-Ti) files according to a standard protocol (Mtwo, VDW, Munich, Germany) with a view to obtaining good visibility of the site. A Ledermix dressing (Haupt Pharma, Wolfratshausen, Germany) was created, and the tooth was temporarily sealed with cement (Havard-Zement, Hofmann & Richter, Berlin, Germany). The presence or absence of cracks was assessed optically using magnifying glasses and a blue-light lamp before and after staining (Mira-2-Ton, Hager and Werken, Duisburg, Germany). No fractures were detected. After the root canal filling was completed, the course of treatment was unremarkable.

3. Discussion

Since the aetiology of barodontalgia is still not completely understood, current dental treatment recommendations for flying and diving personnel are often based on statistical data [11]. A further problem is that barodontalgia can occur irrespective of the type of pressure change, that is, during an increase or a decrease in pressure, and can persist even after pressure equalisation [12]. Possible causative

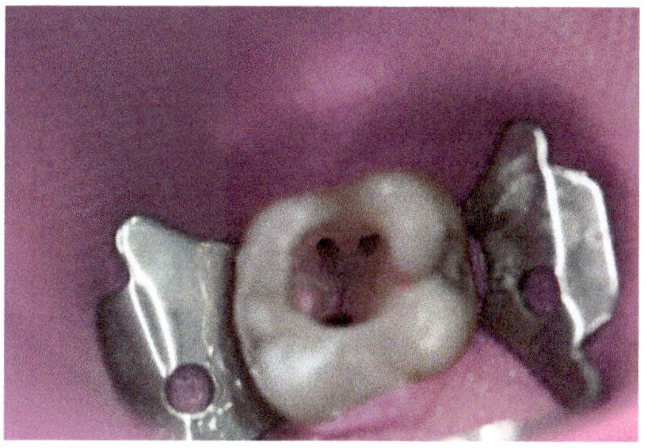

FIGURE 3: Root canal orifices after enlargement during endodontic treatment.

or contributing factors, which, however, are a matter of some controversy, include dentogenic infections, sinusitis, differences in the expansion behaviour of dental enamel and pulp, and pressure-induced movement of fluids from exposed dentine to the pulp [7, 13, 14].

In animal experiments, Carlson et al. [13] showed that fluid moved from the dentine to the pulp chamber after cavity preparation in the enamel under hyperbaric conditions. Retrospective studies showed that most patients with clinically manifest barodontalgia had carious lesions or defective restorations extending into the dentine [15]. The clinical implication of this finding is that patients who have carious lesions or have undergone dental treatment including the exposure of dentine, for example, during prosthetic tooth preparation should avoid exposure to pressure changes until definitive treatment.

In the literature, pulpitis with periapical inflammation or after dental restoration is reported to be the most common cause of barodontalgia. In the case presented here, pain occurred in a tooth with pulp necrosis. The patient was asymptomatic until he was exposed to pressure changes during a flight. In the hypobaric environment, pain developed and persisted even when he was no longer subjected to pressure changes. The pathophysiology of this pain is still not completely understood. It is likely that the clinical symptoms are a result of impaired microcirculation of the pulp.

Apart from dental pain, pressure changes are reported to cause fractures of teeth and dental restorations in pilots and divers [16, 17]. In the case presented here, however, the patient had no such fractures. Gas that is trapped between a tooth and its restoration was long believed to cause fractures of teeth or restorations and lead to barodontalgia. A closer analysis, however, revealed the presence of secondary caries under the fractured restorations. For this reason, a movement of fluids from carious dentine is today believed to be the cause of pulpitis [17].

Indirect pulp capping is currently not recommended in patients exposed to pressure changes. Variations in pressure are believed to adversely affect the regeneration of pulp tissue. In order to avoid possible complications, endodontic treatment or extraction should therefore be performed in cases in which direct pulp capping would be indicated.

As a rule, persons should undergo a thorough dental examination before being exposed to pressure changes. Treatment must include the restoration of all carious lesions, the removal of all defective restorations, and the management of inflammation. Vitality testing of all teeth is required for the detection and treatment of asymptomatic pulp necrosis [18, 19]. Dentists should advise patients to avoid exposure to pressure changes until all necessary surgical, conservative, and prosthetic procedures have been completed.

Conflict of Interests

The authors declare that they have no competing interests.

Authors' Contributions

M. Stoetzer, C. Kuehlhorn, M. Ruecker, D. Ziebolz, N. C. Gellrich and C. V. See conceived of the study and participated in its design and coordination. M. Stoetzer and C. Kuehlhorn made substantial contributions to data acquisition and conception of manuscript. M. Stoetzer, C. Kuehlhorn, D. Ziebolz, N. C. Gellrich and C. V. See drafted and designed the manuscript and contributed equally to this work. MR was involved in revising the manuscript. All authors read and approved the final manuscript.

Consent

Written informed consent was obtained from the patient for publication of this and accompanying images. A copy of the written consent is available for review by the Editor-in-Chief of this journal.

References

[1] Y. Zadik, "Barodontalgia," *Journal of Endodontics*, vol. 35, no. 4, pp. 481–485, 2009.

[2] E. Ferjentsik and F. Aker, "Barodontalgia: a system of classification," *Military Medicine*, vol. 147, no. 4, pp. 299–304, 1982.

[3] M. Hamilton-Farrell and A. Bhattacharyya, "Barotrauma," *Injury*, vol. 35, no. 4, pp. 359–370, 2004.

[4] J. Kieser, "Sinus barotrauma presenting as acute dental pain," *South African Medical Journal*, vol. 87, no. 2, p. 184, 1997.

[5] J. Kressin, "Aviation medicine problems in otorhinolaryngology," *Zeitschrift Fur Arztliche Fortbildung Und Qualitatssicherung*, vol. 93, no. 7, pp. 509–512, 1999.

[6] W. Kollmann, "Incidence and possible causes of dental pain during simulated high altitude flights," *Journal of Endodontics*, vol. 19, no. 3, pp. 154–159, 1993.

[7] Y. Zadik, L. Chapnik, and L. Goldstein, "In-flight barodontalgia: analysis of 29 cases in military aircrew," *Aviation Space and Environmental Medicine*, vol. 78, no. 6, pp. 593–596, 2007.

[8] R. E. Holowatyj, "Barodontalgia among flyers: a review of seven cases," *Journal of the Canadian Dental Association*, vol. 62, no. 7, pp. 578–584, 1996.

[9] D. M. Taylor, K. S. O'Toole, and C. M. Ryan, "Experienced scuba divers in Australia and the United States suffer considerable injury and morbidity," *Wilderness and Environmental Medicine*, vol. 14, no. 2, pp. 83–88, 2003.

[10] M. Del Mar González Santiago, A. Martinez-Sahuquillo Marquez, and P. Bullón Fernández, "Incidence of barodontalgias and their relation to oral/dental condition in personnel with responsibility in military flight," *Medicina Oral*, vol. 9, no. 2, pp. 92–105, 2004.

[11] W. H. G. Goethe, H. Bater, and C. Laban, "Barodontalgia and barotrauma in the human teeth: findings in navy divers, frogmen, and submariners of the Federal Republic of Germany," *Military Medicine*, vol. 154, no. 10, pp. 491–495, 1989.

[12] Y. Zadik, "Aviation dentistry: current concepts and practice," *British Dental Journal*, vol. 206, no. 1, pp. 11–16, 2009.

[13] O. G. Carlson, B. A. Halverson, and R. G. Triplett, "Dentin permeability under hyperbaric conditions as a possible cause of barodontalgia," *Undersea Biomedical Research*, vol. 10, no. 1, pp. 23–28, 1983.

[14] Y. Zadik, "Barodontalgia due to odontogenic inflammation in the jawbone," *Aviation Space and Environmental Medicine*, vol. 77, no. 8, pp. 864–866, 2006.

[15] Y. Zadik, S. Einy, R. Pokroy, Y. B. Dayan, and L. Goldstein, "Dental fractures on acute exposure to high altitude," *Aviation Space and Environmental Medicine*, vol. 77, no. 6, pp. 654–657, 2006.

[16] M. Gunepin, F. Derache, and T. Audoual, "Fracture of a sound tooth in a pilot under hypobaric conditions," *Aviation Space and Environmental Medicine*, vol. 81, no. 7, pp. 691–693, 2010.

[17] I. M. Calder and J. D. Ramsey, "Ondontecrexis-the effects of rapid decompression on restored teeth," *Journal of Dentistry*, vol. 11, no. 4, pp. 318–323, 1983.

[18] K. Woodmansey, "Class II barodontalgia: review and report of a case," *General Dentistry*, vol. 56, no. 7, pp. e39–e42, 2008.

[19] Y. Zadik, "Barodontalgia: what have we learned in the past decade?" *Oral Surgery, Oral Medicine, Oral Pathology, Oral Radiology and Endodontology*, vol. 109, no. 4, pp. e65–e69, 2010.

Accidental Ingestion of Molar Band and Its Management: Maintenance Is Better than Management

Appasaheb Naragond,[1] Smitha Kenganal,[2] K. Rajasigamani,[3] and N. Sathish Kumar[4]

[1] *Department of Orthodontics and Dentofacial Orthopedics, P.M.N.M Dental College and Hospital, Bagalkot, Karnataka, India*
[2] *Department of Conservative Dentistry and Endodontics, P.M.N.M Dental College and Hospital, Bagalkot, Karnataka, India*
[3] *Department of Orthodontics and Dentofacial Orthopedics, Rajah Muthiah Dental College and Hospital, Chidambaram, Tamil Nadu, India*
[4] *Sri Manakula Vinayagar Medical College and Hospital, Kalitheerthalkuppam, Puducherry, Tamil Nadu, India*

Correspondence should be addressed to Appasaheb Naragond; appuinmds@yahoo.co.in

Academic Editors: L. Junquera, A. Kasaj, and E. F. Wright

Ingestion of a broken part of fixed orthodontic appliance is a potential complication during orthodontic treatment. We report a case of accidental ingestion of molar band and its subsequent diagnosis followed by endoscopic retrieval method. Although prevention of such incidence is the best method at the same time management of such an event is also crucial. The objective of this paper is to draw attention to the potentially serious complications that can occur if preventive techniques are not practiced and also the management of such event.

1. Introduction

Management of orthodontic appliance without debonding or fracture is the biggest task for orthodontic patient during treatment. It requires ulmost care, cooperation, and maintenance. Accidental ingestion of orthodontic appliance or a part of it can cause severe problem in the airway or in gastrointestinal tract. Accidental ingestion of an appliance during a chair-side procedure or later, because of inadequate stability or retention of the appliance, can create a medical emergency that can lead to serious complications, like severe breathlessness or internal hemorrhage leading to death from aspiration of the foreign body.

While a wide variety of complications resulting from foreign bodies have been documented in clinical practice, incidence of broken orthodontic appliances or components, dentures, and removable appliance are in majority.

The incidence of aspiration or swallowing dental foreign bodies varies considerably in the literature. Ingestion or aspiration of foreign bodies is recognized as a complication in all clinical specialties of dentistry [1]. Accidental foreign body ingestion or aspiration is usually handled by physicians in the accident and emergency units. A sizeable proportion of those affected are children (80%) below 3 years of age [2]. While food materials constitute the majority of foreign bodies found in the airway in children [2], loose dentures, broken orthodontic appliances, or components and dental instruments are the second most commonly ingested objects in adults [3]. The incidence of aspiration or swallowing dental foreign bodies varies considerably in the literature, in a review article, the range was 3.6% to 27.7% of all foreign bodies, with the number considerably higher in adults than in children [4]. The aspiration or ingestion of orthodontic appliances is less common but not less varied in the types of appliance involved. These include swallowing an expansion appliance key [5], a transpalatal arch [6], a lower spring retainer [7], a fragment of a maxillary removable appliance [8], and a piece of archwire [1]. A rare case of accidental swallowing of a removable quad helix by a 13-year-old boy affected by Down's syndrome, which necessitated surgical removal, has also been reported [9]. A case of accidental ingestion of molar band and its subsequent diagnosis followed by endoscopic retrieval method is being presented. Guidelines for prevention and also management of such event are being discussed.

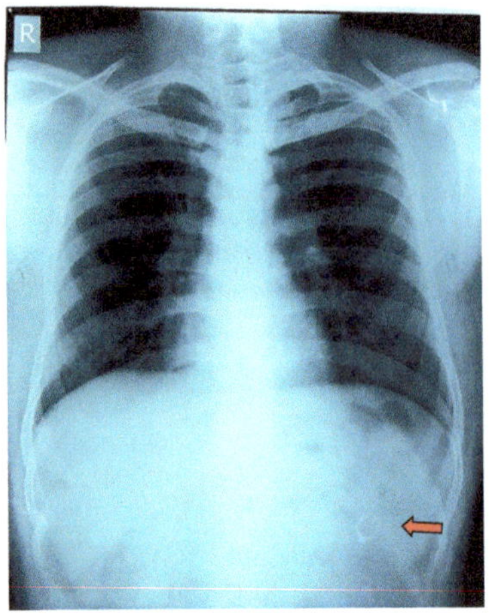

Figure 1: X-ray showing evidence of molar band.

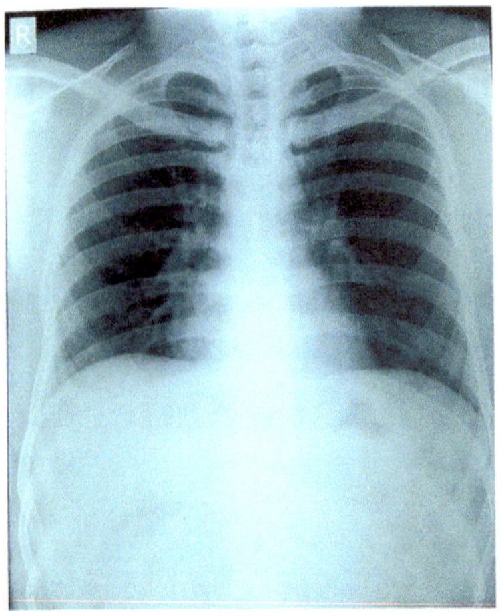

Figure 2: X-ray showing no evidence of molar band.

2. Case Presentation

A 16-year-old boy sought treatment with the chief complaint of proclined upper and lower anterior teeth. To fulfill the objectives of the patient we decided to go for fixed orthodontic appliance therapy along with extraction of all first premolars. All the first and second molars were banded. Upper and lower bonding was done. Patient's followup was done for three months. After that the patient reported to the clinic a complaint of ingestion of some part of the appliance. On examination it has been noticed that second molar band in the upper right side was missing. In search of missing band we did abdominal X-ray. The swallowed band was found in the upper abdomen (Figure 1) with no associated features of perforation or peritonitis. As the patient was asymptomatic we decided to manage him conservatively and use the wait and watch strategy. He was advised to soft diet and laxatives and was admitted for observation. His stools were checked after each act of defecation.

The patient was reevaluated after 72 hours; there had been no passage of molar band along with stool since admission. Repeat abdomen X-ray showed the molar band in the same position as it was in the previous X-ray; this was suggestive of impaction within the gastrointestinal tract. We decided to perform an endoscopy evaluation and attempt endoscopy retrieval of the molar band. At endoscopy it was noted to be in the distal part of stomach and molar tube hook was impacted in the mucosa. Using endoscopic grasper, the molar band was grasped, gently pulling it out of the gastric mucosa fold. The molar band was retrieved along with endoscope (Figure 3). After retrieval of the molar band repeat X-ray was done to rule out bowel perforation and it was normal (Figure 2). He was discharged after one day.

3. Discussion

This paper illustrates the dislodgement of fixed appliance if the patient's cooperation in maintaining the appliance and retention of the appliance is inadequate. Foreign body ingestion or aspiration has the potential to result in acute medical and life-threatening emergencies. Some complications that can arise are bronchial stenosis, bronchiectasis, lung abscess, tissue ulceration or erosion, esophageal perforation with secondary mediastinitis, pneumothorax, intestinal obstruction, perforation with subsequent abscess formation, and hemorrhage or fistula.

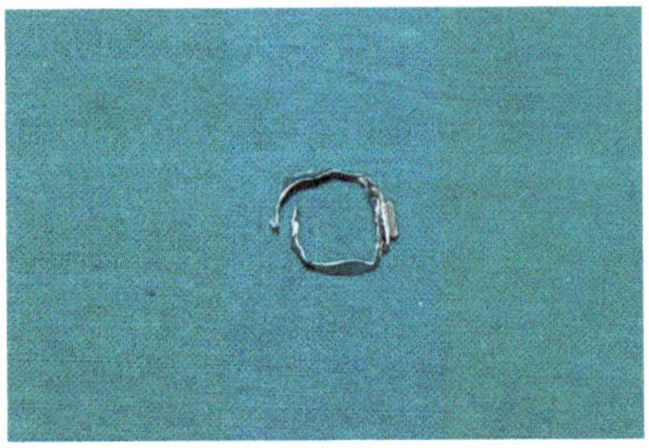

Figure 3: Retrieved molar band.

Early location of an inhaled or ingested foreign body facilitates appropriate and timely treatment management and referral. When a foreign body passes into the gastrointestinal tract, clinical symptoms and signs should be monitored closely until it is excreted or removed. Removable appliance are not the only orthodontic appliance that have given rise to problems. The problem was derived from so many fixed appliances also. Following precautions and recommendations are the outcome of this paper and other authors.

An endodontic file can pass through the gastrointestinal tract asymptomatically and apparently atraumatically within 3 days [10]. When cutting the ends of arch wires with safety distal end wire cutters, the pliers sometimes fails to hold the cut fragment. A cotton wool roll placed over the end of the arch-wire before it is cut will prevent the piece of arch wire becoming displaced in the mouth, or embedded in the soft tissues of the patient or operator [11]. The use of gauze dental napkin as barrier technique can be very successful, when placed behind the orthodontic appliances during adjustment and cutting the distal edge [12]. In some patients, placing second molar bands is difficult. To keep control of bands in case of accidental slip to aid quick retrieval, floss can be tied through the tube. Once the band is cemented on the tooth, the floss can be removed. A similar technique has been recommended for the placement of rubber dam clamps [13].

All the components of removable appliances should be smooth and rounded as far as possible. All cribs and springs should not have sharp ends, and finger springs and stops should be rounded [14]. Keys for turning fixed expansion appliances intraorally should be attached to floss and any open contact on the handle of the key should be soldered to prevent the floss from slipping through the handle [15]. When fitting or removing transpalatal arches and quadhelices, it may be advisable to have a long length of floss tied to the appliance attached via a closed loop on the appliance to avoid its inhalation or swallowing should it be dropped [16]. The choice of archwire material and grade should not only be dictated by the forces required to move teeth, but also by the ability of the wire to withstand masticatory stresses [6]. If a piece of appliance is dropped in the mouth during treatment, the availability of high-speed suction with a pharyngeal tip can help with quick retrieval [17]. The ideal method to locate a swallowed object is by X-ray evaluation. An X-ray helps to localize the site, show evidence of obstruction, onword progression and confirms the passage of swallowed object [1, 3, 10]. Endoscopic removal of foreign bodies is a safe and effective mode of management of swallowed object [1]. Failure at endoscopic retrieval is an indication for proceeding to surgical removal either by open or laparoscopic technique. The use of laxative is not a proven advantage and may increase the chance of perforation [18].

4. Conclusion

Efficiency of the appliance to withstand the masticatory force and retention should be evaluated before delivering. An orthodontic appliance can also be dislodged by patient's negligence to maintain the appliance so it is important to educate the patient to maintain the appliance and mismanagement and also to early report to the doctor when such incidence occurs. Early location of an inhaled or ingested foreign body facilitates appropriate and timely treatment management and referral. It is very important to instruct and educate verbally and in written format regarding management, precautions, adverse effects of loose and broken appliance. When a foreign body passes into the gastrointestinal tract, clinical symptoms and signs should be monitored closely until it is excreted or removed. Noninvasive procedures for managing airway obstruction include the advising laxatives then wait and watch, Heimlich maneuver, abdominal or chest thrusts in pregnant or obese patients, and finger sweeps when the object is located in the oral cavity in unconscious adults. Foreign bodies lodged in the esophagus should be removed endoscopically, but some small, blunt objects may be pulled out using a Foley's catheter and the last option will be surgical removal either by laparoscopy or open technique.

References

[1] T. M. Milton, S. D. Hearing, and A. J. Ireland, "Ingested foreign bodies associated with orthodontic treatment: report of three cases and review of ingestion/aspiration incident management," *British Dental Journal*, vol. 190, no. 11, pp. 592–596, 2001.

[2] A. Aytaç, Y. Yurdakul, C. Ikizler, R. Olga, and A. Saylam, "Inhalation of foreign bodies in children. Report of 500 cases," *Journal of Thoracic and Cardiovascular Surgery*, vol. 74, no. 1, pp. 145–151, 1977.

[3] K. K. Tiwana, T. Morton, and P. S. Tiwana, "Aspiration and ingestion in dental practice: a 10-year institutional review," *Journal of the American Dental Association*, vol. 135, no. 9, pp. 1287–1291, 2004.

[4] N. Tamura, T. Nakajima, and S. Matsumoto, "Foreign bodies of dental origin in the air and food passages," *International Journal of Oral and Maxillofacial Surgery*, vol. 15, no. 6, pp. 739–751, 1986.

[5] A. T. Dibiase, R. H. Samuels, E. Ozdiler, M. O. Akcam, and H. Turkkahraman, "Hazards of orthodontics appliances and the oropharynx," *Journal of Orthodontics*, vol. 27, no. 4, pp. 295–302, 2000.

[6] B. W. Lee, "Case report—swallowed piece of archwire," *Australian Orthodontic Journal*, vol. 12, pp. 169–170, 1992.

[7] W. J. Clark, *Twin-Block Functional Therapy: Applications in Dentofacial Orthopaedics*, Mosby, St Louis, Mo, USA, 2nd edition, 2002.

[8] Choking, "First aid," 2010, http://www.mayoclinic.com/health/first-aid-choking/FA00025.

[9] J. J. Allwork, I. R. Edwards, and I. M. Welch, "Ingestion of a quadhelix appliance requiring surgical removal: a case report," *Journal of Orthodontics*, vol. 34, no. 3, pp. 154–157, 2007.

[10] S. C. Kuo and Y. L. Chen, "Accidental swallowing of an endodontic file," *International Endodontic Journal*, vol. 41, no. 7, pp. 617–622, 2008.

[11] N. Killingback and C. D. Stephens, "A little distal archery," *British Journal of Orthodontics*, vol. 15, no. 2, pp. 121–122, 1988.

[12] W. W. Barkmeier, R. L. Cooley, and H. Abrams, "Prevention of swallowing or aspiration of foreign objects," *The Journal of the American Dental Association*, vol. 97, no. 3, pp. 473–476, 1978.

[13] R. E. Alexander and J. J. Delhom Jr., "Rubber dam clamp ingestion, an operative risk: report of case," *The Journal of the American Dental Association*, vol. 82, no. 6, pp. 1387–1389, 1971.

[14] J. F. McCabe and H. J. Wilson, "A radio-opaque denture material," *Journal of Dentistry*, vol. 4, no. 5, pp. 211–217, 1976.

[15] M. M. Nazif and M. A. Ready, "Accidental swallowing of orthodontic expansion appliance keys: report of two cases," *ASDC Journal of Dentistry for Children*, vol. 50, no. 2, pp. 126–127, 1983.

[16] E. G. Absi and J. G. Buckley, "The location and tracking of swallowed dental appliances: the role of radiology," *Dentomaxillofacial Radiology*, vol. 24, no. 2, pp. 139–142, 1995.

[17] H. A. Israel and S. G. Leban, "Aspiration of an endodontic instrument," *Journal of Endodontics*, vol. 10, no. 9, pp. 452–454, 1984.

[18] C. T. Henderson, J. Engel, and P. Schlesinger, "Foreign body ingestion: review and suggested guidelines for management," *Endoscopy*, vol. 19, no. 2, pp. 68–71, 1987.

8

Aesthetic Rehabilitation of Oligodontia in Primary Dentition with Adhesive Partial Denture

Marília Ferreira Correia,[1] Marianne Nicole Nogueira,[2] Telma Blanca Bedran,[2] and Denise Madalena Palomari Spolidorio[3]

[1] *Department of Pediatric Dentistry, Araraquara Dental School, State University of Sao Paulo, Araraquara, SP, R Humaitá 1680, 14801-903 Araraquara, SP, Brazil*
[2] *Department of Diagnosis and Surgery, Araraquara Dental School, State University of Sao Paulo, Araraquara, SP, R Humaitá 1680, 14801-903 Araraquara, SP, Brazil*
[3] *Department of Physiology and Pathology, Araraquara Dental School, State University of Sao Paulo, Araraquara, SP, R Humaitá 1680, 14801-903 Araraquara, SP, Brazil*

Correspondence should be addressed to Marília Ferreira Correia; mariliafcorreia@gmail.com

Academic Editors: C. Ledesma-Montes, D. Ram, and M. W. Roberts

The primary teeth are essential for bone development and establishment of the arches on occlusion. Thus, the congenitally absence of teeth may trigger a shift in the balance of the occlusion, promoting disharmony in the structures of the maxilla-mandibular system. However, some interventions are possible to be performed in these cases even in pediatric patients, to redirect growth, preventing growth deviations and reestablishing the aesthetic. The aim of this paper is to report the treatment of a 4-year-old child presenting congenitally absence of mandibular central and lateral incisors and maxilla lateral incisors, which consequently compromises aesthetics, occlusal function, and the development and the functional growth of the bones. The oral rehabilitation was performed with an adhesive partial denture, which was able to restore the aesthetic and the occlusal function, therefore being a viable alternative in the treatment of this patient of little age.

1. Introduction

The dental agenesis is a common developmental anomaly that affects approximately 20% of the population and results in a reduction of the number of teeth present in the oral cavity [1, 2]. Dental agenesis is classified according to the number of teeth involved and may be classified into hypodontia, oligodontia, and full anodontia. Thus, hypodontia is defined as the congenital absence of less than six permanent teeth, oligodontia as the congenital absence of more than 6 teeth and full anodontia as the absence of all permanent teeth [3]. The dental agenesis is the result of disturbances in the stages of initiation and proliferation during the formation of teeth. Its etiology is associated with environmental factors such as infections, trauma, chemotherapy, radiotherapy and genetic causes [4, 5].

The most commonly used method of, diagnosis of dental anomalies is clinical examination accompanied by radiographic examination. The periapical and the panoramic radiographs are generally used for the radiographic diagnosis of dental agenesis [6–8].

There are several treatment options for adult and young patients with agenesis, although there are few studies demonstrating treatment in pediatric patients [9]. A specialist with the patient together must make the decision regarding treatment, since it is based not only on which teeth are missing, but also on the arc length, on the position of the incisors and lips, and on the aesthetic profile. The early diagnosis and treatment are important to improve masticatory function, speech, and self-appearance to reduce the psychosocial impact [9, 10]. Thus, this paper reports the oral rehabilitation treatment of a

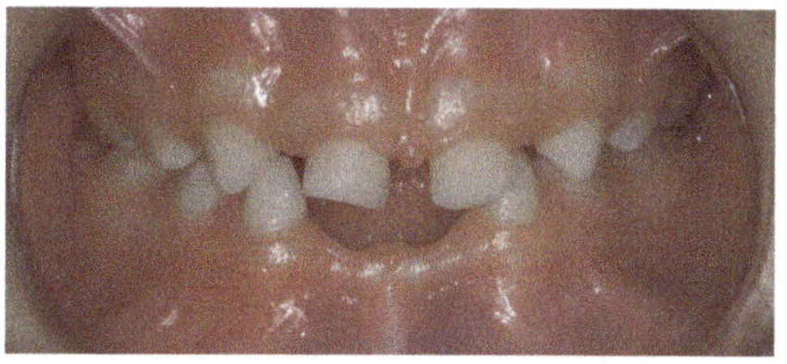

FIGURE 1: Intraoral view of dental agenesis.

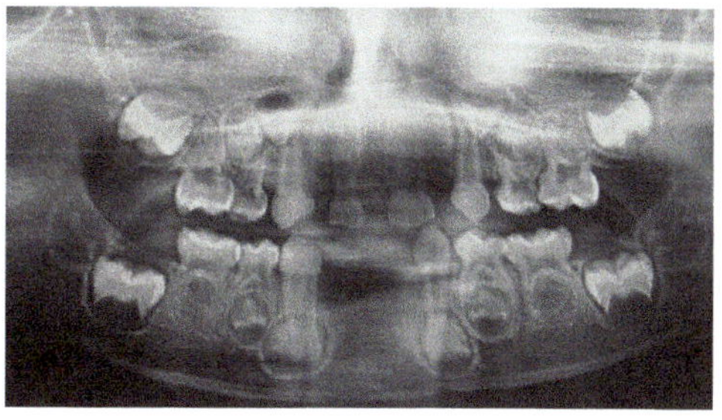

FIGURE 2: Panoramic radiograph demonstrating dental agenesis of 52, 62, 71, 72, 81, 82 (primary dentition) and 12, 22, 31, 32, 41, 42, 15, 25, 35, 45 (permanent dentition).

4-year-old patient with agenesis of six teeth in primary dentition.

2. Case Report

A mother of a girl of 4 years old reported to the pediatric clinic of School of Dentistry in Araraquara (State University of São Paulo) complaining about the aesthetic involvement caused by the absence of primary mandibular incisors of the child. The mother of the patient said during the anamnesis the following statement: "My daughter did not smile anymore and every time she did it, she put the hand in front of the mouth", which demonstrated the social and mental involvement that the absence of teeth was causing.

During clinical examination, besides the absence of mandibular incisors, the absence of upper lateral incisors was noted (Figure 1). The patient was caries-free and had no history of trauma or even any conical tooth, deciduous teeth impacted or delay in eruption of them. In view of those clinical findings, a panoramic radiograph was requested to detect the absence of permanent teeth especially. The analysis of panoramic radiograph detected the agenesis of permanent teeth as lower incisors, upper lateral incisors, and upper and lower premolars (Figure 2). Moreover, the patient had no clinical signs of any syndrome or disorder like ectodermal dysplasia or Down syndrome, which are usually syndromes related with oligodontia in primary dentition.

The treatment plan involved the installation of an adhesive partial denture for restoring only the lower incisors due to the lack of space for construction of an upper dental prosthesis (Figures 1 and 2). The choice of an adhesive prosthesis was due to the difficulty of the patient's adhesion to use a removable appliance.

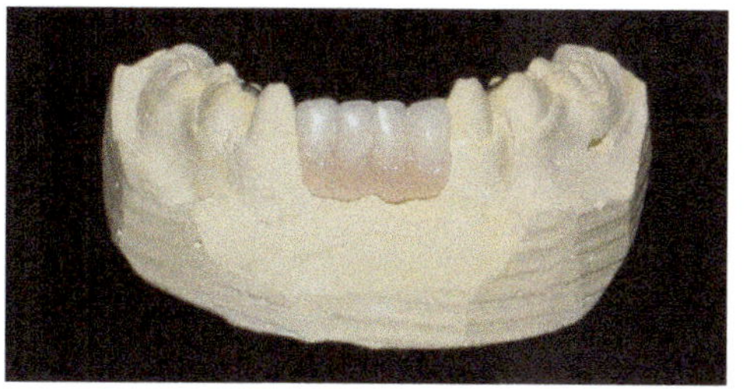

FIGURE 3: Partial dental prosthesis.

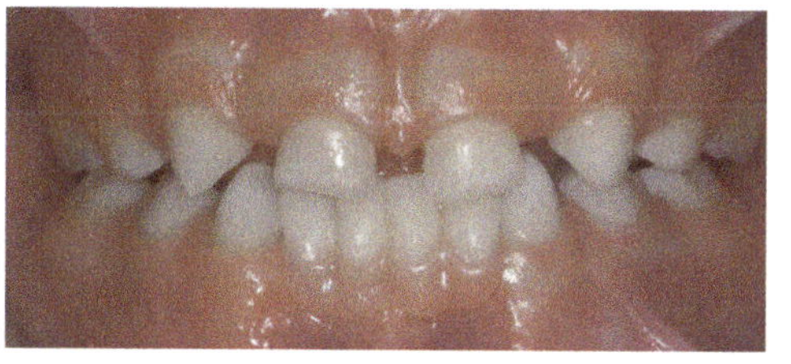

FIGURE 4: Intraoral view of oral rehabilitation.

In the first appointment, the clinical procedure was carried out as follows: upper and lower molding, interocclusal record in wax, and confection of partial dental prosthesis with lower incisors. The partial prosthesis had rods made of metallic steel wire located on each side of their lateral extremity (Figure 3). These rods were designed to be fixed into the lingual surface of the canine and into the first deciduous molar lower with composite resin.

In the second appointment, the partial prosthesis was installed as follows: etching acid of the enamel of canine and first deciduous lower molars with 35% phosphoric acid for 15 seconds, the enamel was rinsed and dried to apply only the Scotchbond Multi-purpose Plus adhesive (3 M/ESPE, USA) according to the manufacturer's directions, and finally, the rods of partial prosthesis were bonded to the surface of these teeth with a thick layer of Z250 (3 M/ESPE, USA) and the occlusion was checked. Figure 4 demonstrated the final result of this case. Adequate care with adhesive dental prosthesis and oral hygiene was given to the mother of the patient.

3. Discussion

The absence of primary teeth is an uncommon condition, being present in 0.5 to 1% of the population [11]. However, when it occurs, it usually affects the upper lateral incisors or the lower incisors and is also generally associated with the absence of the permanent successor [12–14].

The etiology of dental agenesis is related to environmental factors such as rubella [15], different types of traumas to the alveolar processes [12], use of chemical substances or drugs, as thalidomide and chemotherapy [15], radiotherapy [16, 17], and disturbances in the innervation of the jaw [18, 19]. Based on current knowledge of genes and transcription factors that are involved in the development of teeth, it is assumed that different forms of dental agenesis phenotype observed clinically are caused by mutations in different genes which play distinct roles in the intracellular signaling cascade [20].

This knowledge has led us to the understanding of a wide variety of patterns of agenesis. Currently, the list of genes involved in nonsyndromic hypodontia in humans includes genes encoding transforming growth factor beta (TGF-β) and transcription factors (MSX1 and PAX9), which play a critical role during the craniofacial development, as well as genes encoding a protein involved in Wnt signaling pathway (AXIN2) [5, 20]. MSX1 and AXIN2 genes, involved in the early stages of odontogenesis, are associated with tooth agenesis in individuals with disorders such as cleft palate and colorectal cancer [21].

The absence of teeth is a clinical and public health problem [22], since the patients in these conditions may present several signs and symptoms as reduction of the chewing ability, malocclusion, problems in articulating words, and also the aesthetic may be compromised. These complications may affect self-esteem, behavior pattern, and social life of these patients [22, 23].

Regarding the diagnosis of oligodontia, it is normally based on radiographic evidence and routine clinical examination, detecting absence of teeth or delayed eruption of them. The panoramic radiography is the most indicated for the diagnosis and study of agenesis, due to this radiographic exam register all maxilla-mandibular regions as well as the development of the tooth germ of the patient with minimal radiation. This panoramic radiograph may be preferentially requested as soon as possible, that is, around the three and a half years old [7, 8].

The treatment goals are to keep the remaining teeth, recover the masticatory function and aesthetics, improve speech, and reestablish the emotional and psychological wellbeing [9, 11]. Regarding the prosthetic treatment, its objectives include restoring the masticatory function, maintaining the position of adjacent natural teeth preventing undesirable movements, such as inclination, extrusion, or migration, improving aesthetics, avoiding social problems to the patient, especially in adolescence, replace the missing teeth without interfering in the growth of the mandible and maxilla [24]. Considering all possibilities for oral rehabilitation of the referred patient, the prosthetic treatment of choice was the placement of adhesive partial denture due to the difficulty of the patient's adhesion to use a removable appliance. This type of prosthesis allows the restoration of function and aesthetics of missing teeth and does not interfere with bone development.

4. Conclusion

The congenital absence of teeth may occur as an isolated condition or may be associated with a systemic condition or syndrome clinically recognized. The clinical and radiographic examinations are the best way which the clinicians may detect anomalies in primary and permanent dentition. When cases of dental agenesis are diagnosed, treatment should be performed to restore the masticatory function and aesthetics regardless of age or missing teeth. Hence, the following case report summarized an alternative treatment of a 4-year-old patient with agenesis of six teeth in primary dentition. Besides the consequences caused by dental agenesis already mentioned, the emotional and psychological wellbeing of the child in this case was an important factor to perform an early intervention.

Conflict of Interests

The authors declare that there is no conflict of interests regarding the publication of this paper.

References

[1] T. P. Muller, I. N. Hill, A. C. Peterson, and J. R. Blayney, "A survey of congenitally missing permanent teeth," *The Journal of the American Dental Association*, vol. 81, no. 1, pp. 101–107, 1970.

[2] C. J. Larmour, P. A. Mossey, B. S. Thind, A. H. Forgie, and D. R. Stirrups, "Hypodontia—a retrospective review of prevalence and etiology. Part I," *Quintessence International*, vol. 36, no. 4, pp. 263–270, 2005.

[3] K. Bishop, L. Addy, and J. Knox, "Modern restorative management of patients with congenitally missing teeth: 1. Introduction, terminology and epidemiology," *Dental Update*, vol. 33, no. 9, pp. 531–537, 2006.

[4] P. J. Dhanrajani, "Hypodontia: etiology, clinical features, and management," *Quintessence International*, vol. 33, no. 4, pp. 294–302, 2002.

[5] P. J. de Coster, L. A. Marks, L. C. Martens, and A. Huysseune, "Dental agenesis: genetic and clinical perspectives," *Journal of Oral Pathology and Medicine*, vol. 38, no. 1, pp. 1–17, 2009.

[6] K. Haavikko, "Hypodontia of permanent teeth. An orthopantomographic study," *Suomen Hammaslaakariseuran Toimituksia*, vol. 67, no. 4, pp. 219–225, 1971.

[7] R. Pilo, I. Kaffe, E. Amir, and H. Sarnat, "Diagnosis of developmental dental anomalies using panoramic radiographs," *ASDC Journal of Dentistry for Children*, vol. 54, no. 4, pp. 267–272, 1987.

[8] H. Hintze and A. Wenzel, "Longitudinal study of accuracy of clinical examination for detection of permanent tooth aplasia," *Community Dentistry and Oral Epidemiology*, vol. 18, no. 5, pp. 256–259, 1990.

[9] M. A. Derbanne, M. C. Sitbon, M. M. Landru, and A. Naveau, "Case report: early prosthetic treatment in children with ectodermal dysplasia," *European Archives of Paediatric Dentistry*, vol. 11, no. 6, pp. 301–305, 2010.

[10] Z. Kirzioğlu, T. Köseler Sentut, M. S. Ozay Ertürk, and H. Karayilmaz, "Clinical features of hypodontia and associated dental anomalies: a retrospective study," *Oral Disease*, vol. 11, no. 6, pp. 399–404, 2005.

[11] J. H. Nunn, N. E. Carter, T. J. Gillgrass et al., "The interdisciplinary management of hypodontia: background and role of paediatric dentistry," *British Dental Journal*, vol. 194, no. 5, pp. 245–251, 2003.

[12] Y. Schalk-van der Weide, W. H. Steen, and F. Bosman, "Distribution of missing teeth and tooth morphology in patients with oligodontia," *ASDC Journal of Dentistry for Children*, vol. 59, no. 2, pp. 133–140, 1992.

[13] A. H. Brook, "Dental anomalies of number, form and size: their prevalence in British schoolchildren," *Journal of the International Association of Dentistry for Children*, vol. 5, no. 2, pp. 37–53, 1974.

[14] N. N. Nik-Hussein and Z. A. Majid, "Dental anomalies in the primary dentition: distribution and correlation with the permanent dentition," *Journal of Clinical Pediatric Dentistry*, vol. 21, no. 1, pp. 15–19, 1996.

[15] J. S. Gullikson, "Tooth morphology in rubella syndrome children," *ASDC Journal of Dentistry for Children*, vol. 42, no. 6, pp. 479–482, 1975.

[16] A. Maguire, A. W. Craft, R. G. B. Evans et al., "The long-term effects of treatment on the dental condition of children surviving malignant disease," *Cancer*, vol. 60, no. 10, pp. 2570–2575, 1987.

[17] M. Näsman, C.-M. Forsberg, and G. Dahllöf, "Long-term dental development in children after treatment for malignant disease," *European Journal of Orthodontics*, vol. 19, no. 2, pp. 151–159, 1997.

[18] I. Kjær, G. Kocsis, M. Nodal, and L. R. Christensen, "Aetiological aspects of mandibular tooth agenesis—focusing on the role of nerve, oral mucosa, and supporting tissues," *European Journal of Orthodontics*, vol. 16, no. 5, pp. 371–375, 1994.

[19] E. Andersen, L. T. Skovgaard, S. Poulsen, and I. Kjaer, "The influence of jaw innervation on the dental maturation pattern in the mandible," *Orthodontics & Craniofacial Research*, vol. 7, no. 4, pp. 211–215, 2004.

[20] G. Galluccio, M. Castellano, and C. la Monaca, "Genetic basis of non-syndromic anomalies of human tooth number," *Archives of Oral Biology*, vol. 57, no. 7, pp. 918–930, 2012.

[21] I. Bailleul-Forestier, M. Molla, A. Verloes, and A. Berdal, "The genetic basis of inherited anomalies of the teeth. Part 1: clinical and molecular aspects of non-syndromic dental disorders," *European Journal of Medical Genetics*, vol. 51, no. 4, pp. 273–291, 2008.

[22] P. Agarwal, D. P. Vinuth, G. Dube, and P. Dube, "Nonsyndromic tooth agenesis patterns and associated developmental dental anomalies: a literature review with radiographic illustrations," *Minerva Stomatologica*, vol. 62, no. 1-2, pp. 31–41, 2013.

[23] M. Kulkarni, T. Agrawal, and S. Kheur, "Tooth agenesis: newer concept," *Journal of Clinical Pediatric Dentistry*, vol. 36, no. 1, pp. 65–70, 2011.

[24] T. M. S. V. Gonçalves, L. M. Gonçalves, J. R. Sabino-Bezerra, A. R. Santos- Silva, W. J. Silva, and R. C. M. R. Garcia, "Multidisciplinary therapy of extensive oligodontia: a case report," *Brazilian Dental Journal*, vol. 24, no. 2, pp. 174–178, 2013.

9

Three Independent Mesial Canals in a Mandibular Molar: Four-Year Followup of a Case Using Cone Beam Computed Tomography

Adrianne Freire de Paula,[1] Manoel Brito-Júnior,[1] Alex Carvalho Quintino,[1] Carla Cristina Camilo,[1] Antônio Miranda Cruz-Filho,[2] and Manoel Damião Sousa-Neto[2]

[1] *Department of Dentistry, State University of Montes Claros, Avenue Rui Braga s/n, 39401-089, Montes Claros, MG, Brazil*
[2] *Department of Restorative Dentistry, Faculty of Dentistry, University of São Paulo, Avenue Bandeirantes 3900, 14040-900, Ribeirão Preto, SP, Brazil*

Correspondence should be addressed to Manoel Brito-Júnior; manoelbritojr@gmail.com

Academic Editors: J. J. Segura-Egea, K. Seymour, and N. Shah

Endodontic treatment of mandibular molars is challenging because of variable root canal morphology. The nonsurgical endodontic management of a mandibular first molar presenting an independent middle mesial canal is reported. After coronal access, additional clinical inspection of the mesial canals' orifices and their interconnecting groove using an endodontic explorer and 4.5× loupes enabled the identification of the middle mesial canal orifice. All root canals were chemomechanically prepared and filled. The tooth was asymptomatic and functional after 4 years of followup. Cone beam computed tomography (CBCT) images revealed normal periapical status and three-dimensional (3D) anatomical aspects of the root canal system.

1. Introduction

Endodontic treatment of mandibular molars is a constant challenge to the clinician because the number of root canals is highly variable. The root canal system of these teeth consists of fins, accessory, secondary, and lateral canals, as well as transverse anastomosis [1]. Since chemomechanical preparation is a critical step for a successful endodontic outcome, a thorough root canal debridement including additional canals must be achieved [2]. Thus, a better understanding of tooth morphology favoring the search for root canals is essential to attain this purpose.

The first mandibular molars typically have two roots, one mesial with two root canals (mesiobuccal and mesiolingual) and another distal, which contains one or two root canals [1, 2]. Root canal configuration with two distal canals varies from 20% to 46% in different populations [3, 4]. The identification of three [5, 6] or four [7] canals in the mesial root or three canals in the distal root [8] is still anatomical variations reported in the literature.

Regarding the presence of the middle mesial (MM) canal having an independent trajectory in the mesial root of first mandibular molars, a literature search revealed few cases reported over the last decades (Table 1). In addition, the most cases [9–15] were identified by periapical radiographs, which have limitations in describing 3-dimensional (3D) roots and root canal anatomy. Thus, this case report describes the endodontic management of three independent mesial canals in a first mandibular molar where cone beam computed tomography (CBCT) was used at the 4-year followup.

2. Case Report

A 42-year-old male patient with noncontributory medical history was referred for endodontic treatment of the left first mandibular molar. The clinical examination of the tooth revealed no swelling or sinus tract and a slight response to percussion and palpation. The tooth did not respond to thermal or electric pulp tests. A periapical radiograph revealed a deep distal carie and a slight widening of the apical periodontal ligament in the distal and mesial roots (Figure 1(a)). Based on the clinical and radiographic findings, the diagnosis was established as a pulp necrosis. A treatment

TABLE 1: Case reports on three independent mesial canals of first mandibular molar.

Author, year	Evaluation technique	Number of teeth
La et al., 2010 [6]	CBCT	1
Yesilsoy et al., 2009 [9]	PA radiographs	1
Mortman and Ahn, 2003 [10]	PA radiographs	1
Holtzman, 1997 [11]	PA radiographs	1
Ricucci, 1997 [12]	PA radiographs	1
Jacobsen et al., 1994 [13]	PA radiographs	1
Bond et al., 1988 [14]	PA radiographs	1
Martinez-Berna and Badanelli, 1985 [15]	PA radiographs	1

CBCT: cone beam computed tomography, PA: periapical.

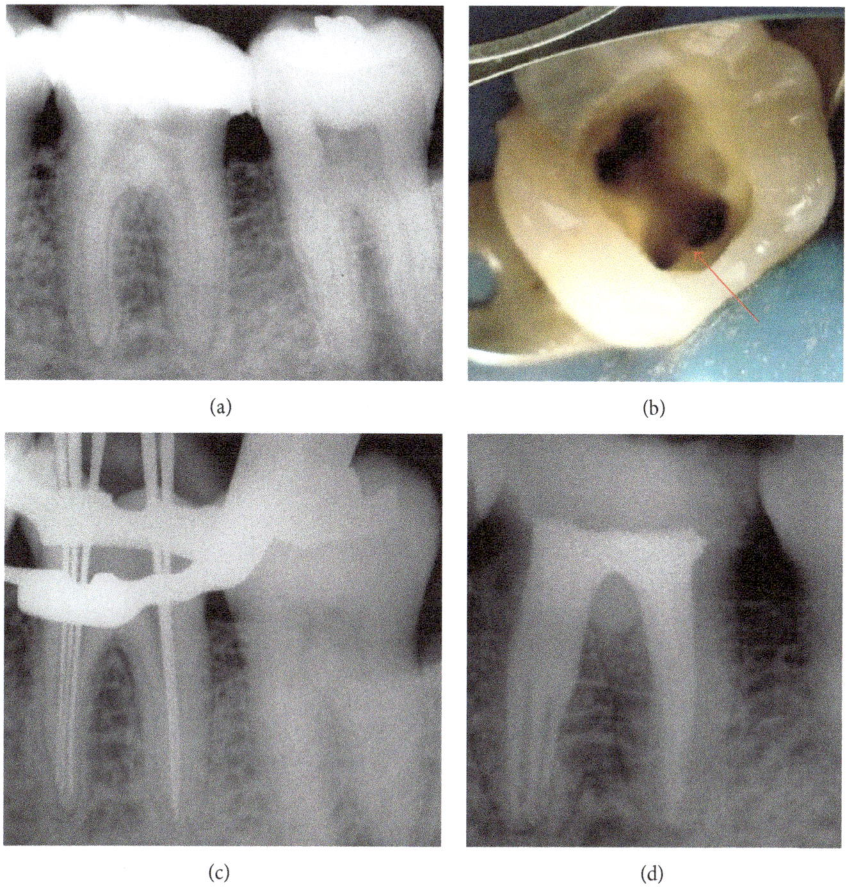

FIGURE 1: (a) Preoperative radiograph. (b) Clinical view of root canal entrances including a middle mesial canal (arrow). (c) Radiograph for working length determination showing three independent mesial canals. (d) Postoperative radiograph.

plan, including nonsurgical root canal therapy of tooth, was presented to the patient. The patient consented to the proposed treatment.

During the first session, local anesthesia was administered, and a rubber dam was applied. Upon access opening, four well-defined root canal orifices were located using an endodontic explorer (Odous, Belo Horizonte, MG, Brazil) on the pulpal floor, two orifices for the distal root, and two separate orifices for the mesial root. The subpulpal groove of the mesiobuccal root was located after removing the excess dentin using an ultrasonic device (Gnatus, Ribeirão Preto, SP, Brazil) with an ultrasonic tip (TU17; Trinity, São Paulo, SP, Brazil). The tip of the explorer attached in the middle mesial canal orifice, which was located closer to the mesiobuccal canal (Figure 1(b)). A 4.5× binocular loupe (Bio-Art Equipamentos Odontológicos, São Carlos, SP, Brazil) was used to facilitate this procedure. The radiograph taken to determine the working lengths showed three independent mesial canals (Figure 1(c)). All root canals were prepared in a crown-down method using ProFile Taper 04/06 rotary NiTi

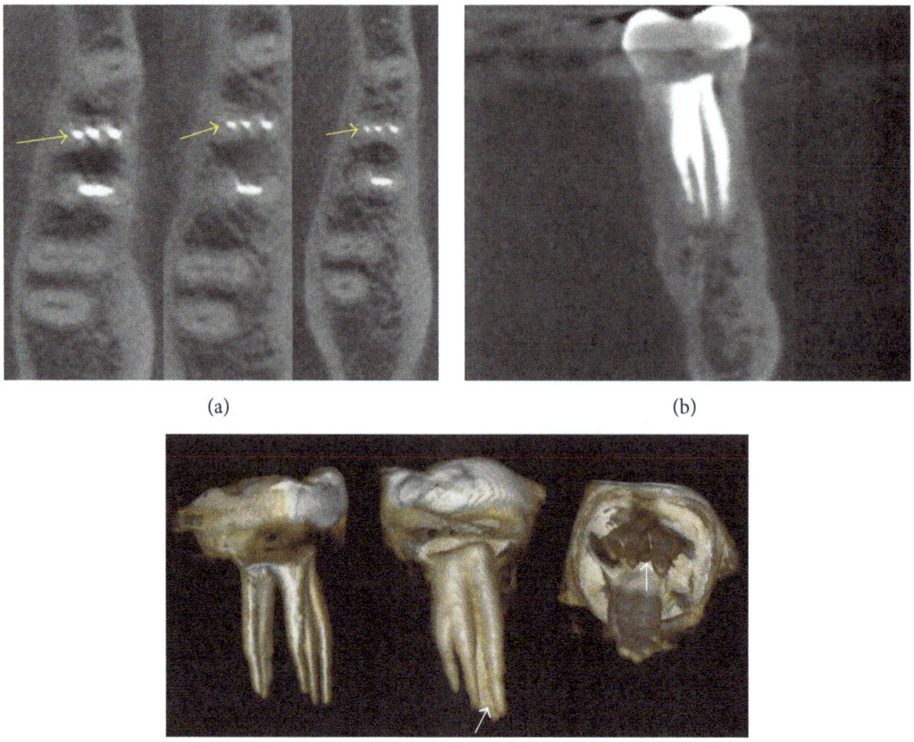

(a) (b)

(c)

Figure 2: (a) Axial CBCT slices on coronal, middle and apical root sections (arrows) showing three independent mesial canals. (b) Coronal CBCT view of mesial root with three filled root canals. (c). 3-Dimensional rebuild illustrating the internal configuration including a filled isthmus between the mesiobuccal and middle mesial canals (arrows).

instruments (Maillefer-Dentsply, Ballaigues, Switzerland). Preparation was always performed under irrigation with 2.5% sodium hypochlorite solution followed by smear layer removal with a 14.3% EDTA solution (pH 7.2) for 3 minutes. Afterward, the root canal was dried with paper points and filled with calcium hydroxide paste (Calen, SS White, Rio de Janeiro, RJ, Brazil) using a lentulo spiral. The cavity entrance was closed with a noneugenol temporary filling material (Coltosol, Vigodent, Rio de Janeiro, RJ, Brazil).

The patient returned for a second appointment 10 days later. The temporary restoration was removed under local anesthesia and rubber dam. The root canals were irrigated with 2.5% sodium hypochlorite, and the intracanal dressing was removed, stirring with a size 15 K-file (Maillefer-Dentsply, Ballaigues, Switzerland), followed by a final rinse with a 14.3% EDTA. The canals were dried and filled with a zinc oxide-eugenol-based sealer (Endofill, Dentsply, Petrópolis, RJ, Brazil) and nonstandardized gutta-percha cones (Odous, Belo Horizonte, MG, Brazil) using cold lateral condensation. A temporary filling was placed and a postoperative radiograph was taken to assess the quality of obturation (Figure 1(d)). The patient was referred for appropriate coronal restoration.

The tooth was asymptomatic and functional after 4 years of followup. The patient was informed about the possibility of CBCT examination, which was unavailable at the time of the initiation of treatment. It was explained that CBCT could be useful to check three-dimensionally the endodontic treatment performed. Thus, CBCT images focused on tooth number 19 were obtained after informed consent of the patient. Axial (Figure 2(a)) and sagittal (Figure 2(b)) slices of 0.076 mm thickness using the CBCT scan (Kodak 9000 3D, Carestream Health, Inc., Rochester, NY, USA) revealed normal periapical status and three independent filled root canals in the mesial root. A three-dimensional rebuild performed from the CBCT images showed in detail the internal configuration of the all filled root canals (Figure 2(c)).

3. Discussion

The present case report describes the treatment of a first mandibular molar with three mesial root canals. A systematic review conducted by de Pablo et al. [16] reported that the overall incidence of this anatomical morphology was 2.6%. They also showed that the confluence of the MM canal with the mesiobuccal or mesiolingual canals having a common apical termination was more frequently observed than a configuration including three distinct, separate apical foramina [16]. This last condition, as presented in this report, is recognized as 3-3 configuration (type 8) by using Vertucci's classification [1]. The entrance of the MM canal was located closer to the mesiobuccal canal, which corresponds to an incidence of 25% according to a previous investigation [17].

The detection of root canal orifices may be influenced by the complexity of the internal anatomy and operator experience [18]. Furthermore, a magnified view of the operating field using dental microscopic or surgical loupes increases the chance of locating hidden canals [5, 7, 17, 18]. The use of a microscope or the use of loupes by practicing endodontists was equivalent in searching for additional canals in first mandibular molars [17]. The endodontic treatment of the present case was performed by an experienced endodontist familiar with the use of loupes for more than 10 years. In addition, a careful examination of the pulpal floor with an endodontic explorer and the use of an ultrasonic tip to remove the dentin coverage over the middle mesial canal orifice were important procedures to ensure the successful treatment [5].

The existence of an MM canal is sometimes observed in angled horizontal radiographs. However, molar cases may require 3D diagnostic images to improve the assessment of root canal systems [6, 8]. In this situation, CBCT provides additional information to detect extra canals. In a vitro study, de Toubes et al. [5] demonstrated that CBCT was an accurate method of identifying accessory mesial canals in mandibular first molars. CBCT also was a helpful imaging tool used by La et al. [6] to detect clinically a challenging case of an independent middle mesial canal.

The presence of three mesial canals that were independent throughout their course in the root was visualized on 3D CBCT images during the follow-up period in the present case. The Kodak 9000 3D used in this report is categorized as a small-volume CBCT based on its scan field of view (FoV), which covers only a few teeth or one jaw. It has been reported that small FoV provides better image quality with lower effective radiation when compared with medium and large FoV devices [19]. In addition, cone beam reconstructions at 0.076 mm obtained with Kodak 9000 3D had a minimal discrepancy compared to histologic sections of extracted teeth with multiple root canal anatomy [20]. The reconstructed images of the root-filled tooth in this particular case showed a similar length of MM and mesiobuccal canals, as well as a filled isthmus between these two canals. The mesiolingual canal presented the smaller dimensions.

In summary, this report corroborates the presence of three independent mesial root canals in a mandibular first molar. Moreover, the details of this internal configuration with filled root canals were displayed on 3D CBCT images.

References

[1] F. J. Vertucci, "Root canal anatomy of the human permanent teeth," *Oral Surgery Oral Medicine and Oral Pathology*, vol. 58, no. 5, pp. 589–599, 1984.

[2] F. J. Vertucci, "Root canal morphology and its relationship to endodontic procedures," *Endodontic Topics*, vol. 10, no. 1, pp. 3–29, 2005.

[3] K. Gulabivala, T. H. Aung, A. Alavi, and Y. L. Ng, "Root and canal morphology of Burmese mandibular molars," *International Endodontic Journal*, vol. 34, no. 5, pp. 359–370, 2001.

[4] S. Sert, V. Aslanalp, and J. Tanalp, "Investigation of the root canal configurations of mandibular permanent teeth in the Turkish population," *International Endodontic Journal*, vol. 37, no. 7, pp. 494–499, 2004.

[5] K. M. de Toubes, M. I. Côrtes, M. A. Valadares, L. C. Fonseca, E. Nunes, and F. F. Silveira, "Comparative analysis of accessory mesial canal identification in mandibular first molars by using four different diagnostic methods," *Journal of Endodontics*, vol. 38, no. 4, pp. 436–441, 2012.

[6] S. H. La, D. H. Jung, E. C. Kim, and K. S. Min, "Identification of independent middle mesial canal in mandibular first molar using cone-beam computed tomography imaging," *Journal of Endodontics*, vol. 36, no. 3, pp. 542–545, 2010.

[7] E. G. Kontakiotis and G. N. Tzanetakis, "Four canals in the mesial root of a mandibular first molar. A case report under the operating microscope," *Australian Endodontic Journal*, vol. 33, no. 2, pp. 84–88, 2007.

[8] S. S. Chandra, M. Rajasekaran, P. Shankar, and R. Indira, "Endodontic management of a mandibular first molar with three distal canals confirmed with the aid of spiral computerized tomography: a case report," *Oral Surgery, Oral Medicine, Oral Pathology, Oral Radiology and Endodontology*, vol. 108, no. 4, pp. e77–e81, 2009.

[9] C. Yesilsoy, O. Porras, and W. Gordon, "Importance of third mesial canals in mandibular molars: report of 2 cases," *Oral Surgery, Oral Medicine, Oral Pathology, Oral Radiology and Endodontology*, vol. 108, no. 1, pp. e55–e58, 2009.

[10] R. E. Mortman and S. Ahn, "Mandibular first molars with three mesial canals," *General Dentistry*, vol. 51, no. 6, pp. 549–551, 2003.

[11] L. Holtzmann, "Root canal treatment of a mandibular first molar with three mesial root canals," *International Endodontic Journal*, vol. 30, no. 6, pp. 422–423, 1997.

[12] D. Ricucci, "Three independent canals in the mesial root of a mandibular first molar," *Endodontics and Dental Traumatology*, vol. 13, no. 1, pp. 47–49, 1997.

[13] E. L. Jacobsen, K. Dick, and R. Bodell, "Mandibular first molars with multiple mesial canals," *Journal of Endodontics*, vol. 20, no. 12, pp. 610–613, 1994.

[14] J. L. Bond, G. R. Hartwell, J. C. Donnelly, and F. R. Portell, "Clinical management of middle mesial root canals in mandibular molars," *Journal of Endodontics*, vol. 14, no. 6, pp. 312–314, 1988.

[15] A. Martinez-Berna and P. Badanelli, "Mandibular first molars with six root canals," *Journal of Endodontics*, vol. 11, no. 8, pp. 348–352, 1985.

[16] O. V. de Pablo, R. Estevez, M. Péix Sánchez, C. Heilborn, and N. Cohenca, "Root anatomy and canal configuration of the permanent mandibular first molar: a systematic review," *Journal of Endodontics*, vol. 36, no. 12, pp. 1919–1931, 2010.

[17] M. Karapinar-Kazandag, B. R. Basrani, and S. Friedman, "The operating microscope enhances detection and negotiation of accessory mesial canals in mandibular molars," *Journal of Endodontics*, vol. 36, no. 8, pp. 1289–1294, 2010.

[18] J. Corcoran, M. J. Apicella, and P. Mines, "The effect of operator experience in locating additional canals in maxillary molars," *Journal of Endodontics*, vol. 33, no. 1, pp. 15–17, 2007.

[19] Z. D. Kajan and M. Taromsari, "Value of cone beam CT in detection of dental root fractures," *Dentomaxillofacial Radiology*, vol. 41, no. 1, pp. 3–10, 2012.

[20] J. Michetti, D. Maret, J. P. Mallet, and F. Diemer, "Validation of cone beam computed tomography as a tool to explore root canal anatomy," *Journal of Endodontics*, vol. 36, no. 7, pp. 1187–1190, 2010.

10

Endodontic Management of Mandibular Second Molar Fused to a Supernumerary Tooth, Using Spiral Computed Tomography as a Diagnostic Aid: A Case Report

Kavitarani Rudagi,[1] B. M. Rudagi,[2] Sandeep Metgud,[3] and Rahul Wagle[3]

[1] *Department of Conservative Dentistry and Endodontics, Sharad Pawar Dental College, Sawangi (Meghe), Maharashtra, Wardha, India*
[2] *Department of Oral and Maxillofacial Surgery, Sharad Pawar Dental College, Sawangi (Meghe), Wardha, India*
[3] *Department of Conservative Dentistry and Endodontics, Rural Dental College, Pravara Institute of Medical Sciences, Loni, India*

Correspondence should be addressed to Kavitarani Rudagi, kavitarudagi_11@rediffmail.com

Academic Editors: R. A. de Mesquita and Y. S. Khader

Fusion is a developmental anomaly characterized by the union of two adjacent teeth. In this paper we report a rare case of fusion involving permanent mandibular second molar with supernumerary tooth. The rarity with which this entity appears, along with its complex characteristics, often makes it difficult to treat. The use of high-end diagnostic imaging modalities such as spiral computed tomography can help the clinician in making a confirmatory diagnosis and determining the treatment plan before undertaking the actual treatment. In the present case, we have used spiral computed tomography (SCT) for better understanding the complicated root canal morphology of the fused tooth and successful management of this rare case.

1. Introduction

Teeth with morphoanatomic changes pose a challenge in endodontic therapy. It is imperative that aberrant anatomy is identified before and during root canal treatment of such teeth. Morphoanatomic changes in teeth may be divided according to the site of their occurrence, that is, tooth crown, roots, and root canals. Fusion and gemination are irregularities in tooth development [1]. Pindborg defined fusion as the union between dentin and/or enamel of two or more separate developing teeth [2]. The incidence of fusion is <1% in the Caucasian population [3]. Clinically, it is often difficult to differentiate between fusion and gemination and it is common to refer these anomalies as "double teeth" [4, 5].

The degree of fusion depends on the stage of tooth development that has occurred at the time of fusion, with the union of dentin being the main criterion. Fused teeth may contain separate pulp canals or share a common pulp canal. Fusion may occur between two normal teeth or between a normal tooth and a supernumerary tooth. Supernumerary tooth is an additional entity to the normal series and is seen in all the quadrants of the jaw [6]. When the supernumerary tooth occurs distal to the molar, it is called a distomolar, and when it erupts buccal or lingual to the molar, it is called a paramolar. Supernumerary teeth might occur singly or might be fused to their normal counterpart [7]. The occurrence of fusion in permanent posterior teeth is rare.

When fusion occurs between a molar and a supernumerary tooth as a result of their abnormal morphology and excessive crown width, problems with crowding, alignment, and occlusal functions can occur [8]. These teeth also tend to be greatly predisposed to caries and periodontal disease [9].

Radiographic examination is an essential component in the management of endodontic problems. However, the conventional intraoral periapical views produce only a 2-dimensional image of a 3-dismensional object, resulting in the superimposition of structures. Conventional multidetector computed tomography (CT) imaging has been widely used in medicine since the 1970s and was introduced in the endodontic field in 1990 [7]. In these areas, spiral computed

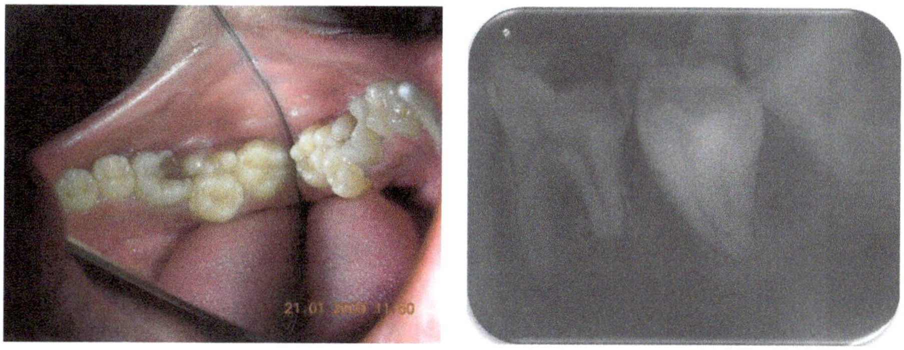

(a) (b)

FIGURE 1: (a) Pre-operative photograph: Occlusal View. (b) Pre-operative radiograph revealing irregular morphology of tooth #20 & istal root resorption with #21.

tomography (SCT) has proved to be a useful diagnostic tool [10, 11].

This paper presents the endodontic management of a fused mandibular second molar with a supernumerary tooth with the use of SCT as a diagnostic aid.

2. Case Report

A 20-year-old male patient presented to the department of conservative dentistry and endodontics with pain to hot and cold food in the left mandibular posterior region. On clinical examination, the mandibular first molar exhibited caries on the distoocclusal aspect and second molar exhibited abnormal crown morphology with 2 large extra cusps on the buccal aspect of the tooth (Figure 1(a)). Distinct developmental occlusogingival grooves between the supernumerary tooth and its normal counterpart were noticed. Despite the presence of the grooves, there was no discernible separation between the 2 teeth. Caries in the developmental groove on the mesial side of the tooth was evident.

There was no previous history of trauma or any hereditary conditions. Medical history was noncontributory. All vital signs were found to be within normal limits. Oral examination revealed a normal set of dentition. The teeth 20 and 21 were not sensitive to palpation or percussion. The tooth responded to an electric pulp tester (Parkell Electronics, Farmingdale, NY, USA) and showed early response to the cold test (R C Ice, Prime Dental products, India). On radiographic examination, tooth 21 showed resorption with the distal root and the exact anatomy of tooth 20 that could not be clearly identified, but it was possible to recognize the complex structure of the pulp (Figure 1(b)). Therefore, to ascertain the complex root canal anatomy of the tooth in a 3-dimensional (3D) manner, dental imaging with the help of spiral computed tomography (SCT) was therefore planned. Informed consent from the patient was obtained, and a multislice SCT of the mandible was performed using the dental software Dentascan (GE Healthcare, Milwaukee, WI, USA). A 3D image of the mandible was obtained. The involved tooth was focused and the morphology was obtained in transverse, axial, and sagittal sections of 0.5 mm thickness (Figure 2).

The images revealed that the mandibular left second molar had 3 root canals and that there was connection between the paramolar and second molar in the pulpal chamber. The paramolar exhibited a type II canal (according to Wiene's classification).

3. Management

Local anesthesia was administered and a rubber dam was applied. The prongs of the rubber dam retainer had to be trimmed to accommodate the unusual anatomy of the tooth. Endodontic access cavity was done on the occlusal surface using a no. 2 round bur and EX 24 bur (nonend cutting tapered fissure; Mani, Tochigi, Japan) (Figure 2(a)). Pulp extirpation was performed using a barbed broach (Denstply-Malliefer, Ballaigues, Switzerland) and K-files (Mani Inc, Tochigi, Japan). The canal was thoroughly debrided with a copious irrigation of sodium hypochlorite (2.5%), followed by saline (0.9%). Coronal flaring of the root canal was done using Gates-Glidden drills no. 1 to 2 (Mani Inc, Tochigi, Japan). The working length was determined using apex locator (Propex, DENTSPLY-Malleifer, Ballaigues, Switzerland) and confirmed radiographically (Figure 2(b)). Cleaning and shaping of the root canal system was completed using Protaper rotary system (Dentsply). Canals were copiously irrigated with sodium hypochlorite (2.5%), followed by saline. The canal was dried with sterile paper points and calcium hydroxide (Ultracal XS, Ultradent, South Jordan, UT, USA) was placed in the root canal and the access cavity was temporized with Cavit G (3 M ESPE, Germany). The patient was recalled after 1 week for obturation.

After a week, the tooth was asymptomatic and the root canal was obturated using thermoplastic obturation technique (E&Q plus Meta Biomed Co ltd, Korea) and AH PLUS as a sealer. The access cavity was then sealed with resin composite (Figure 2(c)).

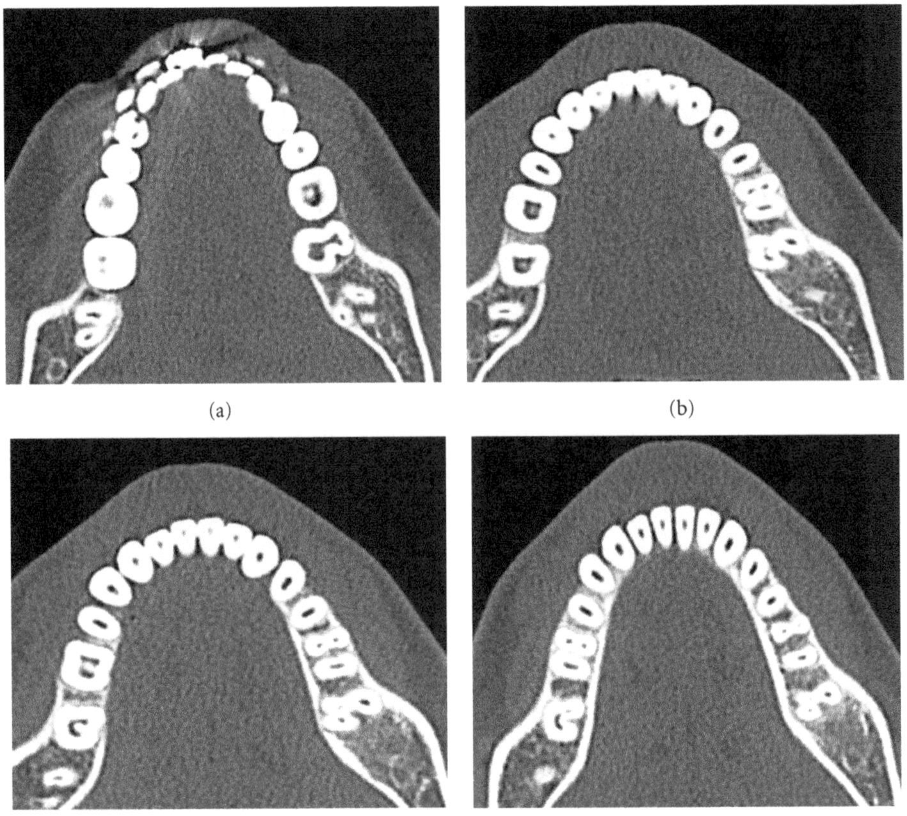

(a) (b) (c) (d)

Figure 2: SCT Images of the Maxilla. (a) Axial view of the coronal third section of the roots of the left mandibular left second molar. (b) Axial view of the cervical third section of the roots of the mandibular left second molar. (c) Axial view of the middle third section of the roots of the left mandibular left second molar. (d) Axial view of the apical third section of the crown of the left mandibular left second molar.

Routine endodontic treatment was carried out with tooth 21. The tooth was totally asymptomatic at a 1-year recall visit (Figures 3 and 4).

4. Discussion

Fused teeth afford a striking clinical manifestation of the differentiable and morphogenetic processes of tooth development. Fusion between supernumerary and permanent teeth occurs less frequently than fusion between other types of teeth. The incidence of unilateral occurrence is estimated in the literature to be 0.5% in the deciduous and 0.1% in the permanent dentition. The incidence of bilateral occurrence is estimated at around 0.02% for both types of dentition [1, 12, 13]. As far as the etiology for fusion is concerned, many theories have been proposed; including genetic factors, local metabolic interference during tooth bud differentiation, traumatic or inflammatory causes [1, 6, 14]. To explain fusion, some authors suggest a lack of space as the cause of deep penetration of the dental follicles. The morphology of fused teeth varies, and complex forms with separated or fused coronal pulp chambers are present. Even separated chambers can meet in the radicular area or can remain separated.

Fusion is a developmental anomaly with inherently unusual and bizarre anatomy. When it occurs, it commonly results in caries, periodontal disease, and crowding [15]. Endodontic treatment is usually problematic, owing to the complex anatomy, tooth positioning, and difficulty in rubber dam isolation [6]. In the present case, we had to trim the prongs of the rubber dam retainer to properly seat the retainer on the tooth. A liquid dam was applied to achieve a fluid tight seal. A prerequisite for endodontic treatment of anomalous teeth is careful examination of radiographs from various angles. The amount of information gained from conventional film and digitally captured periapical radiographs is limited by the fact that the three-dimensional anatomy of the area being radiographed is compressed into a two-dimensional image. As a result of superimposition, periapical radiographs reveal limited aspects of the three-dimensional anatomy. In addition, there may also be geometric distortion of the anatomical structures being imaged [16]. These problems can be addressed by the use of SCT which can produce three-dimensional images of individual teeth and aid in better understanding of the root canal morphology.

A new CT technique, SCT or volume acquisition CT, has been developed that has its inherent advantage. Current CT scanners have a linear array of multiple detectors,

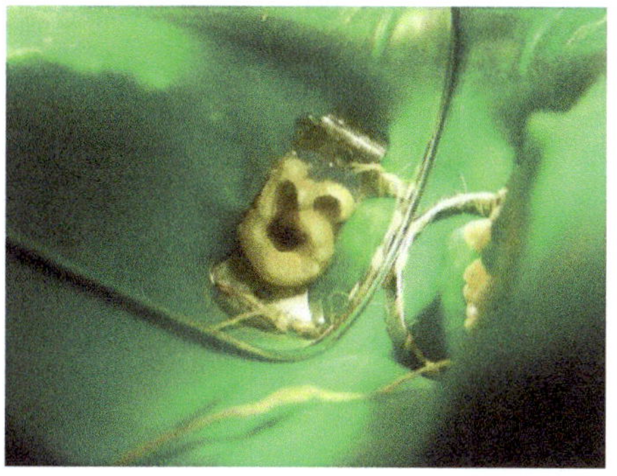

(a)

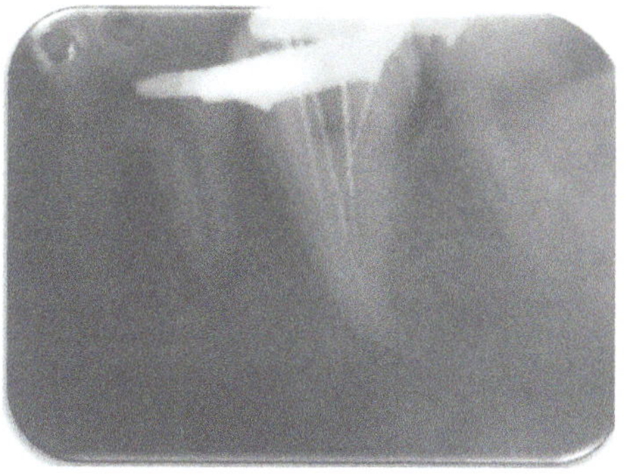

(b)

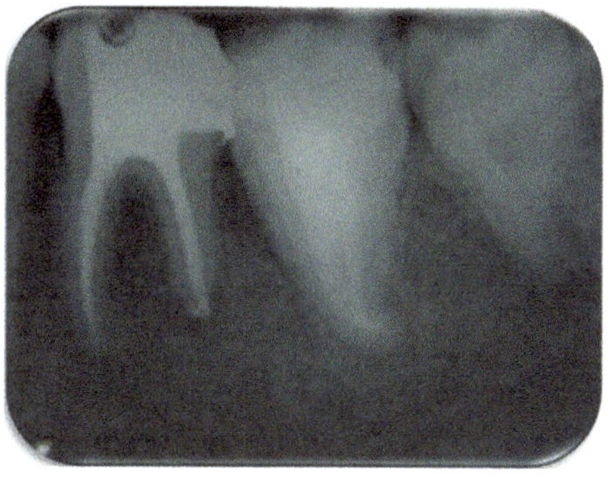

(c)

FIGURE 3: (a) Occlusal view. (b) Working length determination. (c) Postoperative final radiograph.

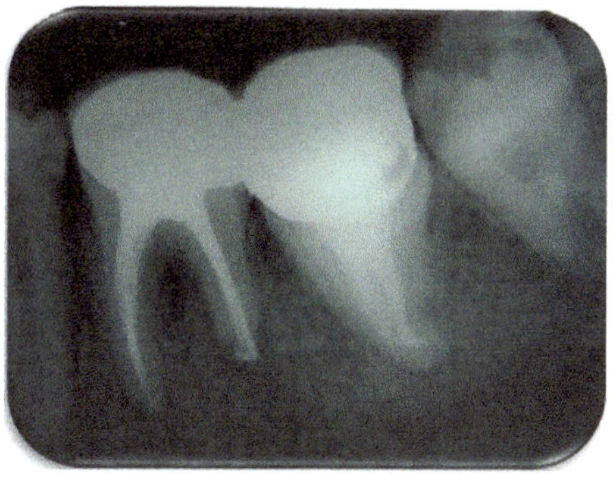

FIGURE 4: Recall radiograph 1-year postoperatively.

allowing multiple slices to be taken simultaneously, resulting in faster scan times and often less radiation exposure to the patient. The slices of data are then "stacked" up and can be reformatted to obtain three-dimensional images [17].

SCT can get a large volume of data in seconds and offer more rapid examination time and with an effective dose in the range of about 1–30 mSv, which is much less than the conventional CT [18]. Christoph et al. [19] have proposed a SCT protocol with a reduced radiation dose (0.56 ± 0.06 mGy) down to the level of a single panoramic radiograph [19]. However, keeping in mind the extra cost associated, its use should be limited to cases with unusual tooth morphology.

In this specific case, a SCT could confirm the complicated morphology of the root canal system of the fused tooth. This technique seems to have the potential to visualize the topography of root canals and offer new perspectives for dental imaging of special clinical cases.

With the advent of newer tomographic scanners like cone beam computed tomography (CBCT) or digital volume tomography (DVT) specifically for maxillofacial and dental use, conventional scanners like SCT will be less preferred for dental imaging purposes. CBCT is advantageous in that it has a low effective dose in the same order of magnitude as conventional dental radiographs [20]. Although there has been enormous interest in the current CBCT technology, it has limitations related to the "cone-beam" projection geometry, detector sensitivity, and contrast resolution. These parameters create an inherent image "noise" that can compromise the quality of the scan and can lead to an inaccurate or false diagnosis [21]. Even though the use of CBCT involves less radiation than conventional CT, the radiation dose is still higher than regular conventional intraoral radiographs [22]. At this point of time, CBCT is limited to major metropolitan areas and is very expensive. Methods and training to improve accessibility and affordability of CBCT should be explored.

5. Conclusion

This paper demonstrates a predictable and successful solution towards the endodontic management of a fused mandibular second molar with a supernumerary tooth by using

SCT as a diagnostic tool to a great effect in understanding the complex root canal anatomy, thus helping a great deal in rendering successful endodontic therapy. Proper diagnosis and treatment planning for endodontic management of fused teeth by using SCT can ensure predictable and successful results.

References

[1] W. K. Duncan and M. L. Helpin, "Bilateral fusion and gemination: a literature analysis and case report," *Oral Surgery, Oral Medicine, Oral Pathology*, vol. 64, no. 1, pp. 82–87, 1987.

[2] J. J. Pindborg, *Pathology of the Dental Hard Tissues*, WB Saunders, Philadelphia, Pa, USA, 1970.

[3] T. M. Bueviaje and R. Rapp, "Dental anomalies in children: a clinical and radiographic survey," *Journal of Dentistry for Children*, vol. 51, pp. 42–46, 1984.

[4] A. H. Brook and G. B. Winter, "Double teeth. A retrospective study of "geminated" and "fused" teeth in children," *British Dental Journal*, vol. 129, no. 3, pp. 123–130, 1970.

[5] S. W. Yuen, J. C. Chan, and S. H. Wei, "Double primary teeth and their relationship with the permanent successors: a radiographic study of 376 cases," *Pediatric Dentistry*, vol. 9, no. 1, pp. 42–48, 1987.

[6] R. Rajenderan and B. Sivapathasundharam, *Shafer's Textbook of Oral Pathology*, Elsevier, New York, NY, USA, 5th edition, 2006.

[7] L. D. Rajab and M. A. M. Hamdan, "Supernumerary teeth: review of the literature and a survey of 152 cases," *International Journal of Paediatric Dentistry*, vol. 12, no. 4, pp. 244–254, 2002.

[8] J. Ghoddusi, M. Zarei, and H. Jafarzadeh, "Endodontic treatment of a supernumerary tooth fused to a mandibular second molar: a case report," *Journal of Oral Science*, vol. 48, no. 1, pp. 39–41, 2006.

[9] E. Nunes, I. G. de Moraes, P. M. de Novaes, and S. M. de Sousa, "Bilateral fusion of mandibular second molars with supernumerary teeth: case report," *Brazilian Dental Journal*, vol. 13, no. 2, pp. 137–141, 2002.

[10] S. Ballal, G. S. Sachdeva, and D. Kandaswamy, "Endodontic management of a fused mandibular second molar and paramolar with the aid of spiral computed tomography: a case report," *Journal of Endodontics*, vol. 33, no. 10, pp. 1247–1251, 2007.

[11] A. K. Rani, S. Metgud, S. S. Yakub, U. Pai, N. G. Toshniwal, and N. Bawaskar, "Endodontic and esthetic management of maxillary lateral incisor fused to a supernumerary tooth associated with a talon cusp by using spiral computed tomography as a diagnostic aid: a case report," *Journal of Endodontics*, vol. 36, no. 2, pp. 345–349, 2010.

[12] G. L. Tasa and J. R. Lukacs, "The prevalence and expression of primary double teeth in western India," *Journal of Dentistry for Children*, vol. 68, no. 3, pp. 196–200, 2001.

[13] M. Tomizawa, A. Shimizu, S. Hayashi, and T. Noda, "Bilateral maxillary fused primary incisors accompanied by succedaneous supernumerary teeth: report of a case," *International Journal of Paediatric Dentistry*, vol. 12, no. 3, pp. 223–227, 2002.

[14] M. Hülsmann, R. Bahr, and U. Grohmann, "Hemisection and vital treatment of a fused tooth—literature review and case report," *Endodontics and Dental Traumatology*, vol. 13, no. 6, pp. 253–258, 1997.

[15] R. Indra, M. R. Srinivasan, H. Farzana, and K. Karthikeyan, "Endodontic management of a fused maxillary lateral incisor with a supernumerary tooth: a case report," *Journal of Endodontics*, vol. 32, no. 12, pp. 1217–1219, 2006.

[16] H.-G. Grondahland and S. Huumonen, "Radiographic manifestations of periapical inflammatory lesions," *Endodontic Topics*, vol. 8, pp. 55–67, 2004.

[17] H. Hu, H. D. He, W. D. Foley, and S. H. Fox, "Four multidetector-row helical CT: image quality and volume coverage speed," *Radiology*, vol. 215, no. 1, pp. 55–62, 2000.

[18] J. Zoetelief and J. Geleijns, "Patient doses in spiral CT," *British Journal of Radiology*, vol. 71, pp. 584–586, 1998.

[19] G. D. Christoph, G. H. E. Wilfried, R. Britta, K. P. Hermann, and J. W. Oestmann, "Must radiation dose for CT of the maxilla and mandible be higher than that for conventional panoramic radiography?" *American Journal of Neuroradiology*, vol. 17, no. 9, pp. 1758–1760, 1996.

[20] S. Patel, A. Dawood, T. Pitt Ford, and E. Whaites, "The potential applications of cone beam computed tomography in the management of endodontic problems," *International Endodontic Journal*, vol. 40, no. 10, pp. 818–830, 2007.

[21] E. Soğur, B. G. Baksi, and H. G. Gröndahl, "Imaging of root canal fillings: a comparison of subjective image quality between limited cone-beam CT, storage phosphor and film radiography," *International Endodontic Journal*, vol. 40, no. 3, pp. 179–185, 2007.

[22] J. B. Ludlow, L. E. Davies-Ludlow, S. L. Brooks, and W. B. Howerton, "Dosimetry of 3 CBCT devices for oral and maxillofacial radiology: CB Mercuray, NewTom 3G and i-CAT," *Dentomaxillofacial Radiology*, vol. 35, no. 4, pp. 219–226, 2006.

11

An Interdisciplinary Approach for Rehabilitating a Patient with Amelogenesis Imperfecta: A Case Report

Niloufar Khodaeian,[1] Mahmoud Sabouhi,[2] and Ebrahim Ataei[3]

[1] *Dental Implant Research Center and Department of Prosthodontics, School of Dentistry, Isfahan University of Medical Sciences, Isfahan, Iran*
[2] *Torabinejad Dental Research Center, Department of Prosthodontics, School of Dentistry, Isfahan University of Medical Sciences, Isfahan 81746-73461, Iran*
[3] *Department of Restorative Dentistry, School of Dentistry, Shahid Sadoughi University of Medical Sciences, Yazd, Iran*

Correspondence should be addressed to Mahmoud Sabouhi, sabouhi@dnt.mui.ac.ir

Academic Editors: D. Cogulu, M. B. D. Gaviao, A. Kasaj, and J. J. Segura-Egea

Amelogenesis imperfecta (AI) has been defined as a group of hereditary enamel defects. It can be characterized by enamel hypoplasia, hypomaturation, or hypocalcification of the teeth. AI may be associated with some other dental and skeletal developmental defects. Restoration for patients with this condition should be oriented toward the functional and esthetic rehabilitation. This clinical report describes the oral rehabilitation of a young patient diagnosed with the hypoplastic type of AI in posterior teeth and hypomatured type of AI in anterior teeth.

1. Introduction

Amelogenesis imperfecta (AI) is a diverse group of hereditary disorders that primarily affect the quantity, structure, and composition of enamel [1]. The inheritance pattern of AI may be autosomal dominant, autosomal recessive, or X-linked [2]. According to the Witkop classification system, there are four main forms of AI: type I hypoplastic enamel, type II hypomatured enamel, type III hypocalcified enamel, and type IV hypomatured-hypoplastic enamel with taurodontism [1]. Clinical presentation of AI varies considerably among the different AI types. In the hypomature type, the affected teeth exhibit mottled, opaque white-brown or yellow discolored enamel, which is softer than normal. The hypocalcified type shows pigmented, softened, and easily detachable enamel. In the hypoplastic type, the enamel is well mineralized but its amount is reduced. Clinically, grooves and pits will be realized on the surface of the fine enamel. The tooth is tapered towards the incisal/occlusal face and has open contact points [3, 4]. AI may be associated with some other dental and skeletal developmental defects or abnormalities, such as unerupted teeth, congenitally missing teeth, taurodontism, pulpal calcification, crown and root resorption, cementum deposition, truncated roots, interradicular dentinal dysplasia, gingival hyperplasia, follicular hyperplasia, constricted maxillary arch (omega-shaped arch), reversed curve of Spee, vertical growth pattern, and dental and skeletal open bite [5–17]. The main clinical problems present in AI patients are tooth sensitivity, unsatisfactory esthetics, and loss of occlusal vertical dimension due to the rapid wearing of dentition [18, 19]. Treatment planning for patients with AI is related to many factors: the age and socioeconomic status of the patient, the type and severity of the disorder, and the intraoral situation. An interdisciplinary approach is necessary to evaluate, diagnose, and resolve AI patient problems using a combination of orthodontic, periodontal, prosthodontics, and restorative treatment [3, 20–22]. This clinical report describes the interdisciplinary approach for rehabilitating a patient with AI.

2. Case Report

A 21-year-old male patient presented with a chief complaint of discolored teeth. He did not complain about tooth

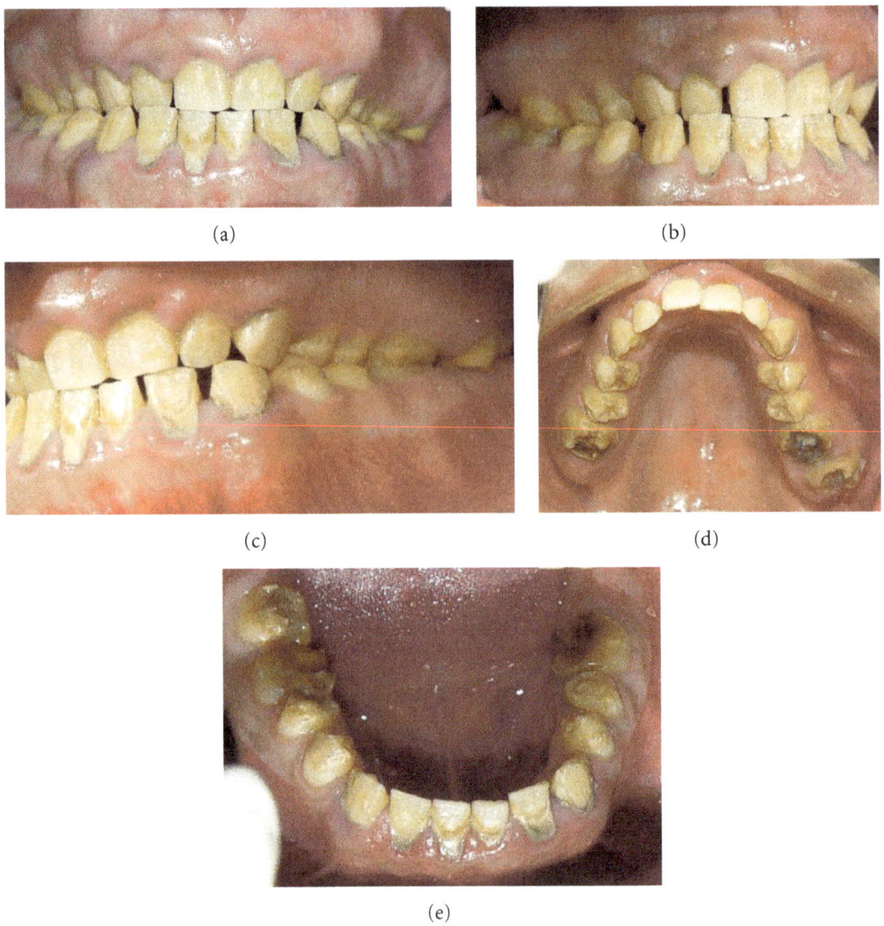

Figure 1: Pretreatment intraoral view: (a) frontal view; (b) right lateral view; (c) left lateral view; (d) maxillary occlusal view; (e) mandibular occlusal view.

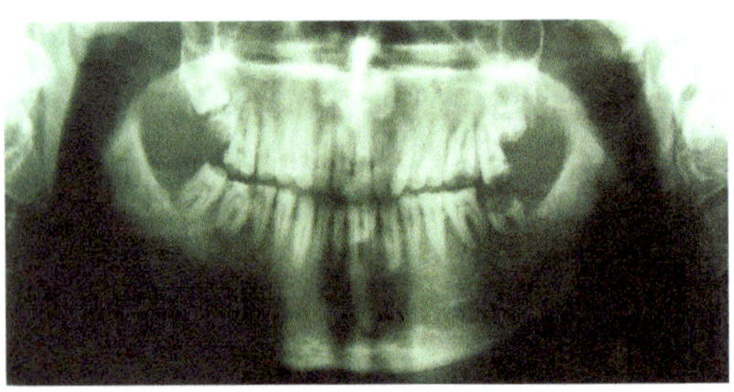

Figure 2: Pretreatment panoramic view.

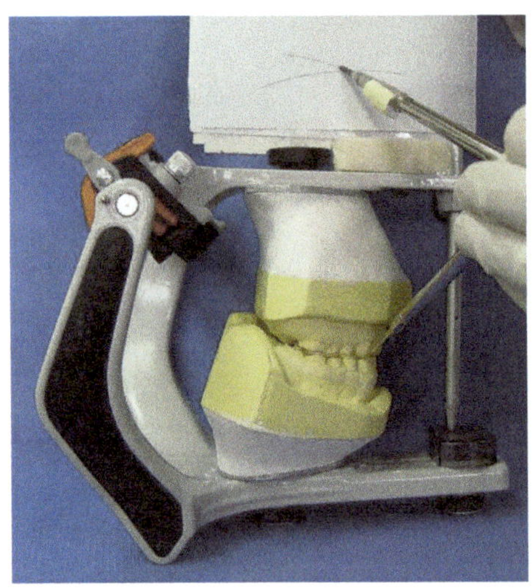

Figure 3: Occlusal plan evaluation using the Broadrick occlusal plane analyzer.

sensitivity and chewing inability. No remarkable findings were identified in his medical records. Among his first-degree family members, only one of his 2 sisters and his brother exhibited the same dental problems and his parents were cousins, so his inheritance pattern of AI was autosomal recessive. He had not received any prior dental treatment. In extraoral examination, the patient had competent lips and showed no facial asymmetry, no muscle tenderness or palpable lymph nodes, and no signs and symptoms of joint disorder. Intraoral examination revealed hypoplastic and hypomature types of AI in posterior and anterior teeth, respectively. The incisal edges were thin and the cuspal structures were aberrant (Figure 1). There were short clinical crowns, especially in the posterior regions. Other findings included posterior teeth wear and caries on teeth

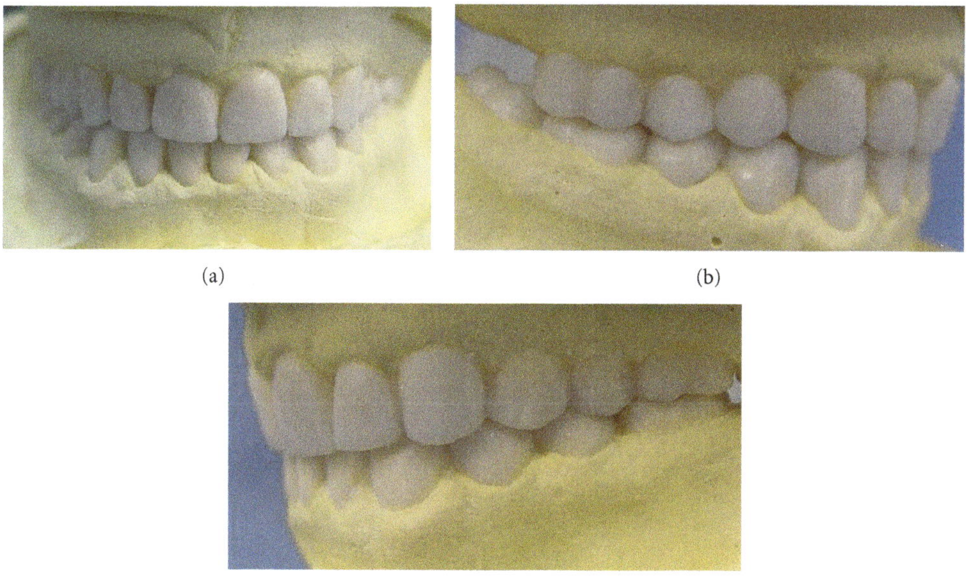

FIGURE 4: Diagnostic wax-up on diagnostic casts. (a) Frontal view; (b) right lateral view; (c) left lateral view.

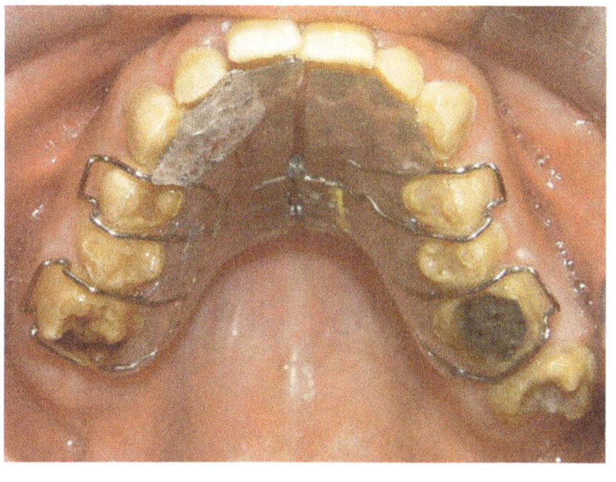

FIGURE 5: Orthodontic treatment with removable appliance.

nos. 14, 15, 29, and 30. The patient had constricted maxillary arch and crossbite relationship in bilateral posterior regions and teeth nos. 6 and 7. The patient suffers from pain on teeth nos. 14 and 29. The patient's oral hygiene was generally poor, as evidenced by bleeding on probing and plaque index findings. No packet deeper than 4 mm was recorded and the gingiva was hyperemic and edematous. Esthetic evaluation revealed a "gummy smile" in anterior maxilla and asymmetry in gingival contours of anterior teeth. The interocclusal distance measured at the premolar region during physiological rest was 3 mm. It was not possible to determine the molar relationship, but a Class I canine relationship was observed. The panoramic radiograph shown in Figure 2 revealed a thin layer of enamel along the top of most erupted teeth. The crown of teeth nos. 2 and 18 were resorbed. The teeth nos. 1, 2, 16, and 18 were impacted and the teeth nos. 17 and 32 were missed. The root of all teeth appeared to be normal in size and shape. Several closely approximated roots were also evident. Pulpal involvement was found on teeth nos. 14, 29, and 30.

3. Treatment Planning

A treatment plan was developed with the aims of pain control for teeth nos. 14 and 29, generally preventive care and improvement in oral hygiene, caries removal and root canal therapy for teeth nos. 14, 29, and 30, extraction of teeth nos. 1, 2, 15, 16, and 18, orthodontic treatment for managing the anterior and posterior crossbite, periodontal correction of gingival contours in anterior sextants and crown lengthening in posterior sextants, and prosthodontic treatment plan that includes porcelain laminate veneer for maxillary and mandibular incisors and metal-ceramic restoration for other teeth.

4. Treatment

Maxillary and mandibular arch primary impressions were obtained using a heavy- and light-body vinyl polysiloxane impression material (Panasil, Kettenbach Dental, Eschenburg, Germany). Two sets of diagnostic casts were made by pouring the impressions twice with a type III dental stone (Fuji Rock, GC Dental Corp., Tokyo, Japan). One cast set was used for the diagnostic wax-up and the other was saved for patient records. A centric relation record was taken according to Dawson's bimanual technique [23] by using anterior deprogrammer. The casts were mounted on a semiadjustable articulator (A_7 Plus articulator, Bio-art, Brazil) using facebow transfer (Professional facebow, Bio-art) and centric relation record. Then, the articulator was adjusted based on excursive records. A Broadrick occlusal plane analyzer showed correct present occlusal plane

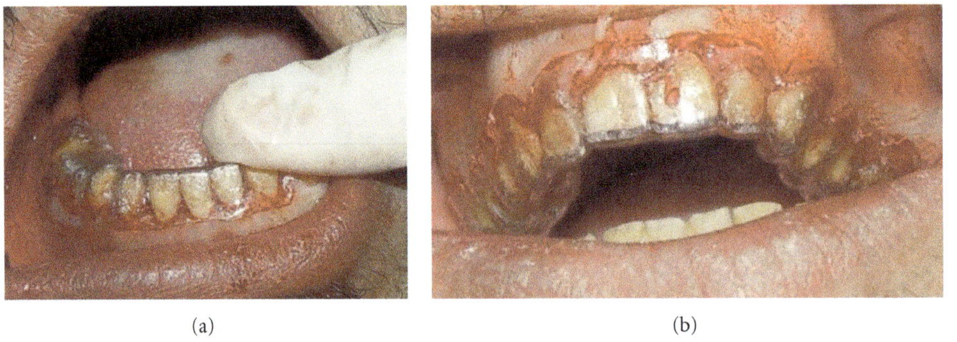

FIGURE 6: Crown lengthening according to fabricated stent: (a) in mandible; (b) in maxilla.

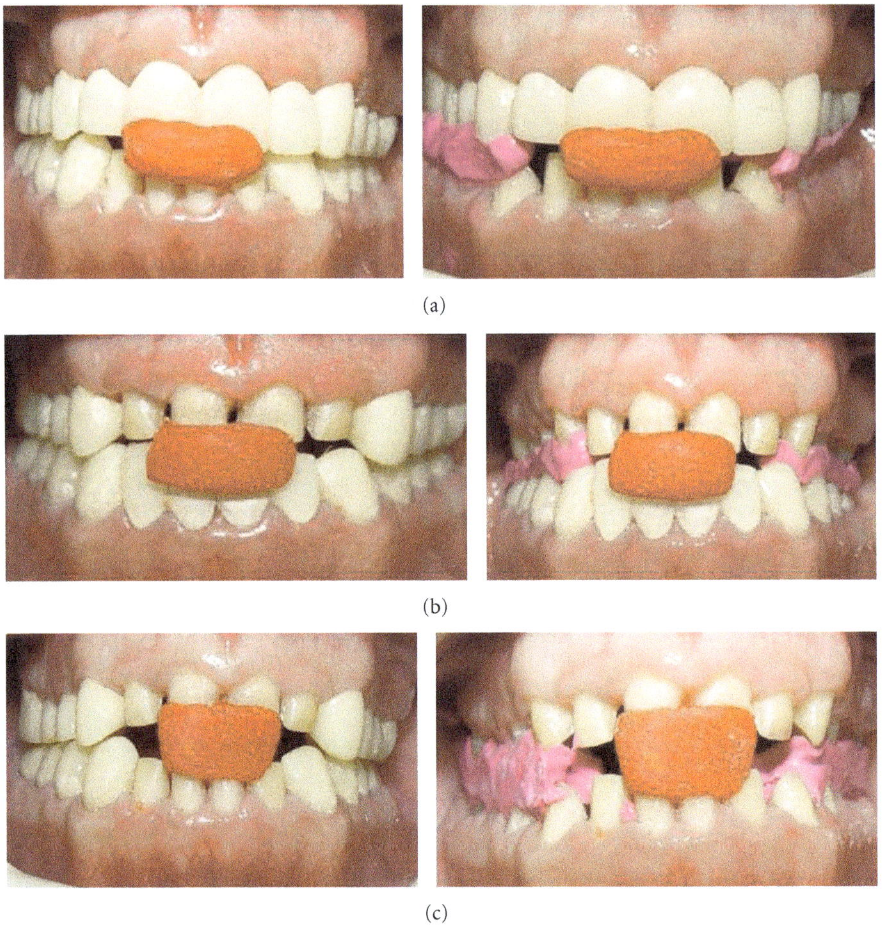

FIGURE 7: Records for cross-mounting: (a) record of maxillary provisional restorations in relation to mandibular prepared teeth; (b) record of maxillary prepared teeth in relation to mandibular provisional restorations; (c) record of maxillary prepared teeth in relation to mandibular prepared teeth.

and curve of spee [24] (Figure 3). The diagnostic wax-up was made according to optimum esthetic and function (Figure 4). After scaling and oral hygiene instruction, the patient adherence to recommended oral health care program was demonstrated after 2 weeks. The gingival edema was resolved and hyperemic appearance of gingival turned to normal. Also, bleeding on probing and plaque index findings became normal. Endodontic treatment for teeth nos. 14, 29, and 30, and extraction of teeth nos. 1, 2, 15, 16, and 18 were done. Amalgam core build up was done on endodontically treated teeth because of adequate coronal structures. Orthodontic treatment using removable appliance lasted about 6 months in active phase and 6 months in passive phase (Figure 5). After completing of orthodontic treatment, periodontal surgery procedures based on fabricated stents were conducted in 4 sessions

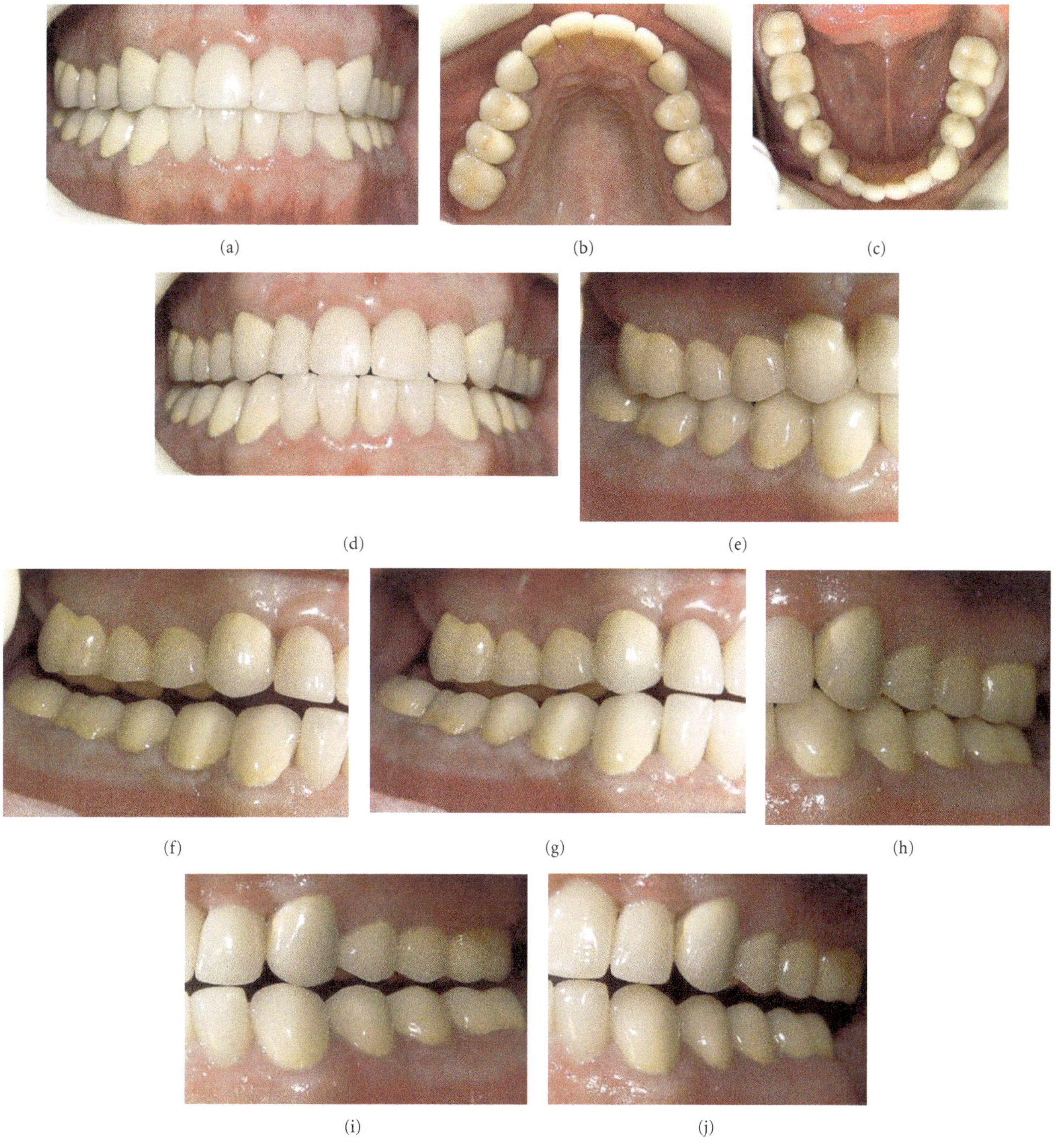

Figure 8: A 1-year posttreatment view of restoration: (a) frontal CR view; (b) maxillary occlusal view; (c) mandibular occlusal view; (d) frontal protrusive view; (e) right-side CR view; (f) right-side nonworking view; (g) right-side working view; (h) left-side CR view; (i) left-side working view; (j) left-side nonworking view.

(Figure 6). After 6 weeks, maxillary and mandibular incisors were prepared for porcelain laminate veneers and other teeth were prepared for metal-ceramic crowns. The amount of reduction was guided by the silicone index of the diagnostic wax-up. Provisional composite veneers (Protemp II, 3 M ESPE, Seefeld, Germany) were fabricated using silicone index for incisors, and laboratory-processed provisional crowns, which were fabricated with the aid of the diagnostic wax-up, were relined (Tempron, GC Dental Products Corp.) for other teeth. The occlusion was adjusted on the provisional restorations to establish a mutually protected scheme in the mouth. Maxillary and mandibular impressions were obtained in vinylpolysiloxane impression material (Panasil, Kettenbach), and irreversible hydrocolloid impressions (Jeltrate, Alginate, Fast set, Dentsply Intl, York, PA, USA) were made to make the cast of temporary restorations after 3 months of periodontal surgery. Cross-mount records were taken to use for mounting of definitive casts and casts of temporary

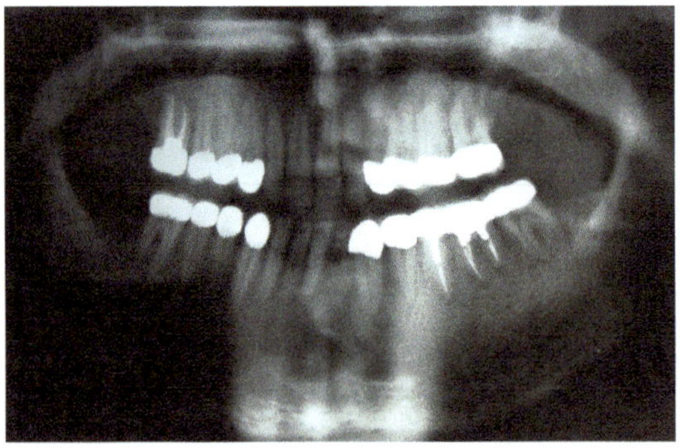

Figure 9: Posttreatment panoramic view.

restorations in the same articulator to serve as a guide for the fabrication of definitive restorations (Figure 7). The metal-ceramic restorations (Ivoclar, Vivadent, Schaan, Liechtenstein), and all-ceramic veneers (IPS Empress II, Vivadent) were evaluated intraorally. Then, veneers were etched with 4.9% hydrofluoric acid (IPS Ceramic gel, Vivadent) for 20 seconds and silanized (Monobond-S, Vivadent). Enamel surfaces of incisors were etched with 37% phosphoric acid (Total etch, Vivadent) for 40 seconds, and the veneers were bonded with a light-cured resin cement (Choice2 veneer cement, Bisco, Inc., Schaumburg, USA). The metal-ceramic restorations were cemented with glass ionomer cement (Ketac Cem, 3 M ESPE). The mutually protected occlusion scheme was preserved for this patient to allow for relatively even distribution and less stress of forces during excursive movement. Follow-up visits were scheduled at 3 months and then at 6 months (Figures 8 and 9). No esthetic and functional problems were seen after the 3 years of follow-up period.

5. Discussion

The marked phenotypic diversity of autosomal recessive AI cases with a hypoplastic phenotype did not permit straightforward classification according to a currently accepted nosology [25]; this patient had hypoplastic and hypomature types of AI in posterior and anterior teeth. Some of dental and skeletal developmental abnormalities in AI patients were also presented in this case. Crown resorption of unerupted teeth in autosomal recessive AI was already investigated [10]. This case showed preeruptive crown resorption on teeth nos. 2 and 18. Edematous and hyperemic gingiva, several closely approximated roots, and omega-shaped maxillary arch, were the other common abnormalities in AI patients which found in this case. Also, the teeth nos. 1, 2, 16, and 18 were impacted. Seow showed that people with AI have 6 times the tendency of unaffected people to have impaction of permanent teeth [26].

Several clinical reports have been presented describing the restorations of individuals affected by AI [22, 27–32]. Several authors prefer full porcelain restorations as the treatment modality of patient with AI [22, 27–31]. Advances in the field of esthetic dentistry, especially in bonding to dentin, help practitioners to restore function and esthetics to an acceptable level [27]. Nevertheless, marginal adaptation and bonding problems have been pointed out as disadvantages of laminate veneers [22]. Several factors may influence the outcome of restorative treatments including acid-etching and bonding of teeth affected by AI. For example, etch pattern of clinically variants of AI enamel may be altered and not produce a good match to normal enamel [33]. Additionally, the morphological pattern of dentin in hypocalcified AI is relatively similar to sclerotic dentin, which responds to acid etch conditioning differently than normal dentin [34, 35]. Newer dentin-bonding systems provide more reliable bonding to dentin and infiltrate more effectively to enamel prism than did the earlier systems. So, they may provide more durable dentin bonding than traditional methods of bonding to abnormal enamel. Despite severe enamel abnormalities, successful bonding of porcelain restorations could be achieved, and there were few adhesion complications in present case and several previously reported cases [22, 24, 29, 30]. The decision as to whether to preserve an enamel layer and use adhesive restorations or to completely remove the enamel and use complete coverage crowns depends on the extension and depth of the patient's enamel lesions [31]. In the present case, it was determined that the enamel should be presented based upon observation of clinically normal enamel during preparation of incisors. But canines and posterior teeth need full coverage restorations. Metal-ceramic restorations were selected because of financial status of this patient. Restoring of a tooth that has undergone crown lengthening is commonly performed in 4 to 6 weeks after the surgical procedure but a clinical study has demonstrated that the biologic width and the position of the free margin of gingiva exhibited no change at 3 to 6 months after surgery [36]. This patient was restored with provisional restoration after 6 weeks of crown-lengthening procedure, and the final restorations were made after 3 months of periodontal surgery.

6. Conclusion

AI is a developmental disorder that can result in reduced oral-health quality of life and causes psychological problems. Thus, these patients need extensive treatment. Coordinated orthodontic, periodontal, prosthodontics, and restorative treatments, with careful consideration of patient expectations, requests, and financial status, were critical for a successful outcome and patient satisfaction. Early treatment of patient with AI disorder can prevent progressive damage of dentition and the psychological impact of this condition.

References

[1] C. J. Witkop, "Amelogenesis imperfecta, dentinogenesis imperfecta and dentin dysplasia revisited: problems in classification," *Journal of Oral Pathology*, vol. 17, no. 9-10, pp. 547–553, 1988.

[2] M. J. Aldred, R. Savarirayan, and P. J. M. Crawford, "Amelogenesis imperfecta: a classification and catalogue for the 21st century," *Oral Diseases*, vol. 9, no. 1, pp. 19–23, 2003.

[3] B. W. Neville, D. D. Douglass, C. M. Allen, and J. E. Bouquot, "Abnormalities of teeth," in *Oral and Maxillofacial Pathology*, pp. 89–94, Elsevier, Philadelphia, Pa, US, 2004.

[4] I. Bailleul-Forestier, M. Molla, A. Verloes, and A. Berdal, "The genetic basis of inherited anomalies of the teeth. Part 1: clinical and molecular aspects of non-syndromic dental disorders," *European Journal of Medical Genetics*, vol. 51, no. 4, pp. 273–291, 2008.

[5] T. Lykogeorgos, K. Duncan, P. J. M. Crawford, and M. J. Aldred, "Unusual manifestations in X-linked amelogenesis imperfecta," *International Journal of Paediatric Dentistry*, vol. 13, no. 5, pp. 356–361, 2003.

[6] M. A. Collins, S. M. Mauriello, D. A. Tyndall, and J. T. Wright, "Dental anomalies associated with amelogenesis imperfecta: a radiographic assessment," *Oral Surgery, Oral Medicine, Oral Pathology, Oral Radiology, and Endodontics*, vol. 88, no. 3, pp. 358–364, 1999.

[7] G. O. Macedo, R. S. Tunes, A. C. F. Motta et al., "Amelogenesis imperfecta and unusual gingival hyperplasia," *Journal of Periodontology*, vol. 76, no. 9, pp. 1563–1566, 2005.

[8] E. Peters, M. Cohen, and M. Altini, "Rough hypoplastic amelogenesis imperfecta with follicular hyperplasia," *Oral Surgery Oral Medicine and Oral Pathology*, vol. 74, no. 1, pp. 87–92, 1992.

[9] M. Nakata, O. Kimura, and D. Bixler, "Interradicular dentin dysplasia associated with amelogenesis imperfecta," *Oral Surgery Oral Medicine and Oral Pathology*, vol. 60, no. 2, pp. 182–187, 1985.

[10] H. M. Korbmacher, R. Lemke, and B. Kahl-Nieke, "Progressive preeruptive crown resorption in autosomal recessive generalized hypoplastic Amelogenesis imperfecta," *Oral Surgery, Oral Medicine, Oral Pathology, Oral Radiology and Endodontology*, vol. 104, no. 4, pp. 540–544, 2007.

[11] J. A. Price, J. T. Wright, S. J. Walker, P. J. M. Crawford, M. J. Aldred, and T. C. Hart, "Tricho-dento-osseous syndrome and amelogenesis inperfecta with taurodontism are genetically distinct conditions," *Clinical Genetics*, vol. 56, no. 1, pp. 35–40, 1999.

[12] M. J. Aldred, R. Savarirayan, S. R. Lamandé, and P. J. M. Crawford, "Clinical and radiographic features of a family with autosomal dominant amelogenesis imperfecta with taurodontism," *Oral Diseases*, vol. 8, no. 1, pp. 62–68, 2002.

[13] G. B. Gertzman, G. Gaston, and I. Quinn, "Amelogenesis imperfecta: local hypoplastic type with pulpal calcification," *The Journal of the American Dental Association*, vol. 99, no. 4, pp. 637–639, 1979.

[14] R. Rowley, F. J. Hill, and G. B. Winter, "An investigation of the association between anterior open-bite and amelogenesis imperfecta," *American Journal of Orthodontics*, vol. 81, no. 3, pp. 229–235, 1982.

[15] B. Bäckman and U. Adolfsson, "Craniofacial structure related to inheritance pattern in amelogenesis imperfecta," *American Journal of Orthodontics and Dentofacial Orthopedics*, vol. 105, no. 6, pp. 575–582, 1994.

[16] T. J. M. Hoppenreijs, R. A. C. A. Voorsmit, and H. P. M. Freihofer, "Open bite deformity in amelogenesis imperfecta. Part 1: an analysis of contributory factors and implications for treatment," *Journal of Cranio-Maxillo-Facial Surgery*, vol. 26, no. 4, pp. 260–266, 1998.

[17] G. Aren, D. Ozdemir, S. Firatli, C. Uygur, E. Sepet, and E. Firatli, "Evaluation of oral and systemic manifestations in an amelogenesis imperfecta population," *Journal of Dentistry*, vol. 31, no. 8, pp. 585–591, 2003.

[18] W. K. Seow, "Clinical diagnosis and management strategies of amelogenesis imperfectavariants," *Pediatric Dentistry*, vol. 15, no. 6, pp. 384–393, 1993.

[19] K. D. Coffield, C. Phillips, M. Brady, M. W. Roberts, R. P. Strauss, and J. T. Wright, "The psychosocial impact of developmental dental defects in people with hereditary amelogenesis imperfecta," *Journal of the American Dental Association*, vol. 136, no. 5, pp. 620–630, 2005.

[20] S. Poulsen, H. Gjørup, D. Haubek et al., "Amelogenesis imperfecta—a systematic literature review of associated dental and oro-facial abnormalities and their impact on patients," *Acta Odontologica Scandinavica*, vol. 66, no. 4, pp. 193–199, 2008.

[21] L. Claman, M. A. Alfaro, and A. Mercado, "An interdisciplinary approach for improved esthetic results in the anterior maxilla," *Journal of Prosthetic Dentistry*, vol. 89, no. 1, pp. 1–5, 2003.

[22] N. Ozturk, Z. Sari, and B. Ozturk, "An interdisciplinary approach for restoring function and esthetics in a patient with amelogenesis imperfecta and malocclusion: a clinical report," *Journal of Prosthetic Dentistry*, vol. 92, no. 2, pp. 112–115, 2004.

[23] P. E. Dawson, "Centric relation. Its effect on occluso-muscle harmony," *Dental Clinics of North America*, vol. 23, no. 2, pp. 169–180, 1979.

[24] J. F. Bowley, J. W. Stockstill, and R. Attanasio, "A preliminary diagnostic and treatment protocol," *Dental Clinics of North America*, vol. 36, no. 3, pp. 551–568, 1992.

[25] M. Nusier, O. Yassin, T. C. Hart, A. Samimi, and J. T. Wright, "Phenotypic diversity and revision of the nomenclature for autosomal recessive amelogenesis imperfecta," *Oral Surgery, Oral Medicine, Oral Pathology, Oral Radiology, and Endodontics*, vol. 97, no. 2, pp. 220–230, 2004.

[26] W. K. Seow, "Dental development in amelogenesis imperfecta: a controlled study," *Pediatric Dentistry*, vol. 17, no. 1, pp. 26–30, 1995.

[27] K. Gokce, C. Canpolat, and E. Ozel, "Restoring function and esthetics in a patient with Amelogenesis imperfecta: a case report," *Journal of Contemporary Dental Practice*, vol. 8, no. 4, pp. 95–101, 2007.

[28] H. Siadat, M. Alikhasi, and A. Mirfazaelian, "Rehabilitation of a patient with amelogenesis imperfecta using all-ceramic crowns: a clinical report," *Journal of Prosthetic Dentistry*, vol. 98, no. 2, pp. 85–88, 2007.

[29] L. Sadighpour, F. Geramipanah, and S. Nikzad, "Fixed rehabilitation of an ACP PDI Class III patient with amelogenesis imperfecta," *Journal of Prosthodontics*, vol. 18, no. 1, pp. 64–70, 2009.

[30] P. M. Yamaguti, A. C. Acevedo, and L. M. De Paula, "Rehabilitation of an adolescent with autosomal dominant amelogenesis imperfecta: case report," *Operative Dentistry*, vol. 31, no. 2, pp. 266–272, 2006.

[31] I. Kostoulas, S. Kourtis, D. Andritsakis, and A. Doukoudakis, "Functional and esthetic rehabilitation in amelogenesis imperfecta with all-ceramic restorations: a case report," *Quintessence International*, vol. 36, no. 5, pp. 329–338, 2005.

[32] E. M. Canger, P. Çelenk, M. Yenísey, and S. Z. Odyakmaz, "Amelogenesis imperfecta, hypoplastic type associated with some dental abnormalities: a case report," *Brazilian Dental Journal*, vol. 21, no. 2, pp. 170–174, 2010.

[33] W. K. Seow, "The effects of acid-etching on enamel from different clinical variants of amelogenesis imperfects: an SEM study," *Pediatric Dentistry*, vol. 20, no. 1, pp. 37–42, 1998.

[34] C. Sánchez-Quevedo, G. Ceballos, I. A. Rodríguez, J. M. García, and M. Alaminos, "Acid-etching effects in hypomineralized amelogenesis imperfecta. A microscopic and microanalytical study," *Medicina Oral, Patología Oral Y Cirugía Bucal*, vol. 11, no. 1, pp. E40–E43, 2006.

[35] S. M. Kwong, F. R. Tay, H. K. Yip, L. H. Kei, and D. H. Pashley, "An ultrastructural study of the application of dentine adhesives to acid-conditioned sclerotic dentine," *Journal of Dentistry*, vol. 28, no. 7, pp. 515–528, 2000.

[36] S. K. Lanning, T. C. Waldrop, J. C. Gunsolley, and J. G. Maynard, "Surgical crown lengthening: evaluation of the biological width," *Journal of Periodontology*, vol. 74, no. 4, pp. 468–474, 2003.

A Novel Approach for Treatment of an Unusual Presentation of Radicular Cysts Using Autologous Periosteum and Platelet-Rich Fibrin in Combination with Demineralized Freeze-Dried Bone Allograft

Veena A. Patil,[1] Manthan H. Desai,[1] Veerendra S. Patil,[2] Hanisha Reddy Kaveti,[2] Kiran Kumar Ganji,[3] and Prasanna M. Danappanavar[4]

[1] *Department of Periodontology, HKES's S.Nijalingappa Institute of Dental Sciences and Research, Sedam Road, Gulbarga, Karnataka 585105, India*
[2] *Department of Endodontics, HKES's S.Nijalingappa Institute of Dental Sciences and Research, Sedam Road, Gulbarga, Karnataka 585105, India*
[3] *Department of Periodontics, Sharad Pawar Dental College & Hospital, Sawangi Meghe Wardha, Maharashtra 442004, India*
[4] *Department of Oral and Maxillofacial Pathology, MNR Dental College & Hospital, Sangareddy, Medak, Andhra Pradesh 502294, India*

Correspondence should be addressed to Veena A. Patil; veenaashokpatil@gmail.com

Academic Editors: R. A. de Mesquita, J. J. Segura-Egea, and K. Seymour

Radicular cysts are the most common cystic lesions affecting the jaws. They are most commonly found at the apices of the involved teeth. This condition is usually asymptomatic but can result in a slow-growth tumefaction in the affected region. The following case report presents the successful treatment of radicular cysts using autologous periosteum and platelet-rich fibrin with demineralized freeze-dried bone allograft.

1. Introduction

Radicular cysts are the most common (52%–68%) cystic lesions affecting the jaw [1]. They are commonly found at the apices of involved teeth and sometimes lateral to accessory root canals. They are a direct sequel of chronic periapical infection [1]. Most of them are asymptomatic and are discovered when periapical radiographs are taken of teeth with nonvital pulps. Patient often complains of slowly enlarging swellings. Radiographically, most radicular cysts appear as round or pear shaped unilocular radiolucent lesions in the periapical region. The cyst may displace adjacent teeth or cause mild root resorption [2].

The following case report presents the successful treatment of radicular cysts using autologous periosteum and platelet-rich fibrin (PRF) with demineralized freeze-dried bone allograft (DFDBA).

2. Case Report

A 17-year-old female patient reported to the Department of Periodontics, HKES's S.Nijalingappa Institute of Dental Sciences and Research, Gulbarga, India, with a chief complaint of pain, swelling ongoing and pus discharge in the lower anterior region since two months. Past history revealed trauma in the lower anterior region 5 years ago with recurrent swelling and pus discharge.

On intraoral examination, inflamed and swollen gingiva was seen in relation to 41, 42, and 43 (FDI notation). A draining fistula was seen on the labial aspect in relation to 41 (Figure 1). 42 had grade I mobility, whereas no mobility was noticed with 31, 41, and 43. Pulp vitality test was negative with 41, 42, and 43, while adjacent teeth showed normal response. Periodontal probing depth was ≤3 mm for concerned teeth, and no clinical attachment loss was seen.

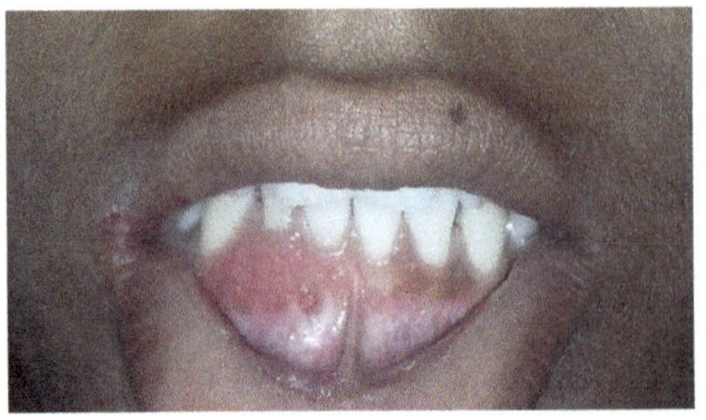

FIGURE 1: Preoperative view of the lesion.

They were also painless on vertical percussion. On radiographic examination, two radiolucent areas of size approximately 2 × 2 mm were seen in relation to 41, 42, and 43 (Figure 2). No root resorption was seen.

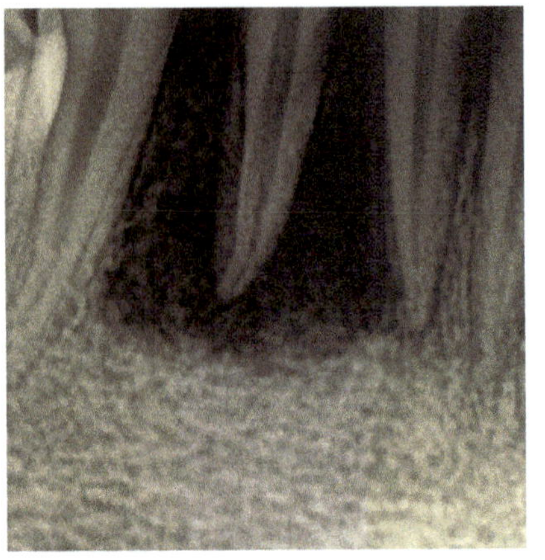

FIGURE 2: Preoperative radiograph.

The treatment plan comprised of endodontic treatment of nonvital teeth followed by surgical enucleation of cystic lesions if necessary. Treatment plan was explained to the patient, and a written informed consent was obtained. In the same visit, root canal treatment was started under rubber dam application followed by working length determination. After complete biomechanical preparation, 2% chlorhexidine gluconate was used as an irrigant and intracanal medicament. In the subsequent visits, root canal treatment was completed. Persistent pus discharge was observed at 3 months after endodontic treatment, and surgical enucleation was planned.

The procedure is as follows: local anesthesia was administered, crevicular incisions were given, and a full thickness mucoperiosteal flap from 41 to 43 and a split thickness flap in 31, 32 region were reflected. The area was degranulated revealing two small perforations of the buccal cortical plate in the regions of 41 to 43 of size 1 × 1 × 1 mm. The remaining buccal cortical covering was carefully removed with rotary and hand instruments to expose the rest of the lesions of size 3 × 3 × 2 mm.

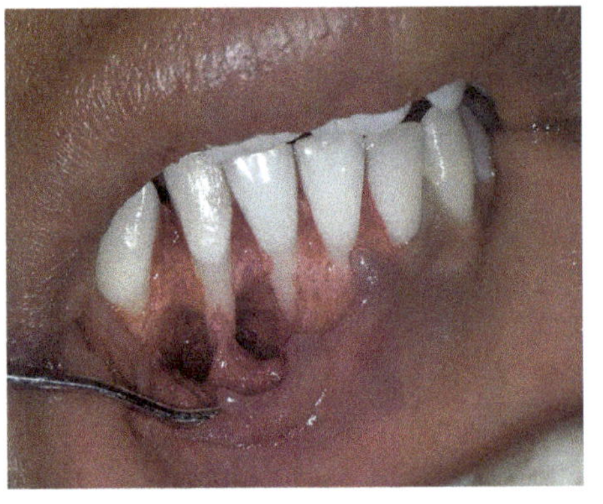

FIGURE 3: Debridement of the lesions.

Fragmented pieces of the lesion were freed from the bone, and complete curettage of the cystic lesions was done (Figure 3). The cystic cavities were thoroughly irrigated, and root biomodification of involved teeth was done using tetracycline. DFDBA was mixed with sterile saline solution and grafted in an attempt to close the defect via osteoconduction (Figure 4). Autologous healthy periosteum was harvested from the 31-32 region (Figure 5), and PRF was prepared from the patient's blood, as described by Choukroun et al. [3]. The lesion was covered with periosteum, over which PRF was placed as a second layer of barrier membrane covering the graft (Figures 6 and 7).

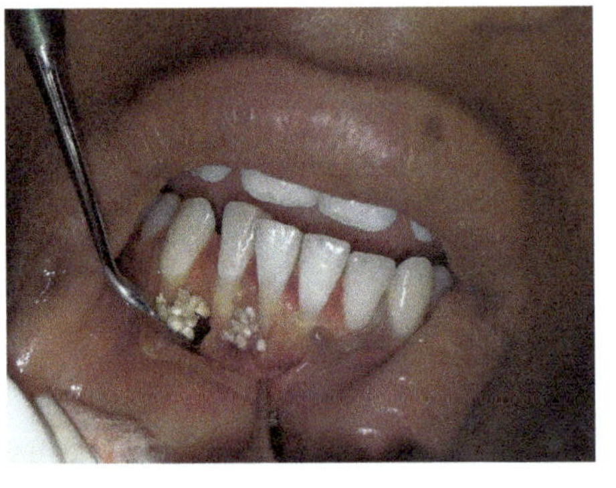

FIGURE 4: DFDBA graft placement.

The flap was coronally advanced and closed with interrupted sutures using 3-0 black braided silk (Figure 8). A periodontal dressing was applied at the surgical site. The patient was prescribed amoxicillin 500 mg TID and diclofenac sodium 50 mg TID both for 5 days with 0.12% chlorhexidine gluconate rinse BD for 7 days. Patient was asked to report after a week for suture removal, and the curetted tissue was submitted for histopathological examination. The patient returned for the postoperative visit, and the healing was uneventful.

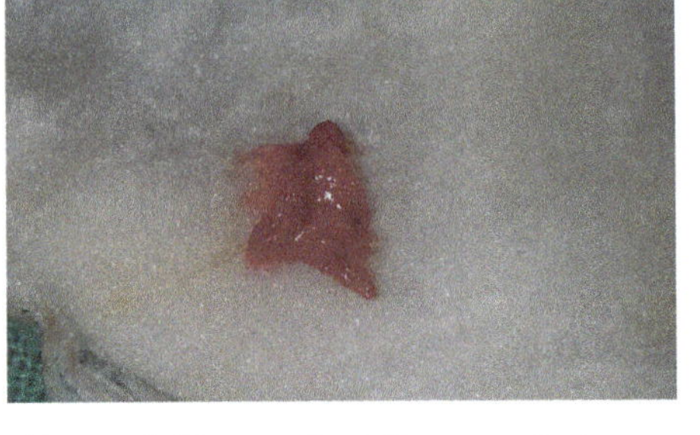

FIGURE 5: Harvested autologous periosteum.

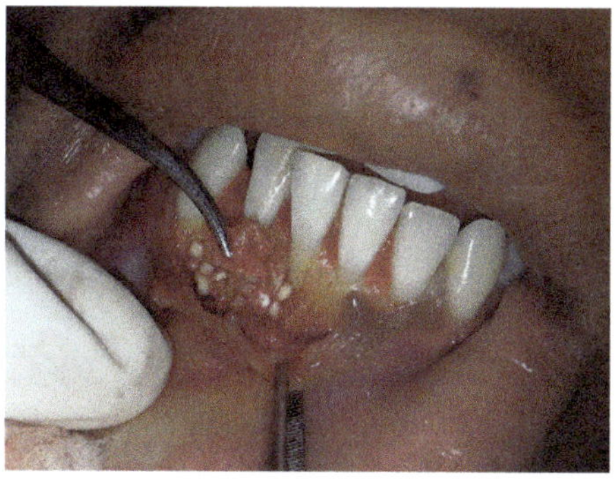

FIGURE 6: Autologous periosteum placed as a barrier membrane.

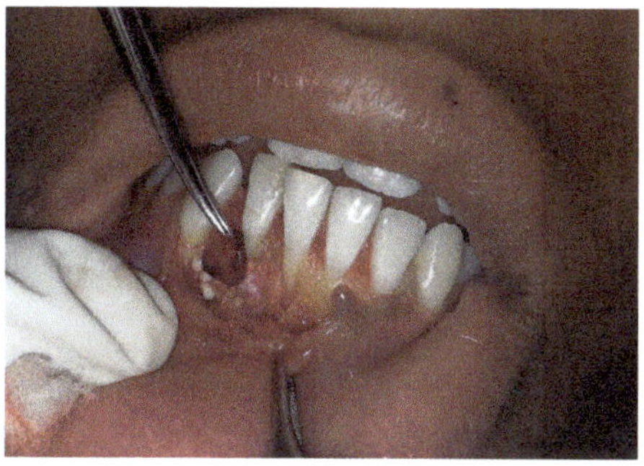

FIGURE 7: PRF placed as a barrier membrane.

Histopathology revealed the presence of a varying thickness of epithelium with fibrocellular connective stroma. The epithelium was disrupted with infiltration of chronic inflammatory cells along with vacuolations within the epithelium. Connective tissue showed dense infiltration of lymphocytes and plasma cells with few macrophages (Figure 9). A diagnosis of radicular cyst was given. Patient was followed up for 9 months. Radiograph at 6 months shows a healing lesion (Figure 10). A subsequent radiograph 9 months after operation (Figure 11) reveals increased radiopacity where the bone graft was placed, and no evidence of recurrence of the lesion was seen (Figure 12).

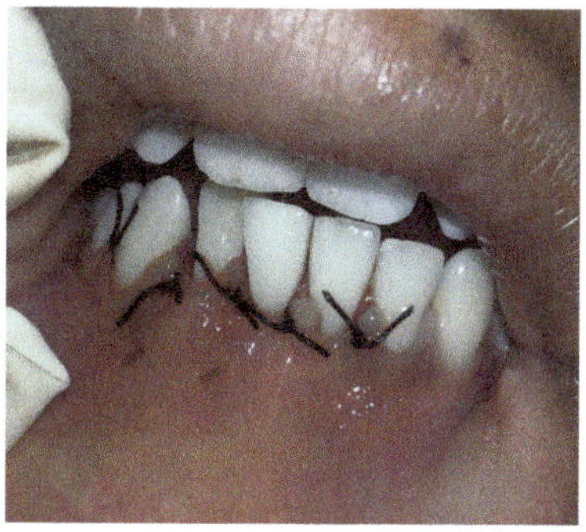

FIGURE 8: Sutured flap with 3-0 silk suture.

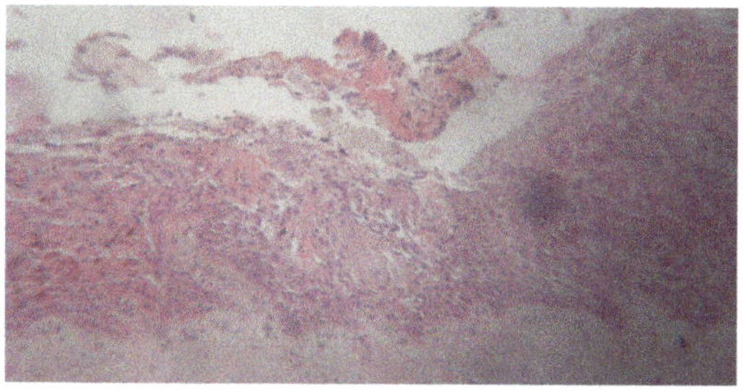

FIGURE 9: Histopathology of excised cyst.

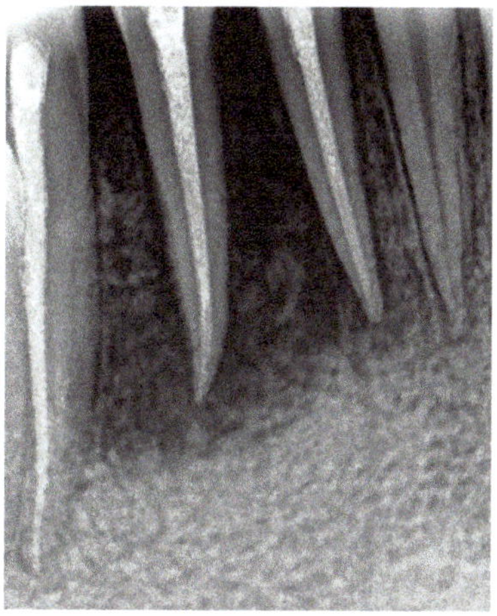

FIGURE 10: 6 months postoperative radiograph.

3. Discussion

A radicular cyst is an odontogenic cyst of inflammatory origin preceded by a chronic periapical granuloma and stimulation of cell rests of Malassez found in the periodontal membrane. The pathogenesis of radicular cysts comprises of three distinct phases: the phase of initiation, the phase of cyst formation, and the phase of enlargement [4]. The initial swellings of these radicular cysts are usually bony hard, but as they increase in size, the covering bone may become very thin despite initial subperiosteal bone deposition. With progressive bone resorption, the swellings exhibit "egg shell crackling." The associated teeth are always nonvital and may show discoloration. Although the associated teeth usually show no root resorption, there may be smooth resorption of root apices. When cysts are intact, cyst cavities may be filled with brown- or straw-colored fluid, giving them a shimmering gold appearance [4]. Radicular cysts are inflammatory lesions leading to bone resorption and can reach great dimensions and become symptomatic when infected or with great size due to nerve compression.

The main cause of failure of endodontic treatment is generally accepted to be the continuing presence of microorganisms in the root canal system that have either resisted treatment or have reinfected the root canal system. *E. faecalis* was the most frequently found microbe in such cases [5]. Chlorhexidine gluconate has been proposed for use both as an irrigant and as a medicament especially in endodontic retreatment. As a medicament, it is more effective than calcium hydroxide in eliminating *E. faecalis* infection inside dentinal tubules [6]. As an irrigant, it appears as effective

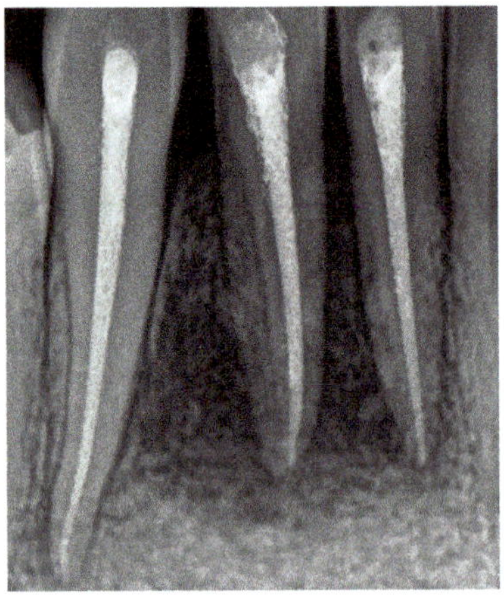

FIGURE 11: 9 months postoperative radiograph.

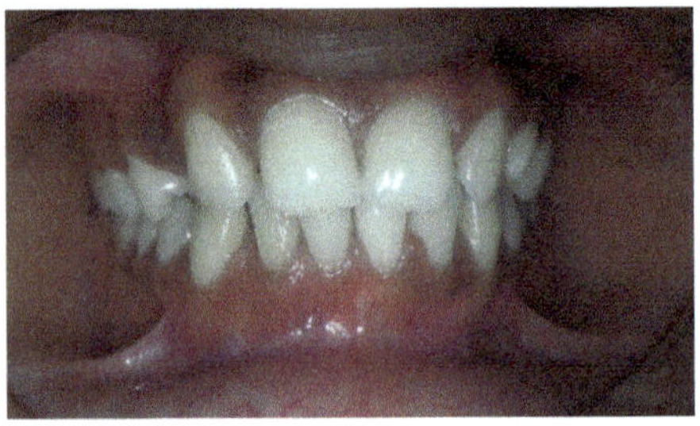

FIGURE 12: Healing at 9 months after operation.

or superior to sodium hypochlorite in the elimination of *E. faecalis* [7].

The adult human periosteum is highly vascular and is known to contain fibroblasts, osteoblasts, and stem cells. Skoog [8] subsequently introduced the use of periosteal flaps for closure of maxillary cleft defects in humans; he reported the presence of new bone in cleft defects within 3–6 months following surgery. Furthermore, animal studies have reported heterotopic ossification in different organs after implantation of free periosteal grafts [9, 10]. In all age groups, the cells of the periosteum retain the ability to differentiate into various cells. [11]. On the basis of these observations, it can be hypothesized that the periosteal membrane can contribute to the stimulation of new bone formation and has an immense potential for regeneration.

PRF belongs to the new generation of platelet concentrates with simplified processing. PRF contains a variety of growth factors, which enhance healing by increasing angiogenesis and matrix biosynthesis [12]. The immense osteoinductive capability of DFDBA is well described in the periodontal literature [13].

The treatments of these cysts are still under discussion, and many professionals opt for a conservative treatment by means of endodontic technique [14]. However, in large or nonhealing lesions, the endodontic treatment alone is not efficient, and surgical treatments like marsupialization or enucleation should be considered [15]. In this case, surgical enucleation was preferred and was performed uneventfully.

4. Conclusion

To conclude, a radicular cyst is a common condition found in the oral cavity. However, it usually goes unnoticed and rarely exceeds the palpable dimension. This case report illustrates the successful management of a radicular cyst with enucleation and endodontic treatment. The use of autologous periosteum and PRF has a promising future in periodontal regeneration.

Conflict of Interests

The authors declare that they have no conflict of interest.

References

[1] P. N. R. Nair, "New perspectives on radicular cysts: do they heal?" *International Endodontic Journal*, vol. 31, no. 3, pp. 155–160, 1998.

[2] M. Shear, "Radicular and residual cysts," in *Cysts of the Oral Region*, pp. 136–162, Wright, Bristol, UK, 3rd edition, 1992.

[3] J. Choukroun, A. Diss, A. Simonpieri et al., "Platelet-rich fibrin (PRF): a second-generation platelet concentrate. Part IV: clinical effects on tissue healing," *Oral Surgery, Oral Medicine, Oral Pathology, Oral Radiology and Endodontology*, vol. 101, no. 3, pp. E56–E60, 2006.

[4] L. Jansson, H. Ehnevid, S. Lindskog, and L. Blomlöf, "Development of periapical lesions," *Swedish Dental Journal*, vol. 17, no. 3, pp. 85–93, 1993.

[5] E. T. Pinheiro, B. P. F. A. Gomes, C. C. R. Ferraz, E. L. R. Sousa, F. B. Teixeira, and F. J. Souza-Filho, "Microorganisms from canals of root-filled teeth with periapical lesions," *International Endodontic Journal*, vol. 36, no. 1, pp. 1–11, 2003.

[6] I. Heling, D. Steinberg, S. Kenig, I. Gavrilovich, M. N. Sela, and M. Friedman, "Efficacy of a sustained-release device containing chlorhexidine and $Ca(OH)_2$ in preventing secondary infection of dentinal tubules," *International Endodontic Journal*, vol. 25, no. 1, pp. 20–24, 1992.

[7] P. Ohara, M. Torabinejad, and J. D. Kettering, "Antibacterial effects of various endodontic medicaments on selected anaerobic bacteria," *Journal of Endodontics*, vol. 19, no. 10, pp. 498–500, 1993.

[8] T. Skoog, "The use of periosteal flaps in the repair of clefts of the primary palate," *The Cleft Palate Journal*, vol. 2, pp. 332–339, 1965.

[9] V. Ritsilä, S. Alhopuro, and A. Rintala, "Bone formation with free periosteum. An experimental study," *Scandinavian Journal of Plastic and Reconstructive Surgery*, vol. 6, no. 1, pp. 51–56, 1972.

[10] J. Cohen and P. Lacroix, "Bone and cartilage formation by periosteum, assay of experimental autogenous grafts," *Journal of Bone and Joint Surgery*, vol. 37, no. 4, pp. 717–730, 1955.

[11] A. Mahajan, "Treatment of multiple gingival recession defects using periosteal pedicle graft: a case series," *Journal of Periodontology*, vol. 81, no. 10, pp. 1426–1431, 2010.

[12] S. Jankovic, Z. Aleksic, P. Klokkevold, V. Lekovic, B. Dimitrijevic, E. B. Kenney et al., "Use of platelet-rich fibrin membrane following treatment of gingival recession: a randomized clinical trial," *International Journal of Periodontics and Restorative Dentistry*, vol. 32, no. 2, pp. 41–50, 2012.

[13] F. Brugnami, P. R. Then, H. Moroi, and C. W. Leone, "Histologic evaluation of human extraction sockets treated with demineralized freeze-dried bone allograft (DFDBA) and cell occlusive membrane," *Journal of Periodontology*, vol. 67, no. 8, pp. 821–825, 1996.

[14] M. M. Hoen, G. L. LaBounty, and E. J. Strittmatter, "Conservative treatment of persistent periradicular lesions using aspiration and irrigation," *Journal of Endodontics*, vol. 16, no. 4, pp. 182–186, 1990.

[15] J. Danin, L. E. Linder, G. Lundqvist, L. Ohlsson, L. O. Ramsköld, and T. Strömberg, "Outcomes of periradicular surgery in cases with apical pathosis and untreated canals," *Oral Surgery, Oral Medicine, Oral Pathology, Oral Radiology, and Endodontics*, vol. 87, no. 2, pp. 227–232, 1999.

13

Regional Aggressive Root Resorption Caused by Neuronal Virus Infection

Inger Kjær,[1] Carsten Strøm,[2] and Nils Worsaae[3]

[1] *Department of Orthodontics, Institute of Odontology, Faculty of Health Sciences, University of Copenhagen, 20 Norre Alle, 2200 Copenhagen, Denmark*
[2] *Private Dental Practice, Lyngbyvej 133, 2100 Copenhagen, Denmark*
[3] *Department of Oral and Maxillofacial Surgery, Copenhagen University Hospital, Rigshospitalet, 2100 Copenhagen, Denmark*

Correspondence should be addressed to Inger Kjær, ik@sund.ku.dk

Academic Editors: R. S. Brown and T. Hata

During orthodontic treatment, root resorption can occur unexplainably. No clear distinction has been made between resorption located within specific regions and resorption occurring generally in the dentition. The purpose is to present cases with idiopathic (of unknown origin) root resorption occurring regionally. Two cases of female patients, 26 and 28 years old, referred with aggressive root resorption were investigated clinically and radiographically. Anamnestic information revealed severe virus diseases during childhood, meningitis in one case and whooping cough in the other. One of the patients was treated with dental implants. Virus spreading along nerve paths is a possible explanation for the unexpected resorptions. In both cases, the resorptions began cervically. The extent of the resorption processes in the dentition followed the virus infected nerve paths and the resorption process stopped when reaching regions that were innervated differently and not infected by virus. In one case, histological examination revealed multinuclear dentinoclasts. The pattern of resorption in the two cases indicates that innervation is a factor, which under normal conditions may protect the root surface against resorption. Therefore, the normal nerve pattern is important for diagnostics and for predicting the course of severe unexpected root resorption.

1. Introduction

Deviations in the dentition can occur regionally (affecting specific teeth) or generally (affecting several teeth in the dentition).

An interesting case was published in 1995 [1] demonstrating a right-sided maxillary underdevelopment of teeth and jaw combined with right-sided hearing loss provoked by mumps virus. This observation motivated the search for clarity regarding jaw innervation. One of the results was an innervation diagram, which was first published in 1998 [2] (Figure 1). In particular, the innervation of the mandible with innervation paths to the different tooth groups, published in 1996 [3], has made it possible to understand that the innervation to the incisors and to the canines/premolars and also to the molars is caused by different nerve paths in the maxilla and mandible. The innervation diagram has made it possible to understand how innervation is involved in eruption [4] showing a close connection between eruption times within the three different tooth groups in each jaw, but not between the tooth groups.

The regional pattern observed in retention of permanent teeth has also been explained from the innervation pattern when regionally affected by virus infection [5]. Furthermore, segmental odontomaxillary dysplasia seems to occur in regions correlated to the innervation patterns [6]. Interrelationship between the central nervous system and the surrounding bone and the relationship between the peripheral nervous system and jaw bone and teeth have been designated neuro-osteology [7]. A relationship between prenatal peripheral nervous tissue and the initial osseous bone formation in the craniofacial skeleton was first described in 1990 [8]. In 1992, Lerner described the interrelationship between neuropeptides and bone metabolism at a molecular level [9]. Thus, the term neuro-osteology is verified in histological as well as molecular studies.

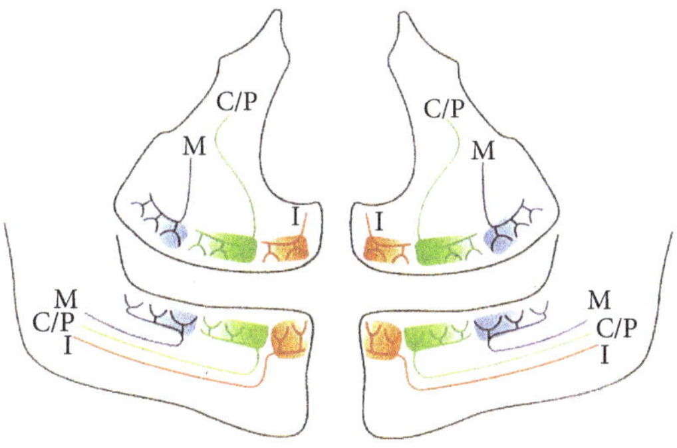

FIGURE 1: Schematic illustration of a panoramic radiograph with peripheral nerves innervating the different tooth groups. Red colour (I) illustrates the innervation of maxillary and mandibular incisors. Green colour (C/P) illustrates the innervation of maxillary and mandibular canines and premolars. Blue colour (M) illustrates the innervation of maxillary and mandibular molars. This illustration is reproduced with permission from Acta Odontologica Scandinavica [7].

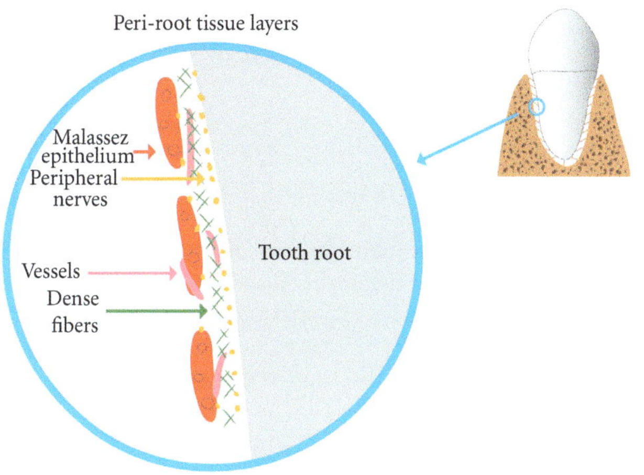

FIGURE 2: The figure in the circle is an enlargement of the area shown on the tooth in the upper right corner. The cell layers close to the root's periodontium, also known as the periroot sheet layers, are demonstrated in the circle. Nerve tissue: yellow. Tense fibre layer: green. Malassez epithelial cells: dark red. Vessels: light red. This illustration is reproduced with permission from Orthodontic Waves [27].

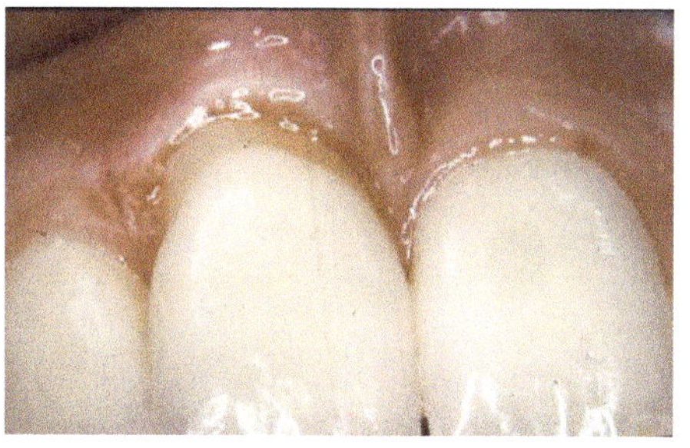

FIGURE 3: Patient 1: gingival retraction at the right maxillary central incisor after acute gingivitis in 1992.

In histological studies of the dental development, it has been shown that the initial dental development may begin without innervation [10], while the innervation is important at the time when the hard dental tissue is formed [11–13]. Recent studies have analyzed tissue components close to the root surface [14–16]. These studies have revealed that an innervation layer exists in close proximity to the root, covered by a layer of tight fibers and cell groups from the Malassez epithelium. It has also been demonstrated that the neuroendocrine cells are located in relation to the Malassez epithelium [17]. Similarly, a study by Yamashiro et al. [18] suggesting that sensory nerve innervation may have a regulatory role in maintenance of the epithelial rests of Malassez [18]. It has been a repeated question if one or all of these layers may offer protection against root resorption. The layers are schematically illustrated in Figure 2.

In Paget's disease, also named osteitis deformans, root resorptions have been observed [19, 20] and a viral aetiology has been discussed in a series of studies [21–25]. The characteristics of Paget's disease are the presence of focal areas of increased bone turnover containing enlarged hyperactive osteoclasts. Also a genetic predisposition has been in focus [26].

In orthodontic literature, a clear distinction has not been made between resorption located within specific regions and resorption occurring generally in the dentition. The distinction between resorption with a known cause and idiopathic root resorption (of unknown cause or spontaneous origin) has not been made. A main problem in orthodontics is that root resorption can occur unexplainably and it is, therefore, important to focus on causes rather than orthodontic forces that may provoke root resorption.

In the present paper, two cases of regional aggressive resorption are described, both seemingly with a viral aetiology.

2. Patient Cases

The paper describes diagnostics and treatment course for two patients referred to the Department of Orthodontics for elucidation and treatment plan.

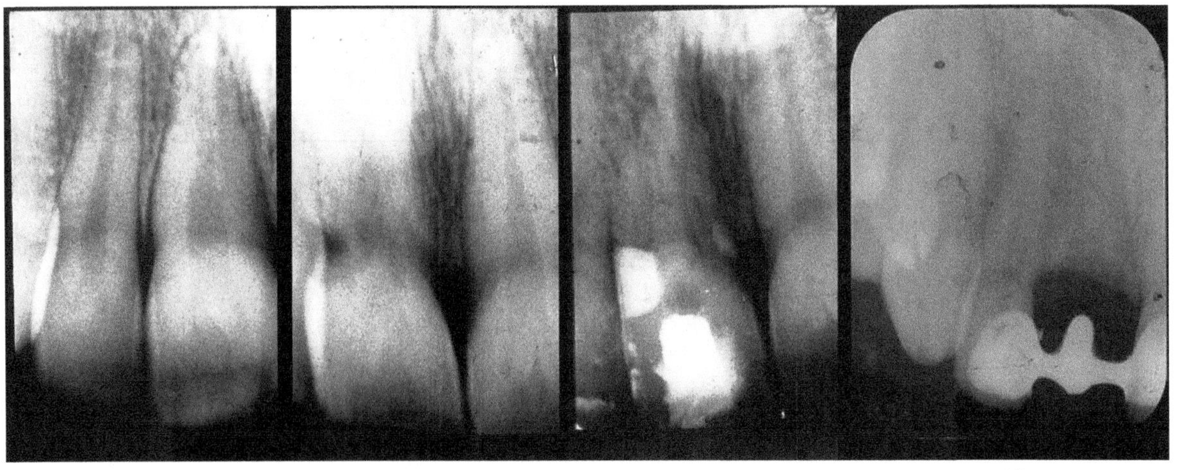

(a) (b) (c) (d)

FIGURE 4: Patient 1: radiographs of the right maxillary central incisor region. (a) 1994. Seemingly normal periodontal conditions in the central incisor region. (b) 1997. Severe cervical resorptions have appeared in the central incisor. (c) August 1999. Severe resorption of the root of the maxillary central incisor. The condition resulted in extraction of the central incisor. (d) December 1999. The maxillary central incisor has been extracted and the alveolar bone level is normal.

2.1. Patient 1. The patient, female born in 1974, is referred in April 2000 for elucidation of a previous severe idiopathic resorption of the right maxillary permanent central incisor that had recently been extracted. For the consultation, the patient brought anamnestic information, a photograph from 1992 (Figure 3) and radiographs from 1994 (Figure 4(a)), 1997 (Figure 4(b)), and 1999 (Figures 4(c) and 4(d)) of the central incisor. The patient had first contacted the dentist in 1992 due to retraction of the gingival level as seen in Figure 3. Examination of the four radiographs revealed severe root resorption starting at the cervical level of the right central incisor gradually progressing to the whole root. In Figure 4(d), the normal alveolar bone level after extraction is seen.

The extraoral examination in 2000 showed a pale scar tissue-like retraction of the upper lip just to the right of the midline in an otherwise normal red prolabium (Figure 5(a)). Furthermore, impaired sensitivity of the skin was observed in an area extending from the right prolabium to the right medial and lateral crus of the external nose. This affected skin area (marked by red colour) is demonstrated in Figures 5(b) and 5(c). Anamnestic information revealed that the patient had meningitis between the age of 8 and 9 and that the change in skin sensitivity began at the same time.

A new radiograph of the incisor region obtained at the consultation in 2000 demonstrated an initial cervical root resorption of the right permanent lateral incisor (Figure 6(a)). The patient has then been followed annually since 2000 and radiographs of the incisor region have revealed a gradual progressive resorption of the root of the lateral incisor as well as of the alveolar bone facing the medial aspects of the root (demonstrated in the examination in 2012, Figure 6(b)). No tumor-like conditions like for instance giant cell granuloma were observed.

2.1.1. Conclusion. It is suggested that the meningitis virus has spread along the right nasopalatine nerve innervating the skin region and the right incisors and that this may be the explanation for the regional root resorption and bone destruction. If this is the explanation, it can be predicted that the destructive process is limited to the right incisor region. For visualization, see the right red nerve path innervating the central and lateral maxillary incisors in Figure 1. Until now, treatment has included a preliminary bridge replacing the central incisor. In the near future, a final treatment must be decided upon replacing both right incisors.

2.2. Patient 2. The patient, female born in 1974, was referred to the Department of Orthodontics in 2002 from a private dental practice for evaluation of resorption of the maxillary left second premolar and left first molar. Furthermore, severe resorption was observed in the mandibular left central and lateral incisors. The referring practitioner presumed that the resorption had occurred as a result of previous orthodontic treatment. The patient had previously received orthodontic treatment with removable appliance in the maxilla, but not with appliance in the lower jaw. Resorption due to orthodontic treatment was, therefore, discarded. The referring dentist requested elucidation of the aggressive resorption and a treatment plan (Figure 7).

Different attempts to excavate and perform endodontic treatment and PA treatment of the two mandibular and two maxillary teeth failed, and in 2004 the maxillary premolar and molar as well as the incisors in the lower jaw were extracted (Figure 8). The extracted teeth were analyzed histologically. Large multinucleated resorptive cells situated in dentine lacunae were observed histologically (Figure 9). Panoramic radiograph from 2004 revealed the beginning of resorption distally in the maxillary left second molar, which was extracted shortly after the radiograph was taken. The left

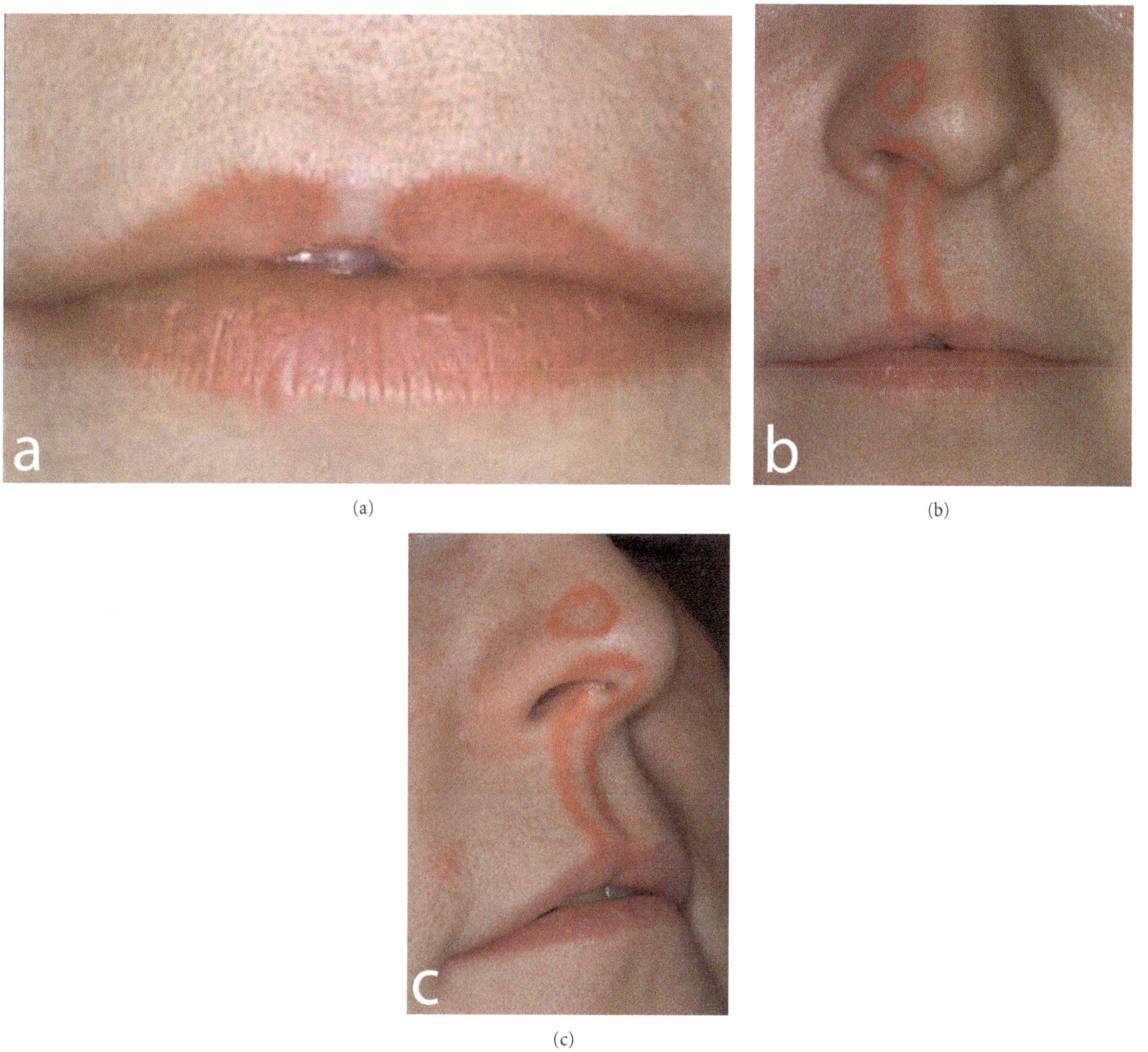

(a)

(b)

(c)

FIGURE 5: Patient 1: extraoral photographs. (a) The photograph shows retraction of the lip in the area of the central incisor. A white fibrous area is seen in the otherwise red prolabium in the same area. (b) and (c) Red colour marks the area of the skin at the upper lip and nose where the sensitivity is different (feeling of dead skin).

mandibular canine showed a slight cervical resorption, which was excavated and filled in 2004.

The patient was examined twice a year since 2004 at the Copenhagen University Hospital. In 2006, the patient informed that she had been severely ill at the age of 9 and hospitalized for three months due to whooping cough and sequelae. No further information was available.

During the following years all remaining maxillary permanent teeth in the left side showed cervical resorptions, which gradually became worse spreading along the entire root (Figure 10). This resulted in extractions. Since 2004, fixed implant supported dental reconstructions have been inserted in the left side of the maxilla, and in the incisor region in the mandible, two single implants have been inserted after bone grafting due to a narrow alveolar process (Figures 11 and 12). The condition around the filling in the left mandibular canine is unchanged since 2004 (Figure 11).

2.2.1. Conclusion. The left-sided severe root resorptions in maxilla and mandible are presumably due to a neurogene spreading of the pertussis virus. According to the innervation pattern (Figure 1), no further destruction will occur in the maxilla. In the mandible, the slight resorption attack on the left canine will be followed, but as it has been unchanged in eight years, there is no reason to presume that further changes will occur here.

3. Discussion

Both cases show signs of neurogene spreading of virus initiating root resorption. In both cases, resorption began as

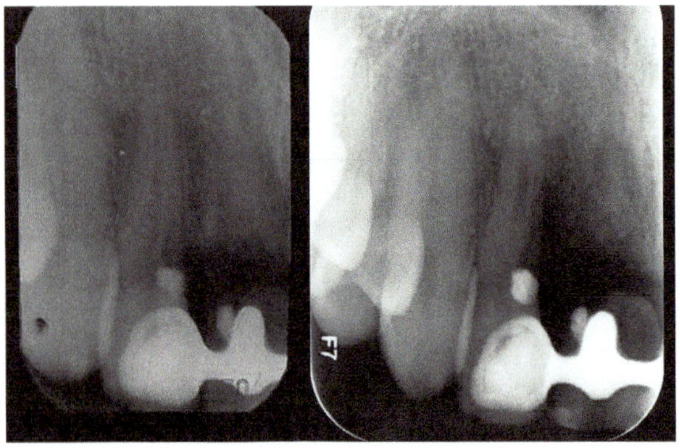

(a) (b)

Figure 6: Patient 1: radiographs of the right maxillary central incisor region. (a) 2000. The radiograph demonstrates a filling in the mesial aspect of the lateral incisor and resorption below this filling. The alveolar bone level has not changed remarkably since the situation demonstrated in Figure 4(d). (b) 2012. The radiograph demonstrates severe bone loss of the alveolar bone mesially to the lateral incisor root. The resorption process below the filling has progressed.

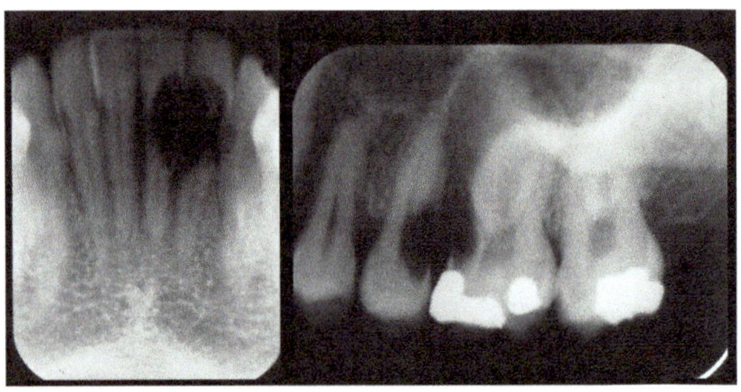

(a) (b)

Figure 7: Patient 2: radiographs demonstrating regional aggressive root resorption in the left mandibular incisors (a) and in the left maxillary second premolar and first molar (b).

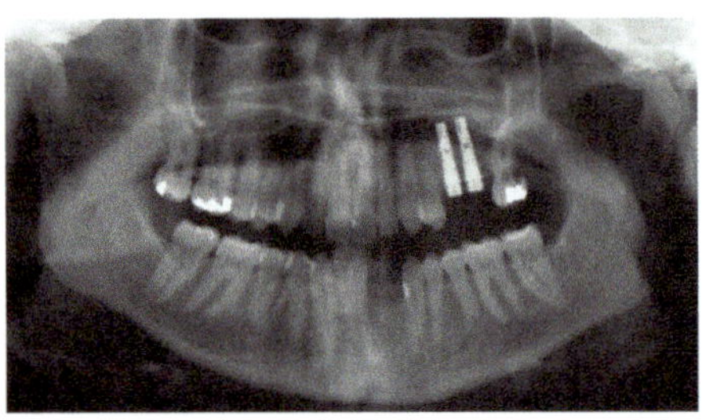

Figure 8: Patient 2: panoramic radiograph from 2004 demonstrating that the left mandibular incisors and left second maxillary premolar and first molar have been extracted. A filling is seen now in the mesial part of the cervical region at the left mandibular canine. Cervical resorption is observed distally in the left maxillary second molar. Implants have been inserted in the left maxillary premolar/molar region.

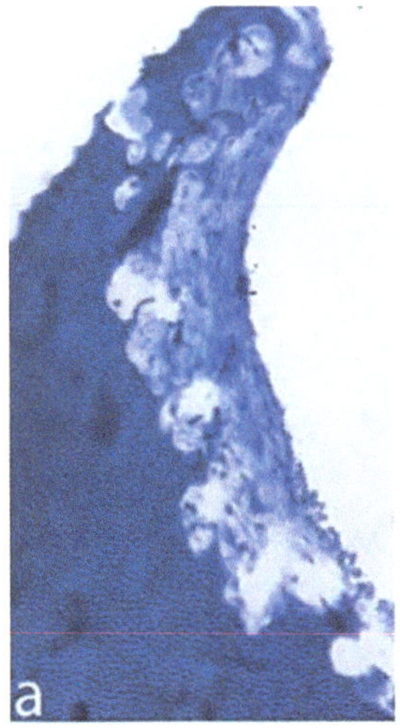

(a)

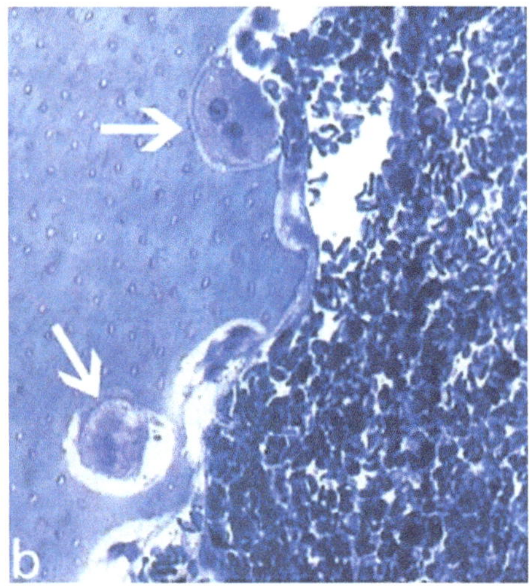

(b)

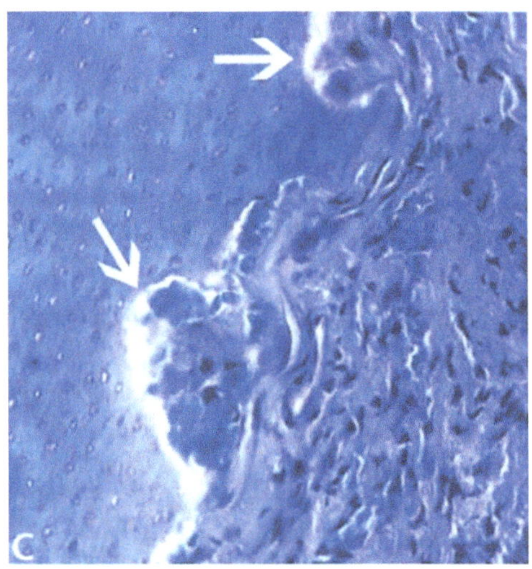

(c)

Figure 9: Patient 2: histological sections of different parts of the extracted mandibular left incisors, demonstrating aggressive multi-lacunary root surface (a). In a larger magnification, multinuclear resorptive dentinoclasts located in the lacunae are demonstrated and marked by arrows ((b) and (c)).

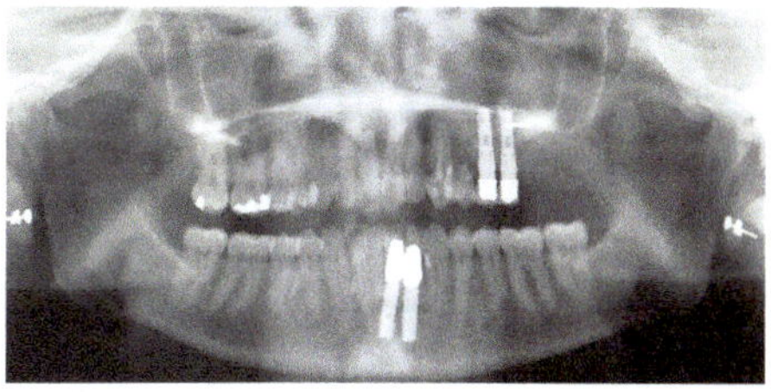

FIGURE 10: Patient 2: panoramic radiograph taken in 2007 demonstrating gradual resorption of the left-sided maxillary teeth when compared to the panoramic radiograph taken in 2004, demonstrated in Figure 8.

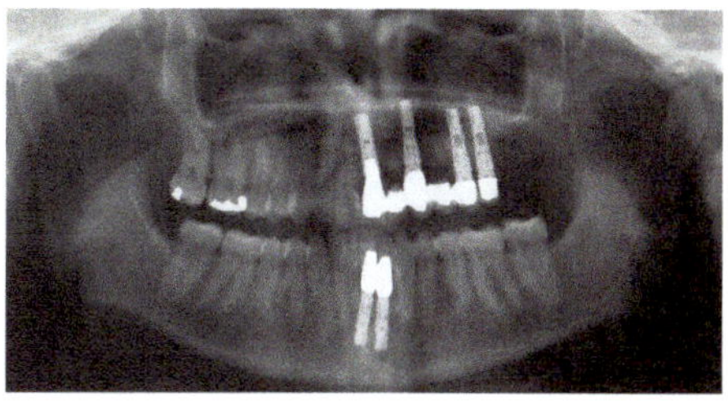

FIGURE 11: Patient 2: panoramic radiograph (from 2012) taken two years after the last implant had been inserted. The treatment has been performed by Chief Surgeon Nils Worsaae. The radiograph demonstrates that the destruction of teeth caused by virus attack on all left-sided maxillary peripheral nerves (illustrated in Figure 1) and on the left mandibular incisor nerve (marked red in Figure 1) has stopped. Also, the condition around the filling in the left mandibular canine is unchanged since 2004 (Figure 8).

invasive low cervical resorptions which later extended apically. Cervical root resorption has previously been described in association with periodontal disease [28].

The study does not demonstrate in which cell layer surrounding the root the resorption begins. The study does reveal that resorption occurs in regions determined by the innervation pattern and accordingly, that innervation seems to play a role in the resorption process. The study also reveals a correlation between the osseous development and root resorption. This is not surprising as it has been demonstrated that the osteoblastic function is regulated by the innervation [9].

The histological findings demonstrated in Patient 2 (Figure 10) are similar to that seen in Paget's disease [20]. However, the difference between Paget's disease and the cases presented in this study is that Paget's disease mostly affects the axial skeleton and has a strong genetic predisposition. In the present case, the root resorption is restricted to the innervation regions [27], and the anamnestic information in both cases suggests that the spreading of virus is the explanation. A regional resorption pattern related to the innervation pattern has not been described in Paget's disease.

It is perhaps the first time that such severe regional resorption processes are shown to be related to virus spreading along peripheral nerve paths.

It is important in odontological diagnostics to distinguish between regional and general resorption because it

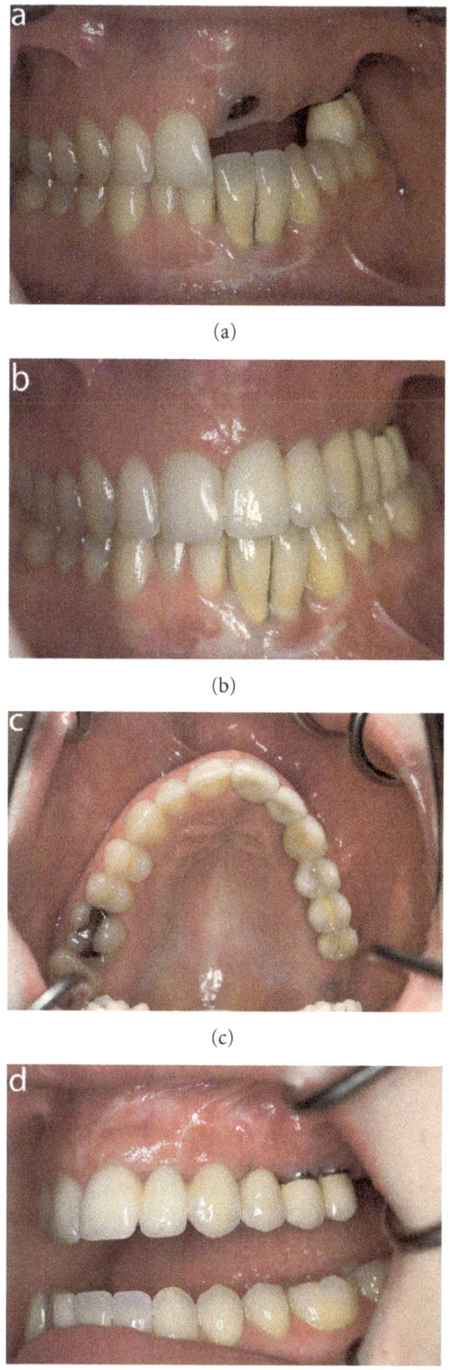

(a) (b) (c) (d)

FIGURE 12: Patient 2: intraoral photographs demonstrating the dentition during and after treatment with dental implants. (a) Frontal view before crowns are inserted on the implants in the left maxillary incisor, canine, and first premolar region. Crowns have been inserted in the left mandibular incisor region. (b) Frontal view after insertion of crowns on the implants. (c) Occlusal view after insertion of crowns on the implants. (d) Lateral view demonstrating the crowns inserted in the implants in the left side of the maxilla.

is decisive for the treatment planning. The present cases demonstrate the importance of early diagnostics and careful registration of anamnestic information. For the orthodontist, it is particularly valuable to focus on idiopathic resorption, as demonstrated in case 2 where the cause behind resorption was wrongfully attributed to the orthodontic treatment.

Registration of such cases may prove helpful for subsequent treatment advice when the number of patients registered has reached a sufficiently quantity.

Acknowledgments

Dorrit Nolting, B.S. degree, is acknowledged for histological tissue preparation. Maria Kvetny, M.A. degree, is acknowledged for linguistic support and paper preparation. The IMK Foundation is acknowledged for financial support.

References

[1] E. Bang, I. Kjær, and L. R. Christensen, "Etiologic aspects and orthodontic treatment of unilateral localized arrested tooth development combined with hearing loss," *American Journal of Orthodontics and Dentofacial Orthopedics*, vol. 108, no. 2, pp. 154–161, 1995.

[2] I. Kjær, "Prenatal traces of aberrant neurofacial growth," *Acta Odontologica Scandinavica*, vol. 56, no. 6, pp. 326–330, 1998.

[3] M. E. Chávez-Lomelí, J. Mansilla Lory, J. A. Pompa, and I. Kjær, "The human mandibular canal arises from three separate canals innervating different tooth groups," *Journal of Dental Research*, vol. 75, no. 8, pp. 1540–1544, 1996.

[4] E. T. Parner, J. M. Heidmann, I. Kjær, M. Væth, and S. Poulsen, "Biological interpretation of the correlation of emergence times of permanent teeth," *Journal of Dental Research*, vol. 81, no. 7, pp. 451–454, 2002.

[5] K. B. Becktor, M. I. Bangstrup, S. Rølling, and I. Kjær, "Unilateral primary or secondary retention of permanent teeth, and dental malformations," *European Journal of Orthodontics*, vol. 24, no. 2, pp. 205–214, 2002.

[6] K. B. Becktor, J. Reibel, B. Vedel, and I. Kjær, "Segmental odontomaxillary dysplasia: clinical, radiological and histological aspects of four cases," *Oral Diseases*, vol. 8, no. 2, pp. 106–110, 2002.

[7] I. Kjær, "Neuro-osteology," *Critical Reviews in Oral Biology and Medicine*, vol. 9, no. 2, pp. 224–244, 1998.

[8] I. Kjær, "Correlated appearance of ossification and nerve tissue in human fetal jaws," *Journal of Craniofacial Genetics and Developmental Biology*, vol. 10, no. 3, pp. 329–336, 1990.

[9] U. H. Lerner, "Effect of kinins, thrombin and neuropeptides on bone," in *Cytokines and Bone Metabolism*, M. Gowan, Ed., pp. 267–298, CRC Press, Boca Raton, Fla, USA, 1992.

[10] I. Thesleff, S. Keränen, and J. Jernvall, "Enamel knots as signaling centers linking tooth morphogenesis and odontoblast differentiation.," *Advances in dental research*, vol. 15, pp. 14–18, 2001.

[11] L. R. Christensen, M. S. Janas, K. Mollgard, and I. Kjær, "An immunocytochemical study of the innervation of developing human fetal teeth using protein gene product 9.5 (PGP 9.5)," *Archives of Oral Biology*, vol. 38, no. 12, pp. 1113–1120, 1993.

[12] P. Kettunen, B. Spencer-Dene, T. Furmanek et al., "Fgfr2b mediated epithelial-mesenchymal interactions coordinate tooth morphogenesis and dental trigeminal axon patterning," *Mechanisms of Development*, vol. 124, no. 11-12, pp. 868–883, 2007.

[13] K. Luukko, I. H. Kvinnsland, and P. Kettunen, "Tissue interactions in the regulation of axon pathfinding during tooth morphogenesis," *Developmental Dynamics*, vol. 234, no. 3, pp. 482–488, 2005.

[14] M. L. B. Bille, B. Thomsen, and I. Kjær, "Apoptosis in the human periodontal membrane evaluated in primary and permanent teeth," *Acta Odontologica Scandinavica*, vol. 69, no. 6, pp. 385–388, 2011.

[15] M. L. B. Bille, B. Thomsen B, and I. Kjær, "The interrelation between epithelial cells of Malassez and vessels studied immunohistochemically in the periodontal membrane of human primary and permanent teeth," *Acta Odontologica Scandinavica*, vol. 70, no. 2, pp. 109–113, 2012.

[16] M. L. B. Bille, B. Thomsen, T. L. Andersen, and I. Kjær, "Immunolocalization of RANK and RANKL along the root surface and in the periodontal membrane of human primary and permanent teeth," *Acta Odontologica Scandinavica*, vol. 70, no. 4, pp. 265–271, 2012.

[17] I. H. Kvinnsland, O. Tadokoro, K. J. Heyeraas, Y. Kozawa, and V. Vandevska-Radunovic, "Neuroendocrine cells in Malassez epithelium and gingiva of the cat," *Acta Odontologica Scandinavica*, vol. 58, no. 3, pp. 107–112, 2000.

[18] T. Yamashiro, K. Fujiyama, T. Fukunaga, Y. Wang, and T. Takano-Yamamoto, "Epithelial rests of Malassez express immunoreactivity of TrkA and its distribution is regulated by sensory nerve innervation," *Journal of Histochemistry and Cytochemistry*, vol. 48, no. 7, pp. 979–984, 2000.

[19] I. B. Bender, "Paget's disease," *Journal of Endodontics*, vol. 29, no. 11, pp. 720–723, 2003.

[20] M. H. Helfrich, "Osteoclast diseases and dental abnormalities," *Archives of Oral Biology*, vol. 50, no. 2, pp. 115–122, 2005.

[21] S. H. Ralston, R. P. Hobson, T. H. Pennington, and M. H. Helfrich, "Does Paget's disease really have a viral aetiology?" *Journal of Bone and Mineral Research*, vol. 12, no. 5, pp. 863–865, 1997.

[22] A. P. Mee, J. A. Dixon, J. A. Hoyland, M. Davies, P. L. Selby, and E. B. Mawer, "Detection of canine distemper virus in 100% of Paget's disease samples by in situ-reverse transcriptase-polymerase chain reaction," *Bone*, vol. 23, no. 2, pp. 171–175, 1998.

[23] A. P. Mee, "Paramyxoviruses and Paget's disease: the affirmative view," *Bone*, vol. 24, no. 5, supplement, 1999.

[24] B. K. Rima, U. Gassen, M. H. Helfrich et al., "The pro and con of measles virus in Paget's disease: con," *Journal of Bone and Mineral Research*, vol. 17, no. 12, pp. 2290–2293, 2002.

[25] S. V. Reddy, "Etiology of Paget's disease and osteoclast abnormalities," *Journal of Cellular Biochemistry*, vol. 93, no. 4, pp. 688–696, 2004.

[26] M. H. Helfrich and L. J. Hocking, "Genetics and aetiology of Pagetic disorders of bone," *Archives of Biochemistry and Biophysics*, vol. 473, no. 2, pp. 172–182, 2008.

[27] I. Kjær, "New diagnostics of the dentition on panoramic radiographs—focusing on the peripheral nervous system as an important aetiological factor behind dental anomalies," *Orthodontic Waves*, vol. 71, no. 1, pp. 1–16, 2012.

[28] W. Beertsen, M. Piscaer, A. J. Van Winkelhoff, and V. Everts, "Generalized cervical root resorption associated with periodontal disease," *Journal of Clinical Periodontology*, vol. 28, no. 11, pp. 1067–1073, 2001.

14

Gorlin-Goltz Syndrome: Case Report of a Rare Hereditary Disorder

Ashutosh Agrawal,[1] Aditi Murari,[1] Sunil Vutukuri,[2] and Arun Singh[3]

[1] *Department of Oral Pathology and Microbiology, Institute of Dental Sciences, Uttar Pradesh, Bareilly 243006, India*
[2] *Department of Oral Pathology and Microbiology, Padmashree Dr. D. Y. Patil Dental College and Hospital, Nerul, Maharashtra, Navi Mumbai 400706, India*
[3] *Department of Oral Pathology and Microbiology, Kothiwal Dental College and Research Centre, Uttar Pradesh, Moradabad 244001, India*

Correspondence should be addressed to Ashutosh Agrawal, drashutoshagrawal@gmail.com

Academic Editors: J. N. dos Santos and M. A. Polack

Introduction. Gorlin-Goltz syndrome is an inherited autosomal dominant disorder with complete penetrance and extreme variable expressivity. *Case Report.* The present paper highlights the importance of diagnostic criteria and histopathology in early and prompt diagnosis which will lead to proper treatment and genetic counseling of the patient. *Discussion.* Gorlin-Goltz syndrome is about multisystem process comprising the triad of basal cell nevi, jaw keratocysts, and skeletal anomalies. A spectrum of other neurological, ophthalmic, endocrine and genital manifestations is known to be variably associated with this triad. Diagnosis of the syndrome is based on major and minor criteria. *Conclusion.* This paper emphasizes the importance of oral and maxillofacial health professionals in the early diagnosis of nevoid basal cell carcinoma syndrome and in a preventive multidisciplinary approach to provide a better prognosis to the patient.

1. Introduction

Gorlin-Goltz syndrome is an infrequent multisystemic disease that is inherited in a dominant autosomal way, which shows a high level of penetrance and variable expressiveness. In 1894, Jarisch and White made the first descriptions of patients with this syndrome, highlighting the presence of multiple basocellular carcinomas. Nevertheless, it was not until 1960 when Gorlin and Goltz established a classical triad that characterises the diagnosis of this syndrome (multiple basocellular epitheliomas, keratocysts in the jaws, and bifid ribs) [1]. A spectrum of other neurological, ophthalmic, endocrine, and genital manifestations are known to be variably associated with this triad. The incidence of this syndrome is estimated to be 1 in 50,000 to 150,000 in general population, but perceived incidence may vary by region. Males and females are equally affected [2].

2. Case Report

A female patient 25 years old come to our department with chief complaint of swelling in bilateral cheeks. The duration of the swelling was 10 month and the growth was slow in nature. She gave a medical history of similar bilateral swellings when she was 12 years old and had underwent surgery for the same. On examination, the swelling was firm and slightly tender on right side. Examination of the face showed frontal bossing, broad nasal bridge, hypertelorism, and mandibular prognathism (Figure 1).

Orthopantomograph revealed multiple multilocular well-defined radiolucencies with sclerotic border located in maxilla and mandible (Figure 2).

The presence of multiple cysts in the jaws and extraoral examination raised a suspicion of Gorlin syndrome and so other relevant investigations were done.

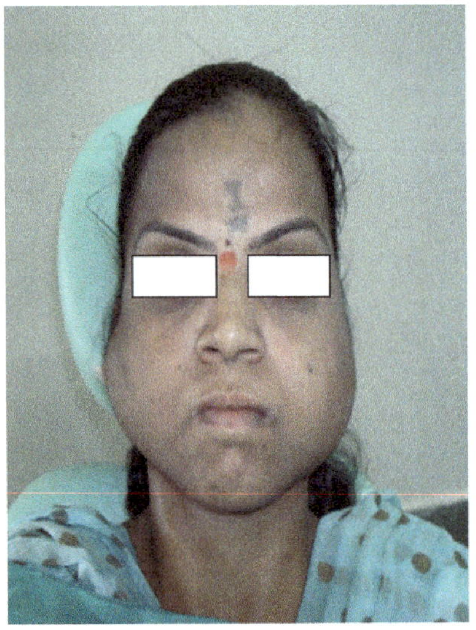

Figure 1: The figure shows frontal bossing, broad nasal bridge, hypertelorism, and mandibular prognathism.

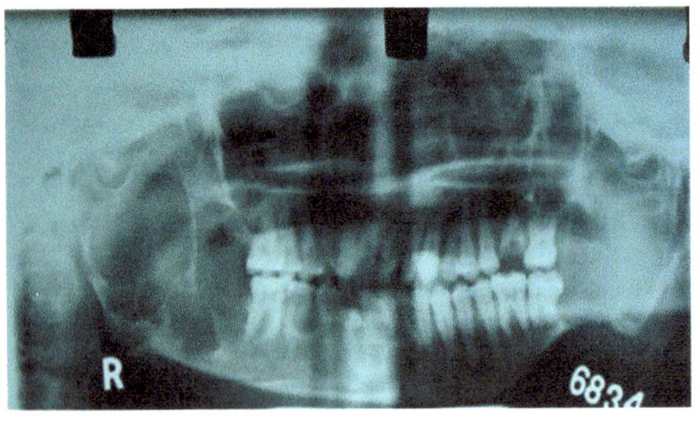

Figure 2: Orthopantomograph showing multiple multilocular well-defined radiolucencies with sclerotic border located in maxilla and mandible.

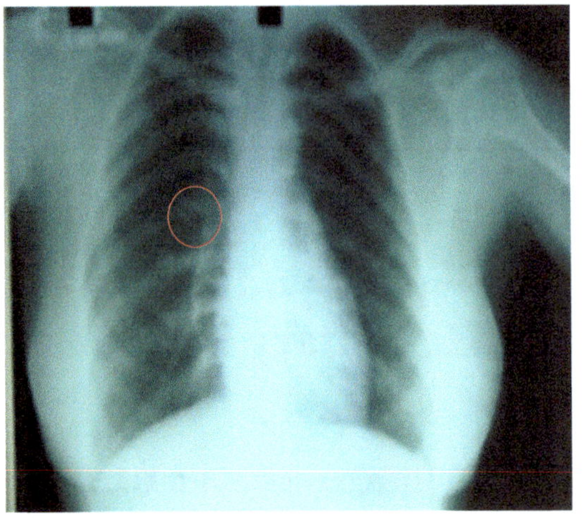

Figure 3: Chest radiograph showing a bifid right fifth rib.

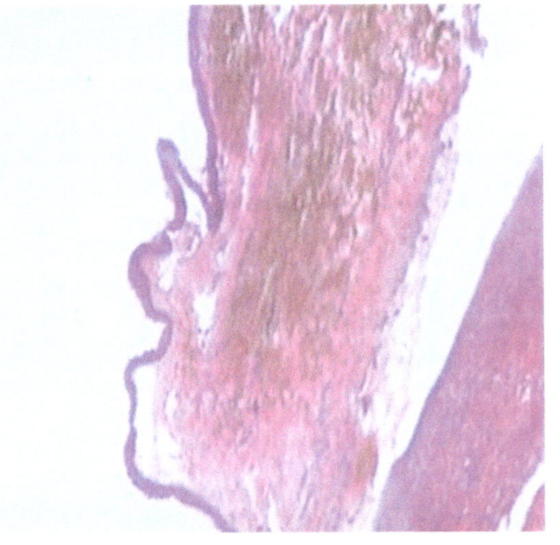

Figure 4: H&E stained section under scanner view shows flat epithelial-connective tissue interface, detachment of epithelial lining due to inflammation and folded epithelial lining.

Chest radiograph showed a bifid fifth rib (Figure 3). The reports of the patient also revealed the presence of nabothian cyst in cervix.

An incisional biopsy of the swelling in left and right side of mandible was advised. Histopathological examination of specimen revealed parakeratinised stratified squamous epithelium with palisading pattern of columnar cells along with keratin flakes with few giant cells and inflammatory cells (found in the specimen of the left side of the mandible) suggestive of odontogenic keratocyst on the right side and an odontogenic keratocyst with secondary infection on the left side (Figures 4 and 5). Surgical enucleation of the cysts was performed in the department of oral surgery. Any skin lesions like basal cell nevus or keratosis were not seen in the patient. Thorough clinical and radiological examination were done for the parents of the patient but they showed no signs of Gorlin-Goltz syndrome.

Based on the clinical, radiographic, and histologic findings, and referring to the diagnostic criteria for nevoid BCC syndrome established by Evans et al. [4], and modified by Kimonos et al. in 1997 [5], the patient was diagnosed as having Gorlin-Goltz syndrome.

3. Discussion

The Gorlin-Goltz syndrome is an autosomal dominant inherited syndrome manifested by multiple defects involving the skin, nervous system, eyes, endocrine system, and bones. It is also known as basal cell nevus syndrome, multiple basal cell carcinoma syndrome, Gorlin syndrome, or hereditary cutaneomandibular polyonocosis, multiple nevoid basal cell epithelioma-jaw cysts, or bifid rib syndrome [3]. The diagnostic criteria for nevoid BCC was established by Evans et al. [4], and modified by Kimonis et al. in 1973 [5, 6]. According to them diagnosis of Gorlin-Goltz syndrome can be established when two major or one major and two minor are present which are described below.

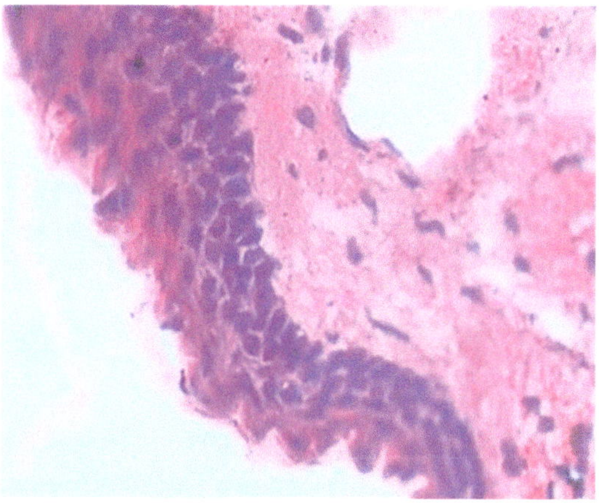

FIGURE 5: H&E stained section under 40X magnification shows 6–8 layers thick epithelial lining which is parakeratinized and corrugated.

Major Criteria are as follows:

(1) more than 2 BCCs or one under age of 20 year,
(2) odontogenic keratocyst,
(3) three or more palmar pits,
(4) bilamellar calcification of falx cerebri,
(5) bifid, fused, or splayed ribs,
(6) first-degree relative with NBCCS.

Minor Criteria are as follows:

(1) macrocephaly adjusted for height,
(2) fontal bossing, cleft lip/palate, and hypertelorism,
(3) sprengel deformity, pectus, and syndactyly of digits,
(4) bridging of sella turcica, hemivertebrae, and flame-shaped radiolucencies,
(5) ovarian fibroma,
(6) medulloblastoma [6, 7].

Odontogenic Keratocysts. Woolgar et al. [8] and Dominiguez et al. [9] found significant differences between syndrome keratocysts and single keratocysts. Syndrome keratocysts were found to have a markedly increased number of satellite cysts, solid islands of epithelial proliferation, odontogenic rests within the capsule, and mitotic figures in the epithelial lining of the main cavity.

There are immunochemical differences between syndromal and solitary keratocysts. Woolgar et al. noted that syndrome keratocysts tend to occur at a much earlier age than single keratocysts [7, 8].

Less than 10% of patients with multiple OKCs have other manifestations of this syndrome; however, it has been suggested that multiple OKCs alone may be the confirmatory of the syndrome. Two types of keratocysts have been distinguished based on differences in the histology and behavior: the more common parakeratotic odontogenic keratocyst (P-OKC) and the less common orthokeratotic odontogenic keratocyst (O-OKC). First, the P-OKC has a more aggressive growth potential and a higher recurrence rate than the O-OKC and other odontogenic cysts. Second, in a minority of patients (particularly, young patients with multiple cysts), the P-OKC is a part of the Jaw cyst-Basal cell nevus-Bifid rib syndrome. Although benign, the recurrence rate of P-OKC is high, ranging from 12% to 62.5% [10].

For apparently isolated cases, detailed examination and X-ray investigation of the relatives should be undertaken before concluding. It is particularly helpful to follow a specific clinical protocol in the examination of these subjects [11] (Table 1).

TABLE 1: Diagnostic protocols in NBCCS.

Family history
Past medical and dental history
Clinical examinations
Oral
Skin
Central nervous system
Head circumference
Interpupillar distance
Eyes
Genitourinary system
Cardiovascular system
Respiratory system
Skeletal system
Genetic testing
X-ray
Chest
A.P. and lateral skull
Panoramic radiograph
Cervical and thoracic spine
Hands (for pseudocysts)
Pelvic (female)

Ovarian ultrasound (female) for ovarian fibroma.
Echocardiogram (children) for cardiac fibroma.
Abbreviations: NBCCS: Nevoid Basal Cell Carcinoma Syndrome.

4. Conclusion

To summarize, it can be said that Gorlin-Goltz syndrome is a dominant autosomal genetic process, which is of particular interest to the oral and maxillofacial health experts. The importance of recognition of this syndrome is because of its malignant potential. In order to be able to establish early diagnosis of NBCCS, specialists should carry out clinical and imaging examinations in early ages of life. The fact that its transmission is autosomal dominant with good penetrance implies the need of genetic counseling.

Conflict of Interests

Authors declare no conflict of interests.

Authors' Contributions

Ashutosh Agrawal was responsiple for conception and design, analysis and interpretation of data, critical revision of the paper, and final approval of the version to be published. Aditi Murari was responsiple for conception and design, drafting the paper, and final approval of the version to be published Sunil Vutukuri was responsiple for analysis and interpretation of data, critical revision of the paper, and final approval of the version to be published Arun Singh. was responsiple for acquisition of data, critical revision of the paper, and Final approval of the version to be published.

References

[1] A. O. G. de Amezaga, O. G. Arregui, S. Z. Nuño, A. A. Sagredo, and J. M. A. Urizar, "Gorlin-Goltz syndrome: clinicopathologic aspects," *Medicina Oral, Patologia Oral y Cirugia Bucal*, vol. 13, no. 6, pp. E338–E343, 2008.

[2] K. Patil, V. G. Mahima, and B. Gupta, "Gorlin syndrome: a case report," *Journal of Indian Society of Pedodontics and Preventive Dentistry*, vol. 23, no. 4, pp. 198–203, 2005.

[3] D. S. Jawa, K. Sircar, R. Somani, N. Grover, S. Jaidka, and S. Singh, "Gorlin-Goltz syndrome," *Journal of Oral and Maxillofacial Pathology*, vol. 13, no. 2, pp. 89–92, 2009.

[4] D. G. R. Evans, E. J. Ladusans, S. Rimmer, L. D. Burnell, N. Thakker, and P. A. Farndon, "Complications of the naevoid basal cell carcinoma syndrome: results of a population based study," *Journal of Medical Genetics*, vol. 30, no. 6, pp. 460–464, 1993.

[5] V. E. Kimonis, A. M. Goldstein, B. Pastakia et al., "Clinical manifestations in 105 persons With nevoid basal cell carcinoma syndrome," *American Journal of Medical Genetics*, vol. 69, pp. 299–308, 1997.

[6] M. Kohli, M. Kohli, N. Sharma, S. R. Siddiqui, and S. P. S. Tulsi, "Gorlin-Goltz syndrome," *National Journal of Maxillofacial Surgery*, vol. 1, no. 1, pp. 50–52, 2010.

[7] R. J. Gorlin, M. M. Cohen Jr., and R. C. M. Hennkem, *Syndromes of Head and Neck*, Chapter12, 4th edition, 2001.

[8] J. A. Woolgar, J. W. Rippin, and R. M. Browne, "A comparative histological study of odontogenic keratocysts in basal cell naevus syndrome and control patients.," *Journal of Oral Pathology & Medicine*, vol. 16, no. 2, pp. 75–80, 1987.

[9] F. V. Dominguez and A. Keszler, "Comparative study of keratocysts, associated and non-associated with nevoid basal cell carcinoma syndrome.," *Journal of Oral Pathology & Medicine*, vol. 17, no. 1, pp. 39–42, 1988.

[10] S. Rai and K. Gauba, "Jaw cyst-Basal cell nevus-Bifid rib syndrome: a case report," *Journal of Indian Society of Pedodontics and Preventive Dentistry*, vol. 25, no. 3, pp. 137–139, 2007.

[11] L. Lo Muzio, "Nevoid basal cell carcinoma syndrome (Gorlin syndrome)," *Orphanet Journal of Rare Diseases*, vol. 3, no. 1, article 32, 2008.

15

Unusual Case of Inflammatory Myofibroblastic Tumor in Maxilla

Jaana Rautava,[1,2] Tero Soukka,[3] Esko Peltonen,[1] Petri Nurmenniemi,[3] Markku Kallajoki,[4] and Stina Syrjänen[1,4]

[1] *Department of Oral Pathology and Oral Radiology, Institute of Dentistry, University of Turku, Lemminkäisenkatu 2, 20520 Turku, Finland*

[2] *Cell Biology Program, Research Institute, Hospital for Sick Children, University of Toronto, Room 7142, 555 University Avenue, Toronto, ON, Canada M5G 1X8*

[3] *Department of Oral and Maxillofacial Surgery, Institute of Dentistry, University of Turku, Lemminkäisenkatu 2, 20520 Turku, Finland*

[4] *Department of Pathology, University of Turku, Kiinanmyllynkatu 4-8, 20520 Turku, Finland*

Correspondence should be addressed to Jaana Rautava; jaana.rautava@utu.fi

Academic Editors: D. W. Boston, L. N. De Souza, A. Markopoulos, and A. Milosevic

Inflammatory myofibroblastic tumor (IMT) is a rare lesion found mostly in children and young adults and originates from the lung, abdominopelvic region, and retroperitoneum. Clinical manifestations of IMT or imaging are nonspecific and diagnosis is based on histopathological and immunohistochemical findings. Minority of all IMTs will metastasize. IMT in the oral cavity is an extreme rarity and this is a first case report of IMT in maxilla causing delayed tooth eruption and multiple cervical root resorption with an 11-year-old child. The IMT reported here was positive for smooth muscle actin, vimentin, and anaplastic lymphoma kinase (ALK1) with immunohistochemistry. Only three IMTs of the jaws have been reported so far and none of them had delayed root eruption and tooth resorption. This unusual case of IMT in a child was also ALK1- positive supporting neoplastic origin of her tumor. The case presented here underscores the importance of histopathological examination of the tissue found in any root resorption especially in the case of multiple resorptions.

1. Introduction

Inflammatory myofibroblastic tumor (IMT, also known as inflammatory pseudotumor, plasma cell granuloma, inflammatory fibrosarcoma, fibrohistiocytoma, etc.) is composed of myofibroblastic cells with inflammatory infiltrate [1, 2]. It is a rare lesion which has a predilection for children and young adults. Most reported cases have been from the lung, abdominopelvic region, and retroperitoneum. Trauma and viral infections such as herpes simplex virus type 8 (HSV-8) and Epstein-Barr virus (EBV), as well as autoimmune reactions, have been suggested as etiological factors. Still, exact etiology remains elusive but more recently neoplastic origin has been suggested as the most likely candidate [3]. IMT may mimic a malignant process. A recent review of the literature reported 22 cases of oral IMT and most of them were observed on buccal mucosa and only three occurred in the jawbones [4]. Since then two more cases of oral IMTs have been reported, one in the tongue and one as a soft tissue mass of the mandibular region [5, 6].

2. Case Report

An 11-year-old previously healthy girl with no medications or allergies had complicated eruption of the left maxillary canine tooth 23 and first premolar 24. A panoramic tomography showed a large resorption of the mesial side of the root of 24 (Figure 1(a)). There was no previous history of trauma to the area. Clinically, marginal gingivitis around the teeth 22–24 was found, both labially and buccally, in addition to external resorption of 24. Six-to-eight millimeter deep gingival pockets were detected adjacent to the teeth 23 and 24. Patient complained of soreness of the area. According to an orthodontic

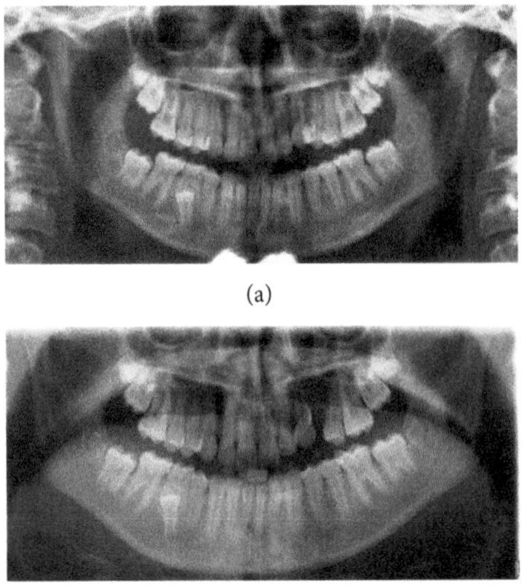

(a)

(b)

FIGURE 1: (a) The first panoramic image shows an osteolytic area on the marginal bone border between 22 and 24. There is a deep vertical bone lesion on the mesial side of 24. It is challenging to see resorption on the coronal part of the roots. (b) Panoramic image three months after the extraction of 24. The healing of the extraction region is in progress. In the region 22-23, the osteolytic area has remained the same compared to the earlier image.

specialist, there was a lack of space and tooth 24 was extracted and granulation tissue was enucleated. At this point, no tissue was obtained for histopathological diagnosis. Twelve weeks later, a significant bone defect was observed and the position of 23 was still in infraocclusion and the patient was referred to the Department of Oral and Maxillofacial Surgery, Turku University Hospital (TUH), Turku, Finland.

At TUH, the bone defect was confirmed. No swelling, deep gingival pockets, or mobility of the teeth in this region were detected on the clinical examination. The adjacent teeth were vital, but there was a slight decrease in vitality related to the second premolar and first molar. The gingiva in the region showed bluish colouring.

Panoramic and intraoral X-rays revealed external resorption in the roots of left maxillary lateral incisor and canine teeth. An osteolytic area in the same region (teeth 22-23) was detected consistently with an image obtained three months earlier (Figure 1(b)). Furthermore, cone beam tomography revealed a cystic, osteolytic area in the left palatal side of the roots from lateral incisor to first premolar in the left side (Figure 2). The palatal cortex was perforated.

The clinical and radiographic pictures were nonspecific. Resorption of multiple teeth and the perforation of palatal cortex suggested locally aggressive lesions. The differential diagnoses included aggressively behaving odontogenic tumors, nodular fasciitis, and malignant lesion. Ameloblastoma is the most common aggressive benign odontogenic tumor but it is rare in children. The resorption of adjacent teeth is common with ameloblastoma but it often presents as a swelling of jaw. Furthermore, the image in panoramic tomography was not lobulated as often found with ameloblastomas. Nodular fasciitis is a benign, reactive process with rapid growth that mimics malignant soft tissue sarcomas. However, also nodular fasciitis is usually diagnosed in adults. Nodular fasciitis is often superficially located at soft tissue mass and is associated with pain.

The likely possible malignancies under consideration were malignant soft tissue sarcomas, malignant bone tumors, and Burkitt's lymphoma. Of the malignant soft tissue sarcomas, rhabdomyosarcoma (especially the embryonic variant) is a relatively common malignant soft tissue tumor in children. Fibrosarcoma is a malignant mesenchymal tumor of fibroblasts that may arise in the jaws, especially the mandible. It usually affects young adults but has been reported also in children. Malignant bone tumors constitute the 6th most common group of malignant neoplasms in children, with osteosarcoma being the most common pediatric bone tumor and Ewing's sarcoma family of tumors being the second. Both may result in an osteolytic image of the jaws in radiographs. Burkitt's lymphoma is related to EBV. It typically affects children and maxilla and may cause tooth displacement or loss, gingival expansion, and pain.

The lesion was treated by enucleation and curettage and the beyond-repair damaged teeth with resorption were extracted and sent for histopathologic examination to the Department of Oral Pathology and Oral Radiology, Institute of Dentistry, University of Turku, Turku, Finland.

Histopathological investigation revealed a compact cellular spindle cell proliferation with collagenous stroma with storiform architecture (Figure 3(a)). The proliferation started directly under the oral mucosal epithelium continuing throughout the tissue samples. The uniform spindle cells contained ovoid nuclei with rather pale eosinophilic cytoplasm. Only mild nuclear pleomorphism was seen. Mitotic activity was low as detected with Ki-67 level (Figure 3(d)). Inflammatory component was minor with single or small groups of lymphocytes scattered around the spindle cell proliferation. With immunohistochemistry (IHC), the tumor tissue was positive for smooth muscle actin (SMA), vimentin, and anaplastic lymphoma kinase (ALK) (Figures 3(b)-3(c)). Calponin, myoglobin, and HHF35 antibodies showed moderate staining in myofibroblasts. Immunostaining of CD34 showed intense vascularisation of the whole tumor. There was no immunoreactivity for S-100, pancytokeratin, desmin, or Myf4. With PCR using the DNA extracted from the paraffin blocks, no HSV-8 or EBV was detected. The final diagnosis was inflammatory myofibroblastic tumor (IMT).

At the department of pediatric oncology, the patient was clinically examined and no symptoms or clinical signs of disease were detected locally or distantly. Furthermore, the complete blood count with C-reactive protein (CRP) and erythrocyte sedimentation rate were within normal limits. Whole body magnetic resonance imaging (MRI) or bone scintigraphy (^{99m}TcHDP) did not reveal signs of occult disease. After three years of followup, there was no recurrence.

3. Discussion

To our knowledge, only three intrabony IMTs of the oral cavity have been reported but none of them had delayed tooth

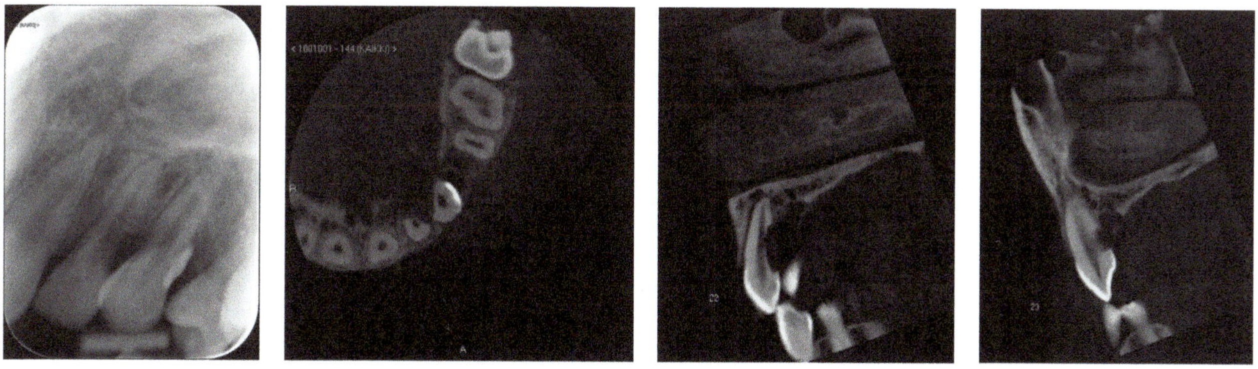

(a) (b) (c) (d)

Figure 2: (a) The root resorption is visible in the intraoral X-ray of 22-23. (b) CBCT axial slice above the marginal bone line. A 6 × 10 mm bone destruction, which is sharply lined, is visible in the region 22-23 on the palatinal side. The roots of the teeth 22-23 have resorption on the palatinal sides. (c) CBCT sagittal slice presenting the root of 22. On palatinal side of the root, there is a 2 × 4 mm deep resorption defect. Lesion on palatinal bone structure can also be seen. (d) CBCT sagittal slice of 23.

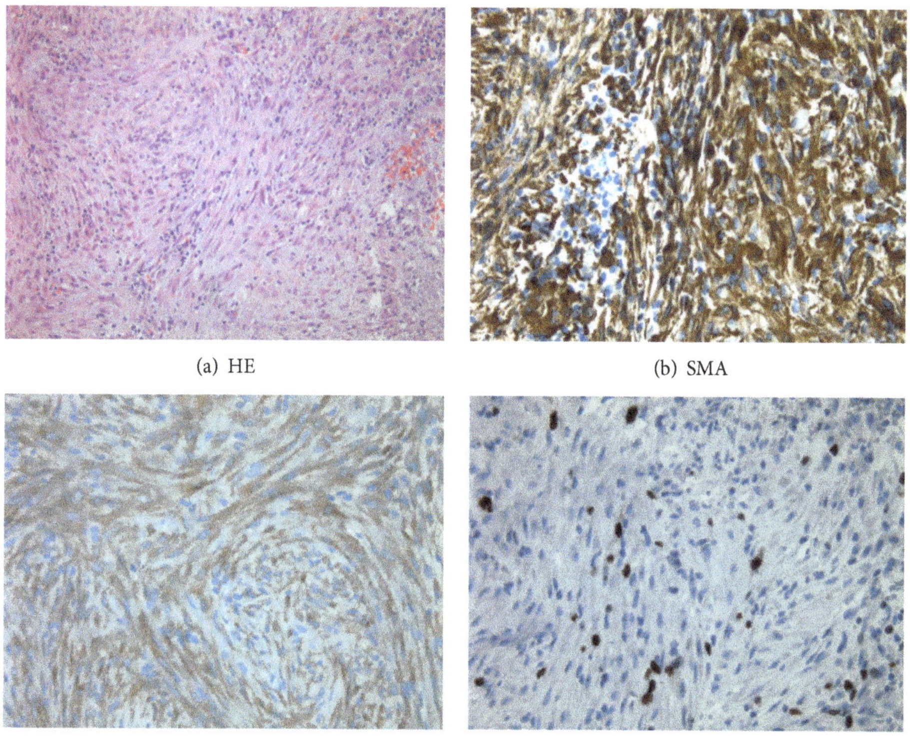

(a) HE (b) SMA

(c) ALK-1 (d) Ki-67

Figure 3: (a) Hematoxylin-eosin staining showed dense aggregates of spindle cells in storiform architecture with scattered lymphocytes. (b) Immunohistochemical staining is strongly positive with smooth muscle actin and (c) with ALK (d) while Ki-67 positivity was low.

eruption and root resoption [3]. The ALK (chromosome band 2p23) gene has been implicated in the pathogenesis of IMT supporting neoplastic origin of tumor [3]. Approximately 50% of all IMTs have been associated with ALK positivity. Most of the previous oral IMT cases have been reported to be ALK negative [4]. Indeed, a question has been raised whether ALK-positive IMTs are a distinct clinicopathologic entity with neoplastic origin with more aggressive behavior and even potential for malignancy. The present case was ALK positive, but within the follow-up time of three years, the tumor has not shown any signs of recurrence.

IMT can present with variable clinical manifestations. Therefore, clinical manifestations of IMT or radiographic images have poor specificity to make a diagnosis, as was shown also with the present case. Diagnosis of IMT is based on histopathological and immunohistochemical findings according to The World Health Organisation (WHO) classification of soft tissue tumors [2]. Histomorphology of IMT has a high degree of overlap with other spindle cell lesions. Differential diagnosis of malignancies such as fibrosarcoma or spindle cell carcinoma is difficult without any immunohistochemistry. Also gingival or periodontal inflammation might easily mask the typical features of the lesion. Collectively, most extrapulmonary IMTs display immunohistochemical reactivity for vimentin, SMA, muscle specific actin, and desmin, but not for S-100 [2].

IMT is classified as a benign lesion but local aggressiveness may be associated with chromosomal aberrations [3]. Aggressive behavior has been associated with high degree of cellular atypia with increased mitotic figures, multinodularity, and presence of ganglion-like cells [7]. In addition, IMTs with ALK positivity, elevated Ki-67 proliferative index (up to 10%), DNA aneuploidy, or oncogenic protein overexpression (p53, bcl-2) exhibit increased risk for recurrence [7]. Among nonoral IMTs, recurrence is seen in 19%–25% of all patients with average of 6 months' time period and in 15% of pediatric patients only. Metastasis is rare and is detected in less than 5% of cases. Moreover, there is a small possibility of malignant transformation to sarcoma. According to the recent literature, oral IMTs seem to run a more favorable clinical course with no likelihood of recurrence or malignant transformation [4].

For oral IMTs which are most likely to display local aggressiveness but not metastasize, management with complete surgical resection and 10-year postoperative reassessment has been suggested [8]. With nonoral extrapulmonary IMTs, where aggressive behavior is more likely to occur, recent reports have found steroid treatments combined with surgery effective at least for pediatric cases. Currently, on-going research attempts to find a molecular therapy against diseases with ALK-driven pathways [9].

The cause of external cervical root resorption is poorly understood. Etiological factors from dental treatment (or trauma) to bruxism and developmental defects have been suggested. It is well established that certain neoplasms or cysts can cause tooth resorption. Multiple idiopathic cervical root resorptions are most frequently seen in young females. In the present case, we suggest that the resorptions were most likely caused by the tumor. Interestingly, a recent publication reported an IMT of a maxillary sinus which caused pulp necrosis of maxillary teeth [10].

4. Conclusion

Maxillary IMTs are extremely rare. Furthermore, oral IMTs with ALK positivity present the minority of the reported cases. The case presented here underscores the importance of histopathological examination of the tissue found in any root resorption cavities especially in the cases with multiple resorptions.

References

[1] L. Barnes, J. W. Eveson, P. Reichart, D. Sidransky, and World Health Organization Classification of Tumours, Eds., *Pathology and Genetics of Head and Neck Tumours*, IARC Press, Lyon, France, 2005.

[2] C. M. Coffin and J. A. Fletcher, "Inflammatory myofibroblastic tumour," in *Pathology and Genetics of Tumours of Soft Tissue and Bone*, C. D. M. Fletcher, K. K. Unni, F. Mertens, and World Health Organization Classification of Tumors, Eds., pp. 91–93, IARC Press, Lyon, France, 2002.

[3] C. M. Coffin, A. Patel, S. Perkins, K. S. J. Elenitoba-Johnson, E. Perlman, and C. A. Griffin, "ALK1 and p80 expression and chromosomal rearrangements involving 2p23 in inflammatory myofibroblastic tumor," *Modern Pathology*, vol. 14, no. 6, pp. 569–576, 2001.

[4] N. O. Binmadi, H. Packman, J. C. Papadimitriou, and M. Scheper, "Oral inflammatory myofibroblastic tumor: case report and review of literature," *Open Dentistry Journal*, vol. 5, pp. 66–70, 2011.

[5] A. Date, K. Yamagata, K. Onizawa et al., "Inflammatory pseudotumor: report of a case in the mandible," *Oral and Maxillofacial Surgery*, vol. 16, no. 1, pp. 65–68, 2012.

[6] S. V. Lourenco, P. Boggio, and M. M. S. Nico, "Inflammatory myofibroblastic tumor of the tongue: report of an unusual case in a teenage patient," *Dermatology Online Journal*, vol. 18, no. 5, article 6, 2012.

[7] J. W. Hussong, M. Brown, S. L. Perkins, L. P. Dehner, and C. M. Coffin, "Comparison of DNA ploidy, histologic, and immunohistochemical findings with clinical outcome in inflammatory myofibroblastic tumors," *Modern Pathology*, vol. 12, no. 3, pp. 279–286, 1999.

[8] L. Ma, K. Wang, W. K. Liu, and Y. K. Zhang, "Is radical surgery necessary to head and neck inflammatory myofibroblastic tumor (IMT) in children?" *Child's Nervous System*, vol. 25, no. 3, pp. 285–291, 2009.

[9] Y. P. Mossé, A. Wood, and J. M. Maris, "Inhibition of ALK signaling for cancer therapy," *Clinical Cancer Research*, vol. 15, no. 18, pp. 5609–5614, 2009.

[10] S. Y. Kim and S. E. Yang, "Inflammatory myofibroblastic tumor of the maxillary sinus related with pulp necrosis of maxillary teeth: case report," *Oral Surgery, Oral Medicine, Oral Pathology, Oral Radiology and Endodontology*, vol. 112, no. 5, pp. 684–687, 2011.

16

Rubinstein-Taybi Syndrome: A Case Report

A. P. Münevveroglu and B. B. Akgöl

Department of Pedodontics, Faculty of Dentistry, Istanbul Medipol University, Fatih, 34093 Istanbul, Turkey

Correspondence should be addressed to A. P. Münevveroglu, apatir@medipol.edu.tr

Academic Editors: A. Epivatianos and A. L. S. Guimaraes

Rubinstein-Taybi syndrome or Broad Thumb-Hallux syndrome is a genetic disorder characterized by facial dysmorphism, growth retardation, and mental deficiency. A seven-year-old girl had come to the Department of Pedodontics, Istanbul Medipol University, Faculty of Dentistry, Turkey, with a complaint of caries and bleeding of gingivae. The patient was mentally retarded. Extraoral features revealed distinctive facial appearance with a broad fore head, hypertelorism, broad nasal bridge, and beaked nose. Intraoral features observed were talons cusps in the upper lateral incisors, carious teeth, and plaque accumulation. Since the patient was mentally retarded, the dental treatment was done under GA. The treatment plan and dental management of this patient are discussed in this case report.

1. Introduction

Rubinstein-Taybi Syndrome (RTS:OMIM 180849), or Broad Thumb-Hallux syndrome, was initially described by Michail et al. in 1957 [1]. In 1963, Rubenstein and Taybi reported on seven cases of this syndrome [2], which included a group of congenital anomalies consisting of short, broad thumbs and great toes, psychomotor retardation, highly arched palates, and histories of recurrent respiratory infections and particular facial abnormalities [3–5]. It is caused by either a microdeletion at 16p13.3 or mutations in the CREB-binding protein (CREBBP or CBP) or EP300 gene (at 22q13) [4–7].

The incidence of the syndrome has been estimated to be 1 in every 300,000 newborns [7]. There is an equal male and female incidence [8–10].

The main distinctive features most commonly linked to this syndrome are downward sloping palpebral fissures, broad thumbs and halluces, growth retardation and psychomotor developmental delay, typical facial dysmorphism, hypertelorism, a prominent forehead, and mental disability [9–11].

One intriguing phenomenon is the fact that RTS patients are prone to develop tumours. These tumours show a pattern of neural and developmental origin, and neuroblastoma, medullablastoma, oligodendroglioma, meningioma, seminoma, odontoma, choristoma, and polimatrixtomas were the reported tumours in RTS patients [3, 12, 13].

Congenital anomalies of cardiovascular system are also described such as ventricular septal defect, patent ductus arteriosus, coarctation and stenosis of the aorta, and pulmonic stenosis [3, 14, 15].

Oral manifestations of this syndrome include limited mouth opening, a pouting lower lip, retro/micrognathia, a high arched and narrow palate, cleft uvula and palate, and rarely a cleft upper lip. Dental abnormalities occur in 67% of individuals with RTS and can include hypodontia, maintenance of deciduous teeth, talon cusps, and enamel hypoplasia. An increased rate of caries and periodontal disease has been reported in these patients. However periodontal disease has not always been associated with this syndrome [7, 11, 16]. Characteristics of RTS are described in Table 1.

Dental treatment is generally complicated due to difficulties in managing the patient's behavior. In most patients with this syndrome, it is necessary to carry out the dental treatment under sedation or general anesthesia. It is important to know that these patients might have upper respiratory obstruction during sleeping or sedation because of the anatomical characteristics of their maxillofacial region [16–18].

Table 1: Characteristics of RTS.

Orthopedic	Broad thumbs, first toes, short stature, vertebral abnormalities
Eye	Strabismus, refractory errors, ptosis, coloboma, ptosis, cataracts, nystagmus
Cardiac	Congenital heart defects
Dental	Crowding teeth, malocclusion, multiple caries, hypodontia, hyperdontia, talon cusps
Tumors	Meningioma, neuroblastoma, medullablastoma, oligodendroglioma, seminoma
Skin	Keloids
Sleep apnea	Obstructive sleep apnea

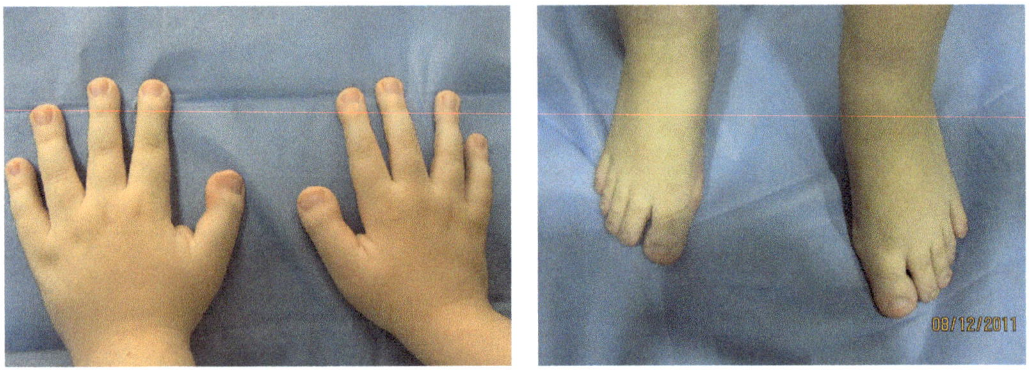

(a) (b)

Figure 1: Hands and feet in RTS. Broad thumbs, broad terminal phalanges were seen.

2. Case Report

A 7-year-old girl accompanied by parents reported to the faculty of Dentistry, Department of Pedodontics, Medipol University, Turkey, with a complaint of caries and bleeding of gingiva. She is the second child of a remote consanguineous couple. Her old sister had no signs of dental anomalies. The patient was born at term, weighing 2 kg 850 g.

The following clinical extraoral findings were observed: short stature with broad thumbs, mental retardation, down slant of the palpebral fissures, strabismus and simple ear (Figures 1(a), 1(b)). The nose has a beaked appearance, broad fleshy bridge, deviated septum, and short low columella (Figure 2) and she had cardiac abnormalities.

Intra-oral findings were high-arched and cleft palate, a small mouth and malocclusion (Figures 3(a) and 3(b)). Talon cusps were present on maxillary central and lateral incisors (Figure 4). The patient also had carious lesions (Figures 3(a), 3(b), 4, 5(a), 5(b)). Upper and lower molar teeth had deep dentinal carious lesions (no. 16, no. 26, no. 36, no. 46, no. 75, no. 85). Heavy calculus and plaque deposition could be noted on all teeth. The marginal gingiva was severely swollen and probing resulted in profuse gingival bleeding.

After the complete clinical examination and investigation, the following dental treatment plan was derived.

(1) Oral prophylaxis and topical fluoride application.

(2) Cavity preparation and composite resin restoration (no. 16, no. 26, no. 36, no. 46, no. 75, no. 85).

(3) Extraction of no. 53, no. 64.

(4) Recall follow-up sessions for every 3 months.

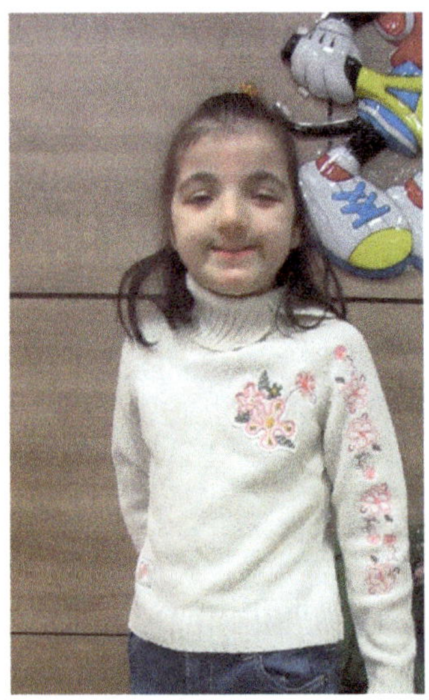

Figure 2: Facial characteristics include slanting palpebral fissures and beaked nose with nasal septum.

Due to difficulties in the patient's behavior and her inability to cooperate during dental treatment because of her mental disability, the treatment was performed under general anesthesia.

Detailed oral hygiene instructions were given to her mother who provided routine care for the patient and the patient recalled follow-up sessions every 3 months. However, because of her incoordination about brushing teeth; evidence

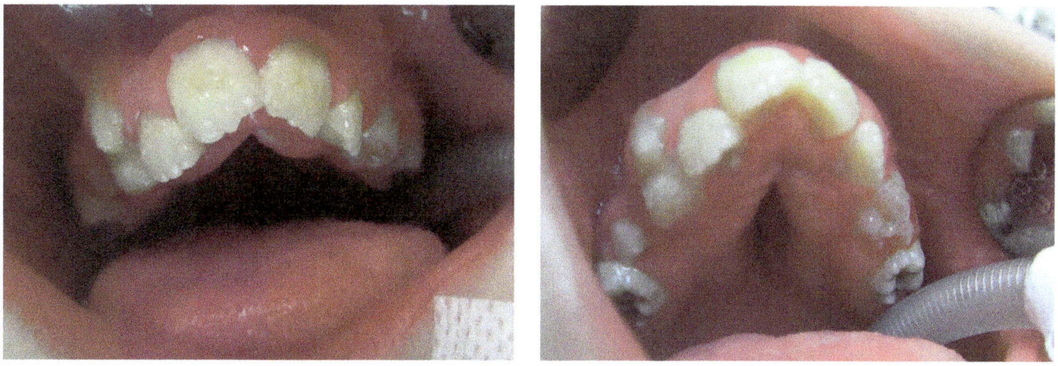

(a) (b)

FIGURE 3: (a) Intraoral findings were a small mouth and malocclusion. (b) In intra-oral findings, high-arched and cleft palate was seen. And upper molar teeth had deep dentinal carious lesions.

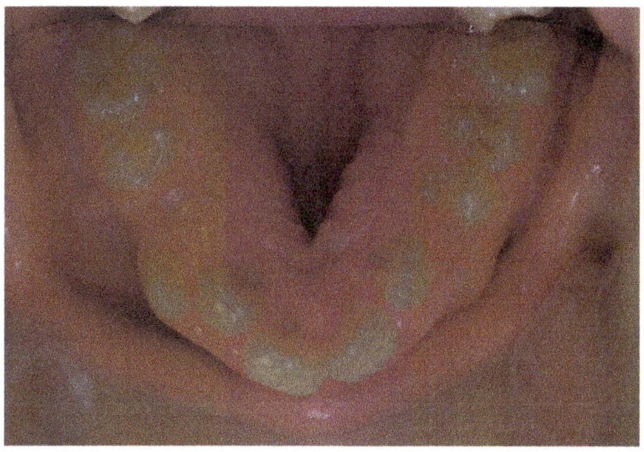

FIGURE 4: Talon cusps were present on maxillary central and lateral incisors.

of unimproved dental hygiene was observed and instead of this no new caries were found. Because of plaque deposition on all teeth, periodontal treatment consisted of scaling, and oral prophylaxis and topical fluoride application were performed under sedation after 6 months later.

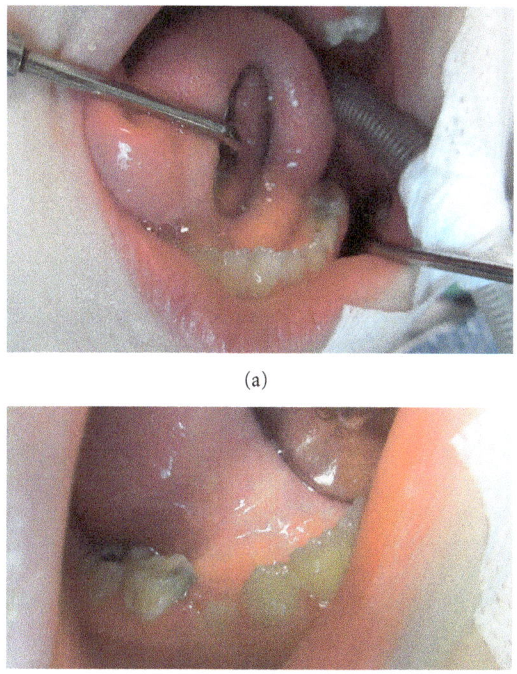

(b)

FIGURE 5: Lower molar teeth had deep dentinal carious lesions.

3. Discussion

The 7-year-old girl described in this paper was diagnosed with RTS associated with a microdeletion at 16p 13.3 chromosome. She had cardiac abnormalities, which are frequently found in 24–38% cases [7, 16, 19].

RTS is a rare multiple congenital anomaly syndrome [20]. Intraoral findings of the patient with RTS were reduced oral opening, a narrow palate, malocclusion, gingivitis, and caries. It was reported that patients with RTS have an increased rate of caries (15% to 36%) because of their poor oral hygiene, which was similar to our patient [7, 12, 21]. Malposition and crowded teeth are present in 62% of patients [7, 22]. In this patient, upper and lower molar teeth had deep dentinal carious lesions (no. 16, no. 26, no. 36, no. 46, no. 75, no. 85). Heavy calculus and plaque deposition could be noted on all teeth. The marginal gingiva was severely swollen and probing resulted in profuse gingival bleeding, and malposition was one of, important problems in our patient.

In most patients with this syndrome, it is necessary to carry out the dental treatment under sedation or general anesthesia. It is important to know that these patients might have upper respiratory obstruction during sleeping or sedation because of the anatomical characteristics of their maxillofacial region [16–18]. The treatment of the patient was performed under general anesthesia by anesthesiologist.

Freitas et al. [19] reported the periodontal and immunological status of a 14-year-old female patient with RTS and possible association between syndrome and periodontal disease was reported in the paper. In this paper, heavy calculus and plaque deposition could be noted on all teeth. The marginal gingiva was severely swollen and probing resulted in profuse gingival bleeding.

Prospects for future good oral and dental status in this patient are questionable because of her extreme lack of cooperation. For this reason, she needs a longer followup.

References

[1] J. Michail, J. Matsoukas, and S. Theodorou, "Arched, clubbed thumb in strong abduction-extension & other concomitant symptoms.," *Revue de Chirurgie Orthopédique et Réparatrice de l'Appareil Moteur*, vol. 43, no. 2, pp. 142–146, 1957.

[2] J. H. Rubenstein and H. Taybi, "Broad thumbs and toes and facial abnormalities. A possible mental retardation syndrome," *American Journal of Diseases of Children*, vol. 105, pp. 588–608, 1963.

[3] J. H. Roelfsema and D. J. M. Peters, "Rubinstein-Taybi syndrome: clinical and molecular overview," *Expert Reviews in Molecular Medicine*, vol. 9, no. 23, pp. 1–16, 2007.

[4] S. H. Kim, B. C. Lim, J. H. Chae, K. J. Kim, and Y. S. Hwang, "A case of Rubinstein-Taybi syndrome with a CREB-binding protein gene mutation," *Korean Journal of Pediatrics*, vol. 53, no. 6, pp. 718–721, 2010.

[5] A. Bloch-Zupan, J. Stachtou, D. Emmanouil, B. Arveiler, D. Griffiths, and D. Lacombe, "Oro-dental features as useful diagnostic tool in Rubinstein-Taybi syndrome," *American Journal of Medical Genetics A*, vol. 143, no. 6, pp. 570–573, 2007.

[6] I. Coupry, C. Roudaut, M. Stef et al., "Molecular analysis of the CBP gene in 60 patients with Rubinstein-Taybi syndrome," *Journal of Medical Genetics*, vol. 39, no. 6, pp. 415–421, 2002.

[7] M. C. Morales-Chávez, "Dental management of a patient with Rubinstein-Taybi syndrome," *Special Care in Dentistry*, vol. 30, no. 3, pp. 124–126, 2010.

[8] D. G. Gardner and S. S. Girgis, "Talon cusps: a dental anomaly in the Rubinstein-Taybi syndrome," *Oral Surgery Oral Medicine and Oral Pathology*, vol. 47, no. 6, pp. 519–521, 1979.

[9] R. L. Cirillo, "Pediatric case of the day. Rubenstein-Taybisyndrome," *Radiographics*, vol. 17, no. 6, pp. 1604–1605, 1997.

[10] J. E. Ming, E. R. Stiehm, and J. M. Graham Jr., "Immunodefiency as a component of recognizable syndromes," *American Journal of Medical Genetics*, vol. 66, no. 4, pp. 378–398, 1996.

[11] R. C. Hennekam, "Bibliography on Rubinstein-Taybi syndrome.," *American Journal of Medical Genetics. Supplement*, vol. 6, pp. 77–83, 1990.

[12] R. W. Miller and J. H. Rubinstein, "Tumors in Rubinstein-Taybi syndrome," *American Journal of Medical Genetics*, vol. 56, no. 1, pp. 112–115, 1995.

[13] C. C. Chuang and H. C. Lin, "Pilomatrixoma of the head and neck," *Journal of the Chinese Medical Association*, vol. 67, no. 12, pp. 633–636, 2004.

[14] M. J. T. Verstegen, P. Van Den Munckhof, D. Troost, and G. J. Bouma, "Multiple meningiomas in a patient with Rubinstein-Taybi syndrome," *Journal of Neurosurgery*, vol. 102, no. 1, pp. 167–168, 2005.

[15] C. A. Stevens and M. G. Bhakta, "Cardiac abnormalities in the Rubinstein-Taybi syndrome," *American Journal of Medical Genetics*, vol. 59, no. 3, pp. 346–348, 1995.

[16] S. Wiley, S. Swayne, J. H. Rubinstein, N. E. Lanphear, and C. A. Stevens, "Rubinstein-Taybi syndrome medical guidelines," *American Journal of Medical Genetics*, vol. 119, no. 2, pp. 101–110, 2003.

[17] L. A. H. Critchley, T. Gin, and J. C. Stuart, "Anaesthesia in an infant with Rubinstein-Taybi syndrome," *Anaesthesia*, vol. 50, no. 1, pp. 37–38, 1995.

[18] J. E. Allanson, "Rubinstein-Taybi syndrome: the changing face," *American Journal of Medical Genetics*, no. 6, pp. 38–41, 1990.

[19] N. M. Freitas, A. V. Imbronito, C. S. K. La Scala, R. F. M. Lotufo, and F. E. Pustiglioni, "Periodontal disease in a Rubinstein-Taybi syndrome patient: case report," *International Journal of Paediatric Dentistry*, vol. 16, no. 4, pp. 292–296, 2006.

[20] A. Stalin, B. Varma, and Jayanthi, "Rubinstein Taybi syndrome," *Journal of Indian Society of Pedodontics and Preventive Dentistry*, vol. 24, supplement 1, pp. S27–S30, 2006.

[21] S. H. Hsiung, "Rubinstein-Taybi syndrome (broad thumb-hallux syndrome)," *Dermatology Online Journal*, vol. 10, no. 3, article 2, 2004.

[22] E. Davidovich, D. Eimerl, and B. Peretz, "Dental treatment of a child with Rubinstein-Taybi syndrome," *Pediatric Dentistry*, vol. 27, no. 5, pp. 385–388, 2005.

Cavernous Hemangioma of the Tongue

Krishna Kripal,[1] Senthil Rajan,[1] Beena Ropak,[2] and Ipsita Jayanti[1]

[1] *Department of Periodontology, Rajarajeswari Dental College & Hospital, Bangalore, Karnataka 560060, India*
[2] *Department of Oral and Maxillofacial Surgery, Rajarajeswari Dental College & Hospital, Bangalore, Karnataka 560060, India*

Correspondence should be addressed to Krishna Kripal; kripalkrishna@yahoo.com

Academic Editors: A. Epivatianos, C. Evans, A. Markopoulos, and A. Milosevic

Hemangioma is a benign tumor of dilated blood vessels. It is most commonly seen in the head and neck region and rarely in the oral cavity. Hemangiomas in the oral cavity are always of clinical importance and require appropriate treatment. We report here a case of a 34-year-old female patient with a swelling on the lateral surface of tongue which did not respond to the sclerosing agent and was finally confirmed as cavernous hemangioma on histological evaluation.

1. Introduction

Hemangioma (Greek: Haima-blood; angeion vessel, omatumor) by definition can be defined as "a benign tumor of dilated blood vessels." Hemangioma of head and neck appear a few weeks after birth and they grow rapidly. It is also known as port-wine stain, strawberry hemangioma, and Salmon patch. They are characterized by hyperplasia of blood vessels, usually veins and capillaries, in a focal area of submucosal connective tissue. It is almost never encapsulated. Whether this condition is a neoplastic or reactive state is uncertain; a reactive cause is favored.

Few of the reactive causes are, namely, hormonal changes, infections, and trauma. Clinically they may manifest as firm, pulsatile, warm masses and the venous malformations appear first in early childhood and clinically manifest as soft and easily compressible mass. According to the classification given by Mulliken and Glovacki in 1982, are divided the vascular deformities, into 2 groups: hemangiomas and the vascular malformations. The hemangiomas can also be classified depending on the vessel type involved or flow types such as the arterial and arteriovenous (high flow) type, capillary or venous (low flow) type [1].

This paper describes a case of a female patient who had a growth on her lateral border of the tongue which was diagnosed as cavernous hemangioma.

2. Case History

A 34-year-old female patient reported to the Department of Periodontology, Rajarajeswari Dental College and Hospital, Bangalore, India, with the chief complaint of swelling on the lateral surface of the tongue. The patient gave a history of trauma at the same site 10 years back. There was no history of associated pain or bleeding from the site. On general examination, the patient was normally built for her age with no defect in stature or gait. No relevant medical history was observed. On intraoral examination, there was a growth measuring about 1.5 cm × 1.5 cm, which was red in colour with a bluish hue present at the left lateral surface of the tongue which appeared to be sessile with no underlying attachment or relation with the muscles (Figure 1). The borders were well defined and there was no ulceration seen on the surface of the lesion. The growth was soft to palpate, and it showed blanching on application of pressure. A provisional diagnosis of capillary hemangioma was given based on the clinical findings.

3. Management

Initially a sclerosing agent was administered topically and the mass was observed for a period of 1 week (Figure 2). No change in the appearance and size of the mass was observed.

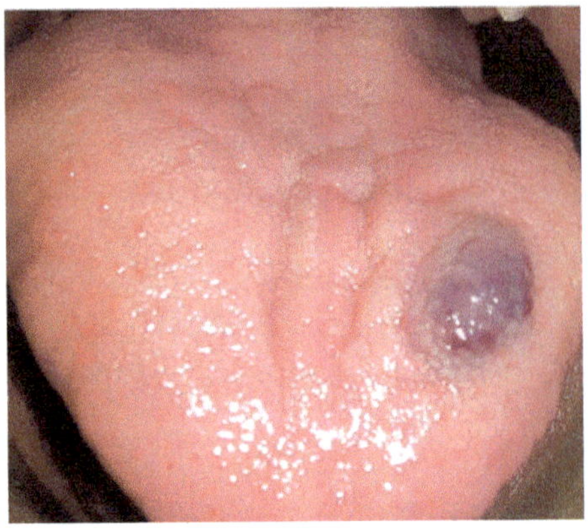

FIGURE 1: Preoperative photograph.

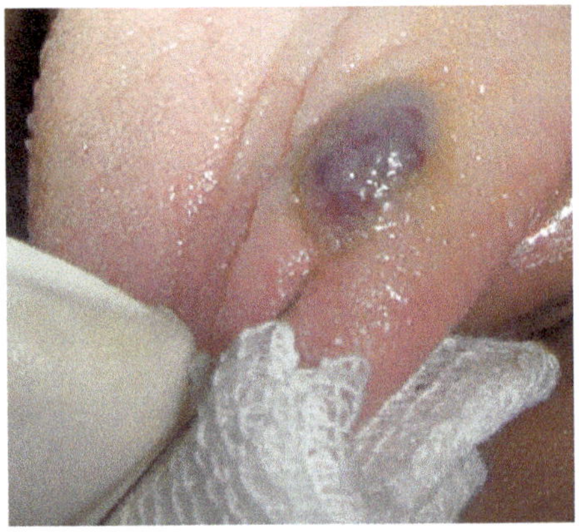

FIGURE 2: Administration of sclerosing agent.

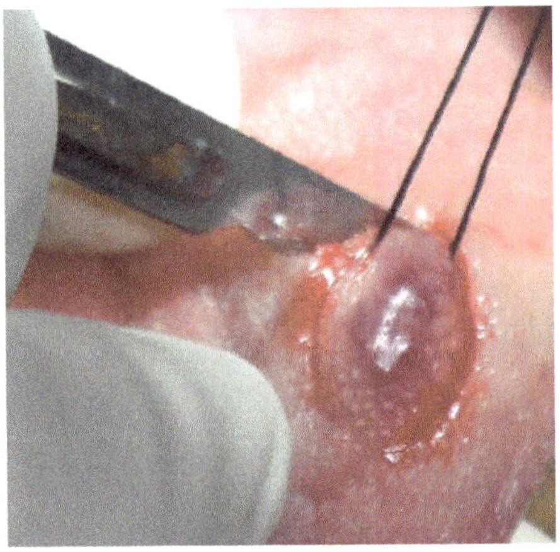

FIGURE 3: Surgical excision.

After a period of 1 week, a surgical excision was carried out under local anesthesia. During the surgical procedure, a thread was tied around the base, and the lesion was stretched in an upward direction in order to get maximum accessibility (Figure 3). The mass was then excised out, and interrupted sutures were placed (Figures 4 and 5). During the surgical procedure, minimal amount of bleeding from the site was

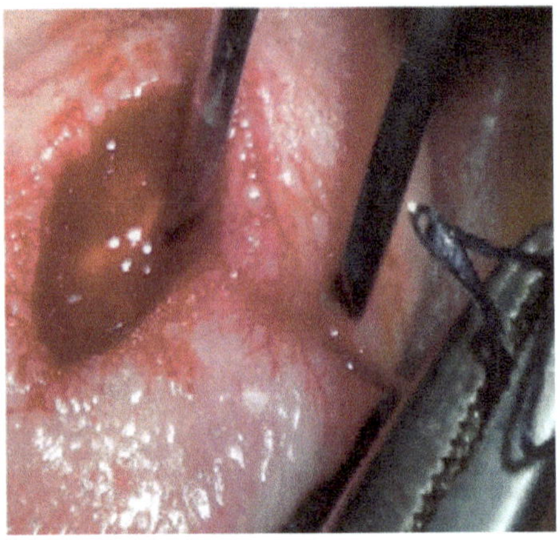

FIGURE 4: Sutures being placed.

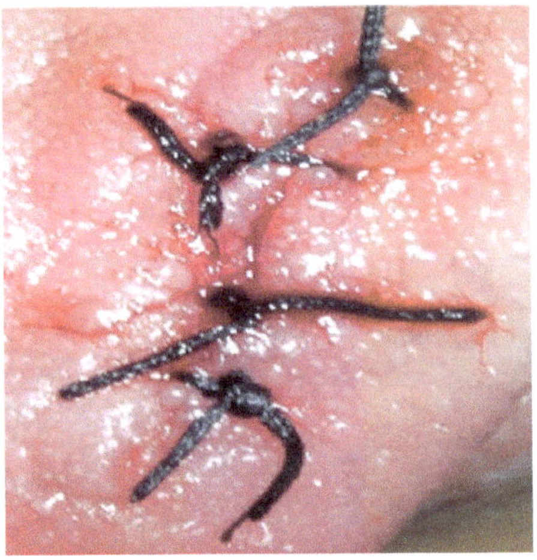

FIGURE 5: Interrupted sutures placed.

observed. The specimen was then sent for a histopathological examination. The healing was uneventful after a period of 1 week (Figure 6) and complete healing was seen after 1 month (Figure 7). The histopathology report confirmed the diagnosis of cavernous hemangioma with void capillary vessel (Figure 8).

4. Discussion

Hemangiomas are the most common benign tumours of the head and neck in children, but their occurrence on the tongue is extremely rare. The tongue requires special consideration because of its susceptibility to minor trauma and consequent bleeding and ulceration, swallowing difficulties, and breathing problem, although the major concern is cosmetic in most cases. The hemangioma appears as soft mass, smooth or lobulated, and sessile or pedunculated and may vary in size from a few millimeters to several centimeters [2, 3]. They are usually deep red and may blanch on the application of pressure and if large in size, it might interfere with mastication [4, 5]. The superficial hemangiomas are often lobulated, and blanch under finger pressure and the deeper lesions tend to

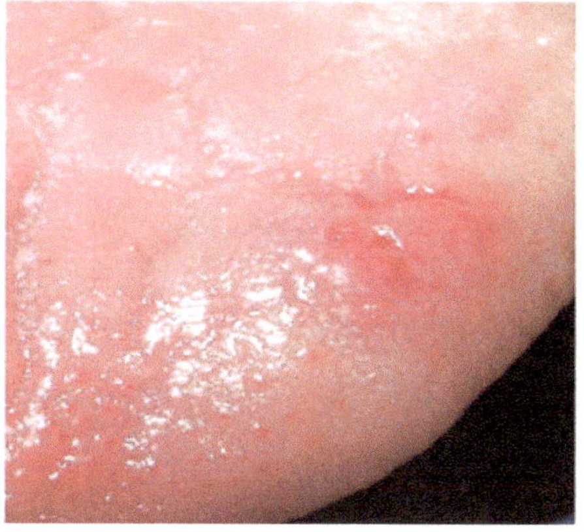

FIGURE 6: 1 week postoperative photograph.

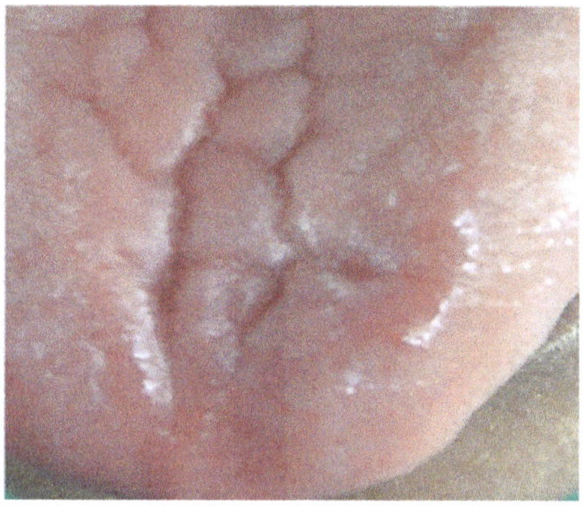

FIGURE 7: 1 month postoperative photograph.

be dome-shaped with normal or blue surface coloration, and they seldom blanch. A lesion with a thrill or bruit or with an obviously warmer surface, is most likely a special vascular malformation, called arteriovenous hemangioma (arteriovenous aneurysm, A-V shunt, arteriovenous malformation), with direct flow of blood from the venous to the arterial system, bypassing the capillary beds.

Various syndromes that are associated with the vascular malformation include the Osler-Weber-Rendu syndrome, Sturge-Weber syndrome, and blue rubber bleb nevus syndrome. A differential diagnosis of granuloma fasciale, insect bite, pyogenic granuloma, and angiosarcoma can be given for this condition.

Clinical diagnosis was based on histopathological evaluation, which was confirmed to be a cavernous hemangioma. Histologically, the appearance of these lesions depends on the stage of the evolution. Early lesions may be very cellular with solid nests of plump endothelial cells and little vascular lumen. Established lesions comprise of well-developed, flattened, and endothelium-lined capillary channels of varying sizes in a lobular configuration. Involuting lesions show increased fibrosis and hyalinization of capillary walls with luminal occlusion [6]. In cavernous hemangioma, there is presence of large dilated blood sinuses with thin walls each showing an endothelial lining. The sinusoidal spaces are

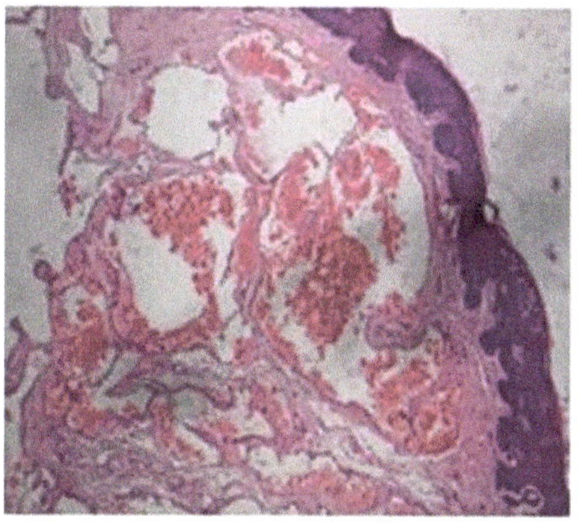

FIGURE 8: Histopathological picture.

usually filled with blood although there might be presence of lymphatic vessels [7].

5. Conclusion

The appearance of cavernous hemangioma is a rare occurrence on the tongue. Early detection and biopsy are crucial in determining the clinical behavior of the tumour and potential complications. The treatment modality should be planned according to the diagnosis and prognosis of the particular vascular malformation.

References

[1] M. S. Greenberg, M. Glick, and J. A. Ship, *Burkett's Oral Medicine*, B. C. Deker, 11th edition, 2008.

[2] A. Werner, A. D. Folz, and R. Rochels, "Current concepts in the classification, diagnosis and treatment of hemangiomas and vascular malformations of the head and neck," *European Archives of Otorhinolaryngology*, vol. 258, pp. 141–149, 2001.

[3] A. Kutluhan, K. Bozdemir, and S. Ugras, "The treatment of tongue haemangioma by plasma knife surgery," *Singapore Medical Journal*, vol. 49, no. 11, pp. e312–e314, 2008.

[4] J. S. Gill, S. Gill, A. Bhardwaj, and H. S. Grover, "Oral haemangioma," *Case Report Med*, vol. 2012, Article ID 347939, 4 pages, 2012.

[5] S. S. Qureshi, D. A. Chaukar, K. A. Pathak et al., "Hemangioma of base of tongue," *Indian Journal of Cancer*, vol. 41, no. 4, pp. 181–183, 2004.

[6] A. Dilsiz, T. Aydin, and N. Gursan, "Capillary hemangioma as a rare benign tumor of the oral cavity: a case report," *Cases Journal*, vol. 2, no. 9, article 8622, 2009.

[7] W. G. Shafer, M. K. Hine, and B. M. Levy, *A Textbook of Oral Pathology*, W. B. Saunders, Philadelphia, Pa, USA, 6th edition, 1983.

18

Rhabdomyomatous (Mesenchymal) Hamartoma Presenting as Haemangioma on the Upper Lip: A Case Report with Immunohistochemical Analysis and Treatment with High-Power Lasers

Aluana Dal Vechio,[1] Edgar Nakajima,[2] Décio Pinto Jr.,[3] Luciane Hiramatsu Azevedo,[2] and Dante A. Migliari[3]

[1] *Department of Stomatology, School of Dentistry, University of São Paulo, 05508-900 São Paulo, SP, Brazil*
[2] *Laboratory for Laser in Dentistry (LELO), School of Dentistry, University of São Paulo, 05508-900 São Paulo, SP, Brazil*
[3] *Department of Stomatology, School of Dentistry, University of São Paulo, Avenida Professor Lineu Prestes 2227, Cidade Universitária, 05508-900 São Paulo, SP, Brazil*

Correspondence should be addressed to Dante A. Migliari; damiglia@usp.br

Academic Editors: L. N. de Souza and C. S. Farah

Rhabdomyomatous hamartoma is a rare disease that occurs predominantly in the skin. This paper describes a congenital lesion in a 17-year-old male, who came to our clinic presenting a circumscribed swelling involving the oral mucosa and vermillion border of the upper lip, purplish in color, and blanching under pressure. The patient reported that he had had lesion since his birth. A clinical diagnosis was of congenital haemangioma, and the patient was treated by photocoagulation using diode laser. When the lesion became smaller, by having its blood content reduced, the upper portion of the lesion was sliced off with CO_2 laser and the tissue was sent for microscopic analysis. Histopathological examination showed an oral mucosa fragment with proliferation of striated muscle bundles admixed with small blood vessels, collagen, and nerve fibres. A supplementary analysis with immunohistochemistry demonstrated positivity for desmin, HHF35, smooth muscle actin, S-100, and CD34. Based on these findings, the lesion was diagnosed as rhabdomyomatous hamartoma. The aesthetic result has been very satisfactory after a 14-month followup.

1. Introduction

Rhabdomyomatous hamartoma (RH) is a rare, congenital lesion with only a few reports (approximately 25 cases), most of them affecting the skin, particularly of the face and neck [1, 2]. Lesions are usually described as a solitary papule or nodule, but they can be multiple and, sometimes, associated with congenital abnormalities [1, 2].

This paper describes a case of RH on the upper lip, diagnosed with the aid of immunohistochemical analysis, followed by largely successful treatment with diode and CO_2 lasers.

2. Report

A 17-year-old male came to our clinic for treatment of a circumscribed swelling on the mucosa and vermillion border of the upper lip (Figures 1(a) and 1(b)), 4 cm in length and purplish in color, which blanched under pressure. The lesion had been present since birth. The patient reported that there was occasional bleeding. His main concern, however, was aesthetic. His general health was good.

A clinical diagnosis of congenital haemangioma was made and the patient was treated under local anesthesia by photocoagulation using diode laser at 830 nm with power

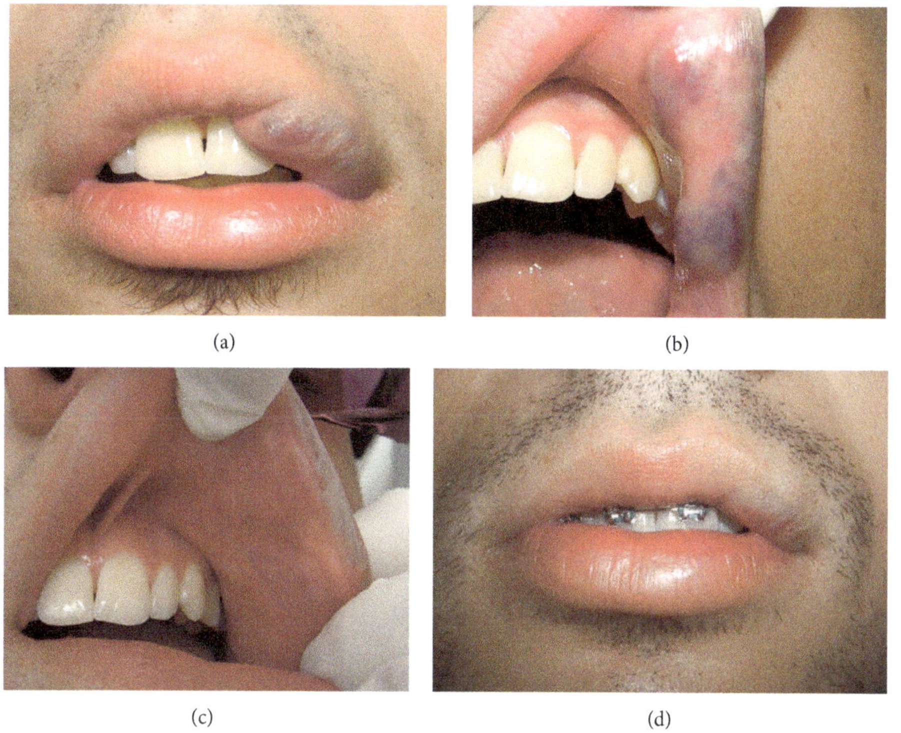

(a) (b) (c) (d)

Figure 1

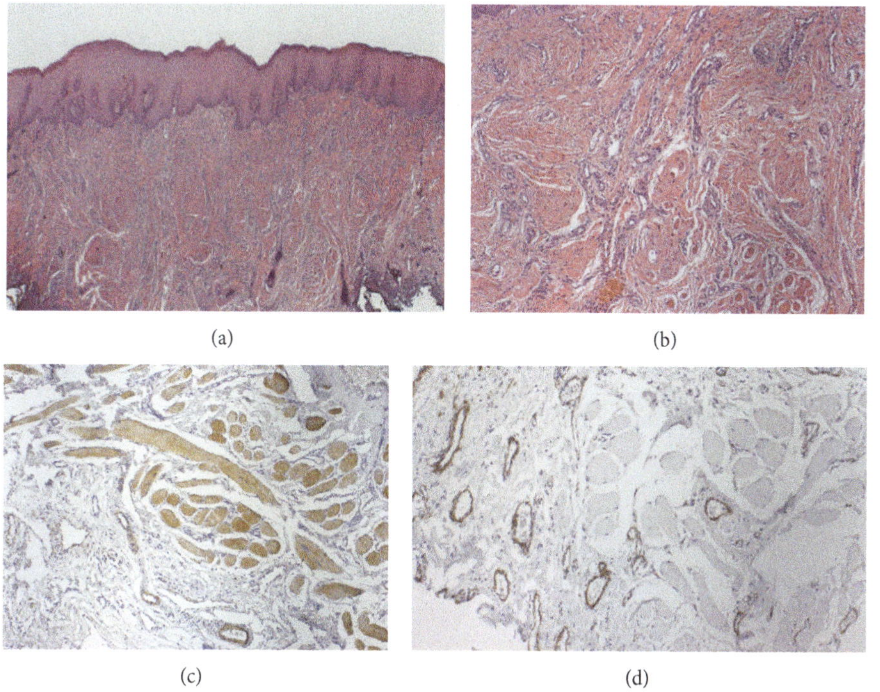

(a) (b) (c) (d)

Figure 2

set at 3.5 W. Irradiation was delivered by means of a flexible quartz fiber that was kept 2-3 mm away from the lesion, in continuous wave mode for 10–20 seconds. This surgical procedure was repeated 3 times at 30-day intervals, thus allowing for recovery of the patient and shrinking of the lesion between sessions. When the lesion became smaller, by having its blood content reduced, the upper portion of the lesion was removed by orienting the CO_2 laser beam parallel with the mucosa surface and sliced off the top of lesion with one single cut. Subsequently, the tissue was sent for histopathological and immunohistochemical examinations.

The aesthetic result has been very satisfactory after a 14-month followup, with only a discrete swelling appearing on the lip (Figures 1(c) and 1(d)).

The histological examination (HE) revealed oral mucosa covered by squamous epithelium with proliferation of striated muscle bundles admixed with small blood vessels, collagen, and nerve fibres. No cytological atypia, necrosis, or mitosis was observed (Figures 2(a) and 2(b)). Immunohistochemical stain was performed by the streptavidin-peroxidase complex technique. Muscular fibres were positive for desmin and HHF35 (Figure 2(c)); smooth muscles of vessel walls were positive for smooth muscle actin (Figure 2(d)); nerve fibres scattered throughout the lesion were positive for S-100, and blood vessels were positive for CD34. Based on these findings, the lesion was diagnosed as RH.

3. Discussion

Hamartoma, a term coined by the Greek (meaning to deviate or miss the goal), is used in the medical literature to describe a disordered arrangement of normal elements forming a tumor-like lesion [2, 3]. Histopathologically, RH is composed of a mixture of mature tissues, haphazardly arranged.

The clinical form most often reported in the literature of RH is a solitary papule or nodule, occurring particularly on the skin in the region of the head and neck [2]. In the present case, the lesion showed an unusual presentation; besides mimicking a typical congenital haemangioma, it had predominantly an oral involvement, which is an exceedingly rare location, there being only 3 cases on the oral mucosa reported in the literature [2, 4, 5].

The treatment yielded a great improvement of the lesion, and the patient felt very pleased with the aesthetic result, reporting little concern about the remaining slightly bluish-swollen aspect of his left upper lip.

In the present case, the histopathological analysis coupled with immunohistochemical assay was highly instrumental for disclosing the congenital origin of the lesion while the high-power lasers treatment provided a safe and effective resolution, largely successful and without scarring.

References

[1] G. Magro, A. Di Benedetto, G. Sanges, F. Scalisi, and R. Alaggio, "Rhabdomyomatous mesenchymal hamartoma of oral cavity: an unusual location for such a rare lesion," *Virchows Archiv*, vol. 446, no. 3, pp. 346–347, 2005.

[2] A. S. Rosenberg, J. Kirk, and M. B. Morgan, "Rhabdomyomatous mesenchymal hamartoma: an unusual dermal entity with a report of two cases and a review of the literature," *Journal of Cutaneous Pathology*, vol. 29, no. 4, pp. 238–243, 2002.

[3] J. C. Steele, A. Triantafyllou, and E. A. Field, "Lingual striated muscle hamartoma or herniation?" *Journal of Oral Pathology & Medicine*, vol. 33, no. 8, pp. 454–455, 2004.

[4] P. de la Sotta, C. Salomone, and S. González, "Rhabdomyomatous, (mesenchymal) hamartoma of the tongue: report of a case," *Journal of Oral Pathology & Medicine*, vol. 36, pp. 58–59, 2007.

[5] P. A. Kreiger, L. M. Ernst, L. M. Elden et al., "Hamartomatosus tongue lesions in children," *The American Journal of Surgical Pathology*, vol. 31, no. 8, 2007.

19

Amelanotic Melanoma Masquerading as a Granular Cell Lesion

Deepak Pandiar, Shaini Basheer, P. M. Shameena, S. Sudha, and Lakshmi J. Dhana

Department of Oral and Maxillofacial Pathology, Government Dental College, Kozhikode, Kerala 673008, India

Correspondence should be addressed to Shaini Basheer; shaini.finoj@gmail.com

Academic Editors: I. El-Hakim, M. O. Sayin, and N. Yarom

Amelanotic melanoma (AM) presents a diagnostic challenge due to its wide clinical presentations, lack of pigmentation, and varied histological appearances. Immunohistochemistry plays a crucial role in the diagnosis of these lesions. Amelanotic melanoma of oral mucosa is an uncommon lesion. We report a case of a 50-year-old male patient with a growth on the anterior mandibular gingiva of seven-month duration. In the present case, histologically, the tumour resembled a granular cell lesion, which has not been reported previously in AM. Diagnosis was possible by a sequential panel of immunohistochemical markers, of which finally vimentin, S100, HMB45, and Melan-A were positive. The tumor was surgically excised, and postsurgical radiotherapy was given.

1. Introduction

Malignant melanomas most commonly occur on skin (over 90%) and less commonly on mucosal surfaces, that is, slightly over 1% [1]. It accounts for approximately 4% of all skin cancers, but it is responsible for 79% of all skin-cancer-related deaths [2]. These lesions are classically pigmented but amelanotic subtype is also well documented in the literature, which is often difficult to diagnose and requires microscopic evaluation aided by immunohistochemistry for correct diagnosis. Thrity-four cases of amelanotic melanomas (AM) have been reported on oral mucosa and only three on the mandibular mucosa. This is to the best of our knowledge of the fourth case. Although different histological subtypes of malignant melanoma are known to occur, PubMed/Medline search did not reveal any previous report of granular cell variant of malignant melanoma.

2. Case Report

A 50-year-old male patient reported to the Department of Oral Pathology and Microbiology, Government. Dental College, Kozhikode, with a chief complaint of a growth on the lower anterior gingiva since 7 months. Medical history revealed that the patient was under medication for epilepsy and hypertension. He is a smoker (1 pack per day for the past 32 years) and occasionally takes alcohol. On examination, a growth of size about $3 \times 2.5 \times 1$ cm was noticed on the labial gingiva extending from 31 to 34 region. The overlying mucosa was slightly erythematous and without any ulceration (Figure 1(a)). The lesion was sessile, nontender, and firm in consistency. There was no bleeding on palpation. Associated teeth were within normal limits. Intraoral periapical radiograph showed mild rarefaction of the alveolar bone in the 33–35 region (Figure 1(b)). Lymph nodes were not palpable. A provisional diagnosis of pyogenic granuloma was given. Incisional biopsy was done.

Microscopically, the specimen showed sheets of large ovoid to polygonal tumor cells with pale eosinophilic granular cytoplasm and eccentrically placed nuclei in most of the cells (Figure 2(a)). Nuclear pleomorphism with increased nuclear cytoplasmic ratio was noticed (Figure 2(b)). Some cells showed vesicular nuclei with prominent nucleoli, and mitotic activity was high (Figure 2(c)). At some areas tumor cells showed spindling (Figure 2(d)). H&E staining and Masson-Fontana staining did not demonstrate melanin pigments (Figure 3). Immunohistochemically, the tumor cells were positive for vimentin, desmin, S100, HMB-45, and Melan-A and negative for cytokeratin, NSE, and CD68 (Figures 4(a)–4(i)). Based on these findings, diagnosis of amelanotic melanoma was given. The patient was referred to the Regional Cancer Center, Thiruvananthapuram. The lesion was surgically excised, and postsurgical irradiation therapy was given.

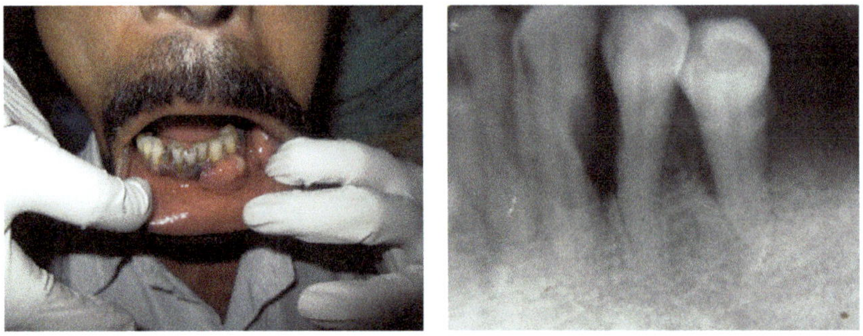

(a) (b)

Figure 1: (a) Intraoral view of lesion in anterior mandibular region. (b) IOPA showing mild rarefaction and bone loss in the 33–35 region.

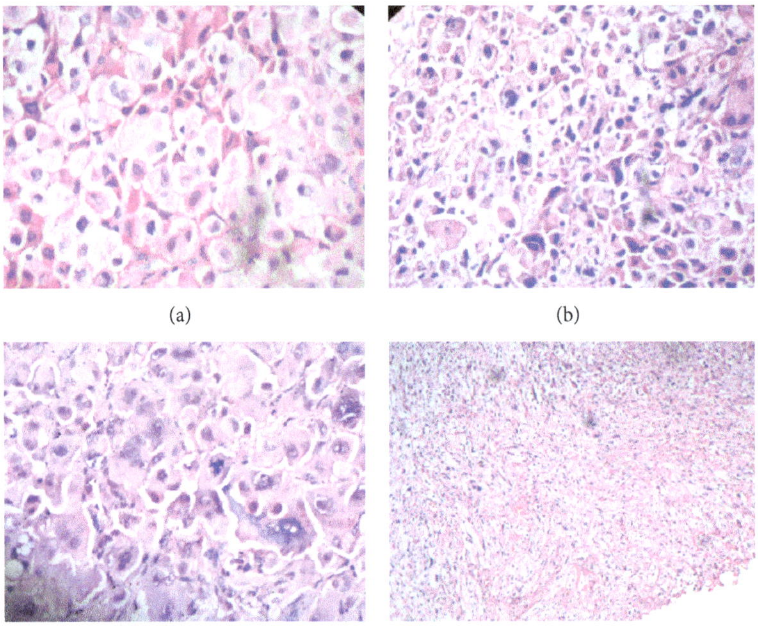

(a) (b)

(c) (d)

Figure 2: (a) Photomicrograph of amelanotic melanoma shows diffuse proliferation of large ovoid to polygonal tumor cells with pale eosinophilic granular cytoplasm and eccentrically placed nucleus (H&E 40x). (b) Nuclear pleomorphism and increased nucleocytoplasmic ratio (H&E 40x). (c) Abnormal mitotic figures (H&E 40x). (d) Tumor cells showing spindling (H&E 10x).

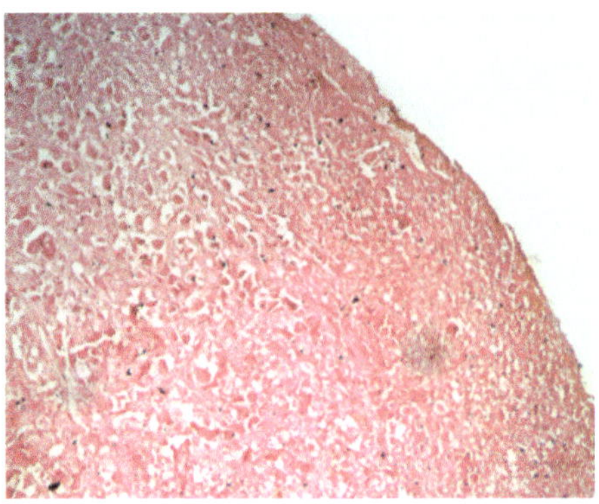

Figure 3: Masson-Fontana staining showing no positive cells (20x).

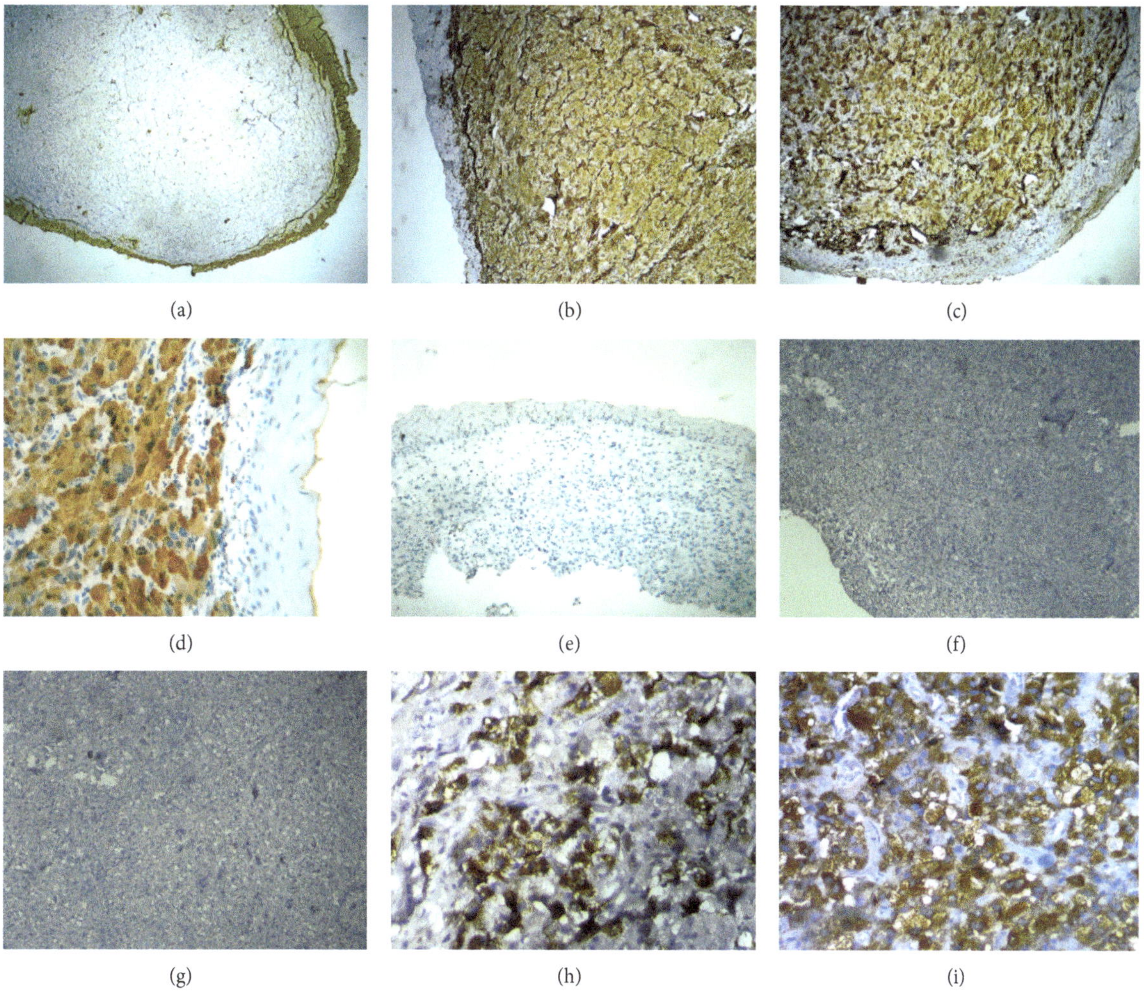

FIGURE 4: (a) Immunohistochemistry for pan cytokeratin showing no expression in tumour cells (5x). (b) Immunohistochemistry for desmin showing diffuse positivity (10x). (c) Immunohistochemistry for vimentin (diffusively positive (10x)). (d) Immunohistochemistry for S100 showing diffuse nuclear and cytoplasmic expression (40x). (e) Immunohistochemistry for CD 68 (negative, (10x)). (f) Immunohistochemistry for neuron-specific enolase (negative, (10x)). (g) Immunohistochemistry for myoglobin (negative, (5x)). (h) Immunohistochemistry showing positivity for HMB-45 (40x). (i) Immunohistochemistry for Melan-A; granular localization is observed in the cytoplasm (40x).

3. Discussion

In the literature, amelanotic melanoma has been described under the term "the great masquerader" as clinical and histological features are often deceptive [3]. Medline search revealed 34 cases of AM in the oral cavity [4–24]. Three cases have been described in mandibular gingival area, but none of the case, has the presentation of granular cell lesion. The sites in those cases were palatal ($n = 17$), maxillary gingiva ($n = 13$), upper lip mucosa ($n = 1$), and mandibular gingiva ($n = 3$).

Based on the histological presentation, differential diagnosis included poorly differentiated squamous cell carcinoma, malignant granular cell tumor (MGCT), rhabdomyosarcoma, and malignant peripheral nerve sheath tumor (MPNST). Granular cell presentation of malignant melanoma being never reported was not included in the differential diagnosis. An initial immunohistochemical panel of pancytokeratin, vimentin, desmin, and S100 excluded tumours of epithelial origin (Figures 2(a)–2(d)) and narrowed down the possible diagnoses to MPNST, MGCT, and rhabdomyosarcoma. The next panel of immunomarkers consisted of CD68, NSE (neuron specific enolase), and myoglobin (Figures 2(e)–2(g)). However, when all of them turned out to be negative, we then considered AM, taking into consideration the S100 positivity of the tumour cells. The tumor cells were found to be positive for HMB45 and Melan-A, based on which the lesion was diagnosed as AM (Figures 2(h) and 2(i)).

For differential diagnosis of AM, immunohistochemistry is generally used and the standard melanoma immunohistochemical antigens include S-100 protein, HMB-45, and Melan-A/MART1. Thirteen of fifteen cases of AM were positive for S-100 protein (Gibson and Goellner) [25]. In a study, Wick et al. found 92% melanomas to be positive for

HMB-45 [26]. Together with Melan-A, immunostaining of HMB-45 and S100 increases the sensitivity and specificity for melanomas. Recently, microphthalmia transcription factor, tyrosinase, and Melan-A immunostains have been used to highlight melanocytes. The inclusion of these in a panel of stains for melanoma should be beneficial. Gazit and Daniels in their study showed a high immunoreactivity of oral melanoma to protein S-100 (46 cases out of 50) and HMB-45 (especially in the epithelioid variations) [27].

Several variants of AM are presently recognized, and these usually parallel the subtypes of pigmented melanoma. The more commonly known growth patterns are superficial spreading, acral lentiginous, nodular, neurotropic, and desmoplastic types/melanomas. Some unusual variants of the AM reported are adenoid/pseudopapillary, small cell, myxoid, hemangiopericytoid, and signet-ring cell melanomas [28]. In the present case, tumor cells did not reveal melanin pigment by H&E and Masson-Fontana staining. Histologically, the tumor most closely resembled the malignant granular cell tumor. Immunostaining is an essential diagnostic tool where diagnosis based merely on H&E staining becomes difficult.

Ethnicity and sun exposure appear to play a major role in the development of cutaneous melanomas while mucosal melanomas have no association with sun exposure. Cigarette smoking, alcohol consumption and denture irritation are some of the risk factors for oral melanomas [29]. The history of smoking and alcohol consumption could be possible risk factors in the present case.

At present, the recommended treatment is wide excision in combination with chemotherapy and, to a lesser extent, immunotherapy or irradiation therapy.

4. Conclusion

The diagnosis of amelanotic melanoma can be very challenging especially when they present with unusual histological appearances. Proper documentation of such cases and the role of immunohistochemistry are emphasized in this paper.

Consent

Written informed consent was obtained from the patient for publication of this paper and any accompanying images. A copy of the written consent is available for review by the Editor-in-Chief of this journal.

Conflict of Interests

The authors declare that they have no conflict of interests.

Authors' Contribution

D. Pandiar drafted the paper. S. Basheer did the immunohistochemical assays and contributed to the drafting of the manuscript. P. M. Shameena revised the manuscript critically for important intellectual content. S. Sudha revised the manuscript and supervised the immunohistochemical assays.

References

[1] M. J. Hicks and C. M. Flaitz, "Oral mucosal melanoma: epidemiology and pathobiology," *Oral Oncology*, vol. 36, no. 2, pp. 152–169, 2000.

[2] W. Franke, N. J. Neumann, T. Ruzicka, and K. W. Schulte, "Plantar malignant melanoma: a challenge for early recognition," *Melanoma Research*, vol. 10, no. 6, pp. 571–576, 2000.

[3] P. Sbano, N. Nami, L. Grimaldi, and P. Rubegni, "True Amelanotic melanoma: the great Masquerader," *Journal of Plastic, Reconstructive & Aesthetic Surgery*, vol. 63, no. 3, pp. e307–e308, 2010.

[4] T. Furuhashi, H. Kuno, M. Teramoto et al., "A case of amelanotic melanoma originating in the area of mandibule," *Japanese Journal of Oral and Maxillofacial Surgery*, vol. 25, no. 6, pp. 1509–1513, 1979.

[5] G. Kawasakia, S. Yanamoto, I. Yoshitomi, A. Mizuno, S. Fujita, and M. Umed, "Amelanotic melanoma of the mandible: a case report," *Oral Science International*, vol. 8, no. 2, pp. 60–63, 2011.

[6] S. Y. Kao, J. C. C. Yang, W. Y. Li, and R. C. S. Chang, "Maxillary amelanotic melanoma: a case report," *Journal of Oral and Maxillofacial Surgery*, vol. 59, no. 6, pp. 700–703, 2001.

[7] T. Saku, H. Takahashi, H. Okabe, N. Tsuda, H. Okumura, and M. Sasaki, "Oral amelanotic melanoma–report of a case with desmoplastic changes at the site of lymph node metastasis," *Japan Journal of Cancer Clinics*, vol. 29, no. 5, pp. 424–432, 1983.

[8] M. Usui, K. Shirasuna, T. Morimoto et al., "Malignant melanoma in the upper alveolus: report of a case," *Japanese Journal of Oral and Maxillofacial Surgery*, vol. 31, pp. 1233–1240, 1985.

[9] H. Akizuki, K. Ohno, H. Yoshida et al., "A case of bilateral Warthin's tumors of parotid gland associated with amelanotic malignant melanoma of maxilla," *Japanese Journal of Oral and Maxillofacial Surgery*, vol. 32, pp. 461–465, 1986.

[10] M. Umeda, O. Teranobu, K. Nakanishi, and K. Shimada, "Treatment and prognosis of primary malignant melanoma of the oral cavity. An analysis of 12 our and 96 reported cases," *Journal of Japan Society for Cancer Therapy*, vol. 25, no. 10, pp. 2499–2510, 1990.

[11] L. Chu, A. Abdul, T. Takahashi et al., "Amelanotic melanoma of the oral cavity," *The Journal of Nihon University School of Dentistry*, vol. 35, no. 2, pp. 124–129, 1993.

[12] R. I. van der Waal, G. B. Snow, A. B. Karim, and I. van der Waal, "Primary malignant melanoma of the oral cavity: a review of eight cases," *British Dental Journal*, vol. 176, no. 5, pp. 185–188, 1994.

[13] K. Ohshima, A. Ohtawa, K. Yoshiga et al., "A case of amelanotic malignant melanoma in the maxilla," *Japanese Journal of Oral and Maxillofacial Surgery*, vol. 40, pp. 1006–1008, 1994.

[14] R. Tani, T. Okamoto, A. Sakamoto et al., "A case of an amelanotic malignant melanoma successfully treated with LAK therapy," *Japanese Journal of Oral and Maxillofacial Surgery*, vol. 40, pp. 825–827, 1994.

[15] B. F. Barker, W. M. Carpenter, T. E. Daniels et al., "Oral mucosal melanomas: the WESTOP Banff workshop proceedings. Western Society of Teachers of Oral Pathology," *Oral Surgery, Oral Medicine, Oral Pathology, Oral Radiology and Endodontology*, vol. 83, no. 6, pp. 672–679, 1997.

[16] K. Shimazu, M. Mohri, M. Nishio, M. Kamata, and I. Morimoto, "Amelanotic malignant melanoma in the palatal mucosa," *Practica Otologica*, vol. 90, no. 3, pp. 331–338, 1997.

[17] Y. Shibuya, T. Yoshikawa, M. Umeda et al., "A case of amelanotic malignant melanoma of the maxillary gingiva," *Japanese Journal of Oral and Maxillofacial Surgery*, vol. 44, pp. 814–816, 1998.

[18] Y. Kimijima, M. Mimura, N. Tanaka et al., "A difficult-to-diagnose case of amelanotic malignant melanoma in the anterior alveolar of the maxilla," *Japanese Journal of Oral and Maxillofacial Surgery*, vol. 45, pp. 703–705, 1999.

[19] J. Ohno, S. Fujita, I. Tohjyo et al., "A case of amelanotic malignant melanoma of the oral mucosa that temporarily responded to a continuous intraarterial infusion of interferon-β," *Journal of Japan Society for Oral Tumors*, vol. 12, no. 4, pp. 327–331, 2000.

[20] Y. Ducic and D. A. Pulsipher, "Amelanotic melanoma of the palate: report of case," *Journal of Oral and Maxillofacial Surgery*, vol. 59, no. 5, pp. 580–583, 2001.

[21] T. Kuwazawa, T. Okamoto, T. Yamamura et al., "A case of the multiple primary cancer involving maxillary amelanotic malignant melanoma and gastric cancer," *Japanese Journal of Oral and Maxillofacial Surgery*, vol. 47, pp. 243–246, 2001.

[22] M. Katsuno, T. Kubota, K. Matsui et al., "A case of amelanotic malignant melanoma in the hard palatal mucosa successfully treated with intra-tumoral injection of interferon," *Stomato-Pharyngol*, vol. 13, no. 2, pp. 203–207, 2001.

[23] K. Notani, M. Shindoh, Y. Yamazaki et al., "Amelanotic malignant melanomas of the oral mucosa," *British Journal of Oral and Maxillofacial Surgery*, vol. 40, no. 3, pp. 195–200, 2002.

[24] N. Tanaka, M. Mimura, Y. Kimijima, and T. Amagasa, "Clinical investigation of amelanotic malignant melanoma in the oral region," *Journal of Oral and Maxillofacial Surgery*, vol. 62, no. 8, pp. 933–937, 2004.

[25] L. E. Gibson and J. R. Goellner, "Amelanotic melanoma: cases studied by Fontana stain, S-100 immunostain, and ultrastructural examination," *Mayo Clinic Proceedings*, vol. 63, no. 8, pp. 777–782, 1988.

[26] M. R. Wick, P. E. Swanson, and A. Rocamora, "Recognition of malignant melanoma by monoclonal antibody HMB-45. An immunohistochemical study of 200 paraffin-embedded cutaneous tumors," *Journal of Cutaneous Pathology*, vol. 15, no. 4, pp. 201–207, 1988.

[27] D. Gazit and T. E. Daniels, "Oral melanocytic lesions: differences in expression of HMB-45 and S-100 antigens in round and spindle cells of malignant and benign lesions," *Journal of Oral Pathology and Medicine*, vol. 23, no. 2, pp. 60–64, 1994.

[28] R. E. Nakhleh, M. R. Wick, A. Rocamora, P. E. Swanson, and L. P. Dehner, "Morphologic diversity in malignant melanomas," *American Journal of Clinical Pathology*, vol. 93, no. 6, pp. 731–740, 1990.

[29] F. Femiano, A. Lanza, C. Buonaiuto, F. Gombos, F. D. Spirito, and N. Cirillo, "Oral malignant melanoma: a review of the literature," *Journal of Oral Pathology and Medicine*, vol. 37, no. 7, pp. 383–388, 2008.

20

Peripheral Cemento-Ossifying Fibroma: Case Series Literature Review

Kiran Kumar Ganji,[1] ArunKumar Bhimashankar Chakki,[2] Sharanbasappa Chandrashekar Nagaral,[3] and Esha Verma[4]

[1] *Department of Periodontics, Sharad Pawar Dental College, Datta Meghe Institute of Medical Sciences (Deemed University), Nagpur, India*
[2] *Department of Oral and Maxillofacial Pathology, Guru Gobind Singh College of Dental Sciences, Devi Ahilya University, Burhanpur, Indore, India*
[3] *Department of Prosthodontics, Al-badar Dental College and Hospital, Near PDA Engineering College, Rajiv Gandhi University of Health Sciences, Gulbarga, Bangalore, India*
[4] *Department of Periodontics, College of Dental Sciences & Hospital, Devi Ahilya University, Rau, Indore, India*

Correspondence should be addressed to Kiran Kumar Ganji; kiranperio@gmail.com

Academic Editors: A. Kasaj, Y. S. Khader, and M. Machado

The concept of fibroosseous lesions of bone has evolved over the last several decades and now includes two major entities: fibrous dysplasia and ossifying fibroma. Peripheral cemento-ossifying fibroma is a relatively rare tumour classified between fibroosseous lesions. It predominantly affects adolescents and young adults, with peak prevalence between 10 and 19 yrs. The cemento-ossifying fibroma is a central neoplasm of bone as well as periodontium which has caused considerable controversy because of confusion regarding terminology and the criteria for its diagnosis. The cemento-ossifying fibroma is odontogenic in origin, whereas ossifying fibroma is of bony origin. Lesions histologically similar to peripheral ossifying fibroma have been given various names in existing literature. Therefore, we present and discuss in this paper a series of cases of peripheral cemento-ossifying fibroma emphasizing the differential diagnosis.

1. Introduction

Benign fibroosseous lesions of the jaws present problems in diagnosis and classification. The 1992 WHO classification groups under a single designation (cemento-ossifying fibroma) two histologic types (cementifying fibroma and ossifying fibroma) that may be clinically and radiographically undistinguishable [1]. Cemento-ossifying fibroma is a relative rare lesion considered as an osteogenic tumor (nonodontogenic) with variable expressiveness. It is defined as a well-demarcated and occasionally encapsulated lesion consisting of fibrous tissue containing variable amounts of mineralized material resembling bone (ossifying fibroma), cementum (cementifying fibroma), or both [2, 3].

Peripheral cemento-ossifying fibroma (PCOF) accounts for 3.1% of all oral tumors [4] and for 9.6% of gingival lesions [5]. The pathogenesis of this tumor is uncertain. Due to their clinical and histopathological similarities, some PCOFs are believed to develop fibrous maturation and subsequent calcification. PCOF is frequently associated with irritant agents such as calculus, bacterial plaque, orthodontic appliances, ill adapted crowns, and irregular restorations. The mineralized product probably originates from periosteal cells or from the periodontal ligament [6]. PCOF affects both genders, but a higher predilection for females has been reported in the literature [4]. With respect to race, there is a predominance in Whites (71%) compared to Blacks (36%) [7]. It may occur at any range, but exhibits a peak incidence between the second [8] and third decades [7]. However, Neville et al. [9] say that it predominantly affects adolescents and young adults, with a peak prevalence between 10 and 19 years.

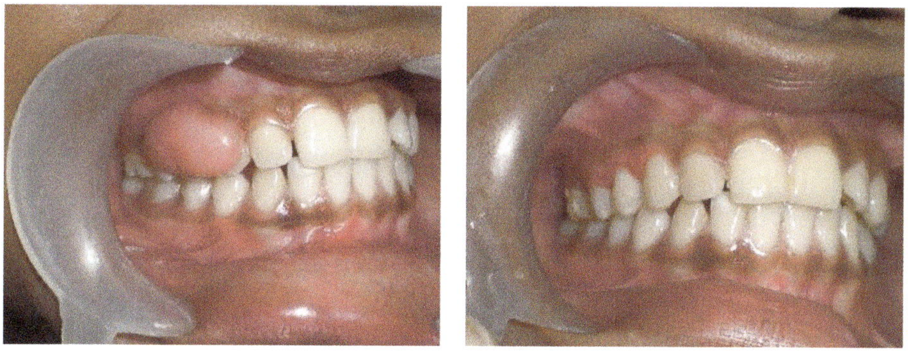

(a) (b)

FIGURE 1: (a) Clinical view of lesion. (b) Postoperative view.

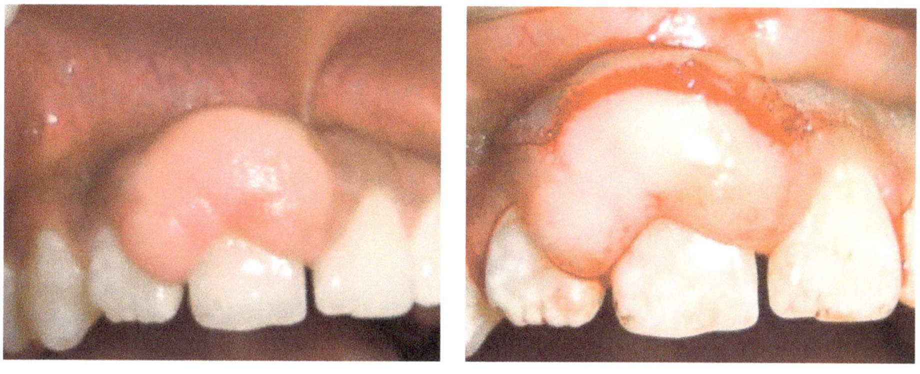

(a) (b)

FIGURE 2

Clinically, PCOF manifests as a pediculate or sessile nodular mass, which usually originates in the interdental papilla. Its color is similar to that of the mucosa unless the lesion is ulcerated. Most tumors measure less than 2 cm in diameter, although lesions larger than 10 cm are occasionally observed. About 60% of the tumors occur in the maxilla and more than 50% of all cases affect the region of the incisors and canines. A potential of tooth migration PCOF has been reported [6]. Hence, the purpose of this paper is to present a series of cases of PCOF lesions and emphasize the importance of discussion of the reasonable differential diagnosis with the patient.

2. Case Description

Case 1. A 21-year-old male reported to College of Dental Sciences & Hospital, Rau, Indore, India, with his slow growing, painless growth that had been present facial in upper right premolar to molar region. Lesion started as a small papule approximately 1 year earlier. According to the patient, there was no bleeding and pain except difficulty in mastication. Examination revealed approximately 2 × 1.5 cm pedunculated nontender, firm, pinkish red growth present on the buccal gingival in relation to maxillary right canine to 1st molar. The lesion extended up to the level of occlusal plane and revealed indentations made by the occluding mandibular premolar. The surface of the occlusal plane was pinkish red in color (Figure 1).

Case 2. A healthy 25-year-old male reported to College of Dental Sciences & Hospital, Rau, Indore, India, with a lump in his back teeth. According to the patient, the reddish purple lump has been present for approximately 6 months and the lump was interfering with his bite and felt uncomfortable. Occasionally bleeding occurred when he brushed his teeth. Clinical examination revealed erythematous interdental papilla in relation to maxillary central incisors 11,12 visible from facial aspect with no evidence of lesion palatally. The lesion appeared exophytic and nodular with irregular surface. It measured approximately 10 mm laterally and 8 mm in anterior-posterior direction and 6 mm thick. It was slightly pedunculated with what appeared to be a broad-based attachment. The lesion was neither fluctuant nor did it blanch on pressure, but had a rubbery consistency. It was tender (Figure 2).

Case 3. A 26-year-old male patient was referred by his general dental practitioner for gingival swelling in relation 15 to 16 region. The past dental history revealed presence of swelling since last one and half year duration. On examination, the associated soft tissue was slightly swollen but there was no

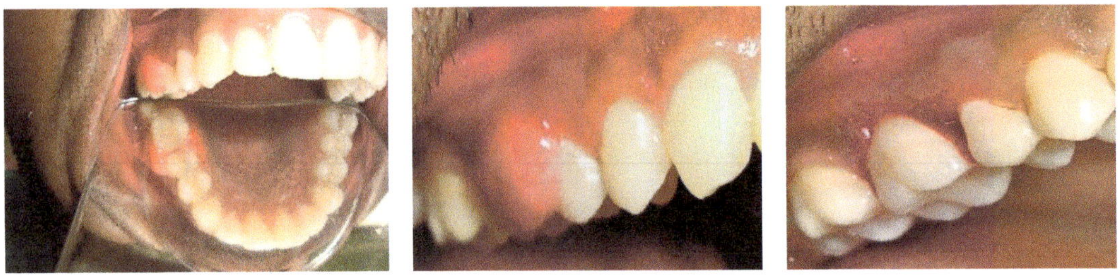

(a) (b) (c)

Figure 3: (a) Clinical view. (b) Clinical view. (c) View after excision.

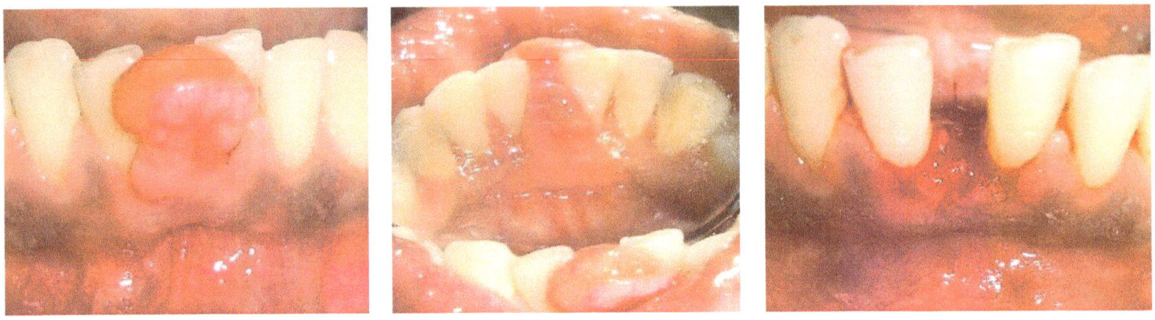

(a) (b) (c)

Figure 4: Clinical view.

ulceration, on palpation the swelling was soft rubbery in consistency, but no tenderness. The lesion was well demarcated and pedunculated measuring approximately 1.5 × 2 cm (Figure 3).

Case 4. A 31-year-old male reported to the College of Dental Sciences & Hospital, Rau, Indore, India complaining of inability to chew food since 6 to 8 months. The patient was apparently asymptomatic 18 months back when he developed a small swelling in the mandibular anterior labial region in 31, 41 which gradually increased in size. On examination, a uniform rounded swelling was present in mandibular anterior region due to which the patient could not chew the food. The size of the lesion was 2.5 × 2 cm and the shape was ovoid. The overlying mucosa was pinkish in color and firm in consistency. The texture was smooth. There was no compressibility or depressibility (Figure 4).

3. Diagnosis

Differential diagnosis consisted of irritational fibroma, pyogenic granuloma, peripheral giant cell granuloma, peripheral cemento-ossifying fibroma.

A confirmatory diagnosis of peripheral cemento-ossifying fibroma is made by histopathologic evaluation of biopsy specimens. The following features were observed during microscopic examination:

(1) ulcerated stratified squamous surface epithelium;

(2) benign fibrous connective tissue with varying numbers of fibroblasts;

(3) sparse-to-profuse endothelial proliferation;

(4) mineralized material consisting of mature, lamellar or woven osteoid, cementum like material, or dystrophic calcifications;

(5) acute or chronic inflammatory cells in lesion (Figure 5).

4. Discussion

Peripheral ossifying fibroma is thought to be either reactive or neoplastic in nature. Considerable confusion has prevailed in the nomenclature of peripheral ossifying fibroma with various synonyms being used, such as peripheral cementifying fibroma, ossifying fibroepithelial polyp, peripheral fibroma with osteogenesis, peripheral fibroma with cementogenesis, peripheral fibroma with calcification, calcifying or ossifying fibroma epulis, and calcifying fibroblastic granuloma [10]. Ossifying fibromas elaborate bone, cementum and spheroidal calcifications, which has given rise to various terms for these benign fibroosseous neoplasms. When bone predominates, "ossifying" is the appellation, while the term "cementifying" has been assigned when curvilinear trabeculae or spheroidal calcifications are encountered [11]. When bone and cementum-like tissues are observed, the lesions have been referred to as cemento-ossifying fibroma [11]. Cementifying fibromas may be clinically and radiographically impossible to separate from ossifying fibromas [12]. An attempt has been made by Endo et al. to distinguish cementifying fibroma from ossifying fibromas and fibrous dysplasias by using immunohistochemical analysis for keratin sulfate and

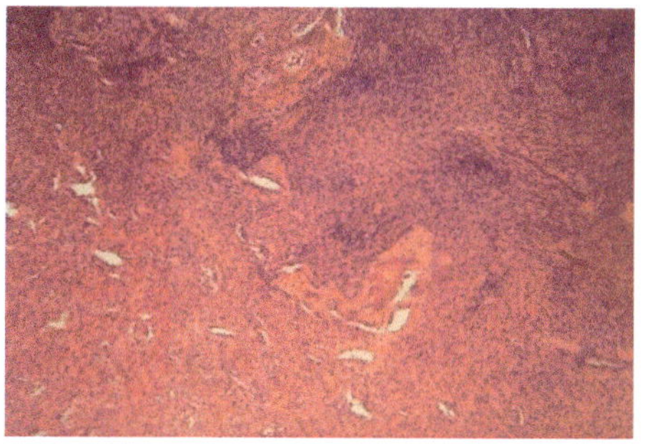

(a)

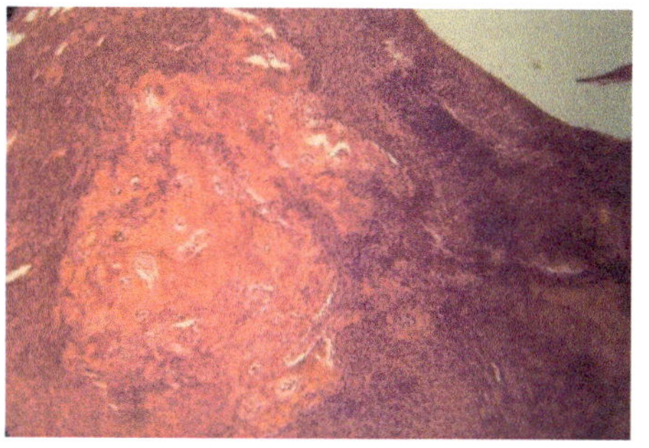

(b)

FIGURE 5: Histologic view of the lesion under 20x magnification.

chondrotoin-4 sulfate in which the cementifying fibromas showed significant immunoreactivity for keratan sulfate and ossifying fibromas, and fibrous dysplasias showed intensive immunostaining for chondroitin-4-sulfate [12].

The term cemento-ossifying has been referred to as outdated and scientifically inaccurate [13] because the clinical presentation and histopathology of cemento-ossifying fibroma are the same in areas where there is no cementum, such as the skull, femur, and tibia. These are all ossifying fibromas; those that happen to occur in the jaws should not be termed cement ossifying fibromas merely because of the presence of teeth. Moreover, there is no histologic or biochemical difference between cementum and bone. Cemento-ossifying fibroma is the term given mainly due to presence of dysmorphic round basophilic bone particles within ossifying fibroma, which have arbitrarily been called cementicles. However, these so-called cementicles are not from cementum but instead represent a dysmorphic product of this tumour analogous to the keratin pearls, which are a dysmorphic product of squamous cell carcinoma [13].

Though the etiopathogenesis of peripheral ossifying fibroma is uncertain, an origin from cells of periodontal ligament has been suggested [10]. The reasons for considering periodontal ligament origin for peripheral ossifying fibroma include exclusive occurrence of peripheral ossifying fibroma in the gingiva (interdental papilla), the proximity of gingiva to the periodontal ligament, and the presence of oxytalan fibres within the mineralized matrix of some lesions [10]. Excessive proliferation of mature fibrous connective tissue is a response to gingival injury, gingival irritation, subgingival calculus, or a foreign body in the gingival sulcus. Chronic irritation of the periosteal and periodontal membrane causes metaplasia of the connective tissue and resultant initiation of formation of bone or dystrophic calcification. It has been suggested that the lesion may be caused by fibrosis of the granulation tissue [14].

Lesions involving the gingival soft tissues are rare compared to the lesions appearing within bone [12]. Mesquita RA found higher numbers of argyrophilic nucleolar organizer regions (AgNORs) and proliferating cell nuclear antigen-(PCNA-) positive cells in ossifying fibroma than in peripheral ossifying fibroma, indicating higher proliferative activity in ossifying fibroma [15]. X-ray diffraction analysis indicated that the mineral phase of both central and peripheral tissues consists of apatite crystals and that the crystallinity of the apatites might improve progressively with the development of the lesion, possibly to the same degree as that of bone apatite [16]. Peripheral ossifying fibroma tends to occur in the 2nd and 3rd decades of life, with peak prevalence between the ages of 10 and 19.

Eversole and Rovin [17] stated the similar sex and site predilection of pyogenic granuloma. Gardner [18] stated that peripheral ossifying fibroma, cellular connective tissue is so characteristic that a histologic diagnosis can be made with confidence, regardless of the presence or absence of calcification. Buchner and Hansen [19] hypothesized that early POF presents as ulcerated nodules with little calcification, allowing easy misdiagnosis as a pyogenic granuloma. Although it is also important to maintain a high index of suspicion, discussion with family members should be tactful to prevent undue distress during the waiting period between differential diagnosis and definitive histopathologic diagnosis. Because the clinical appearance of these various lesions can be remarkably similar, classification is based on their distinct histologic differences. The POF must be differentiated from the peripheral odontogenic fibroma (PODF) described by the World Health Organization [18, 19]. Histologically, the PODF has been defined as a fibroblastic neoplasm containing odontogenic epithelium [20]. Despite a preponderance of the literature supporting differentiation, some authors continue to argue that the POF (or peripheral cemento-ossifying fibroma) is the peripheral counterpart of the central cemento-ossifying fibroma [21]. The POF, as discovered in this case, is a focal, reactive, nonneoplastic tumour-like growth of soft tissue often arising from the interdental papilla [19]. It is a fairly common lesion, comprising nearly 3% of oral lesions biopsied in 1 study 1 approximately 1%-2% in other studies [21]. In 1993, S. Das and A. Das [8] obtained similar results, with 1.6% POFs among 2,370 intraoral biopsies.

POFs are believed to arise from gingival fibers of the periodontal ligament as hyperplastic growth of tissue that is unique to the gingival mucosa [17, 18]. This hypothesis is based on the fact that POFs arise exclusively on the gingiva, the subsequent proximity of the gingiva to the periodontal ligament, and the inverse correlation between age distribution of patients presenting with POF and the number of missing teeth with associated periodontal ligament [20]. The POF lesion is generally small and does not require imaging beyond radiographs [18]. Treatment consists of conservative surgical excision [20] and scaling of adjacent teeth [18]. Therefore, regular followup is required. Although peripheral ossifying fibroma is benign, reactive lesion, the recurrence rate is fairly high. Therefore, the patients are still under follow-up period.

5. Conclusions

POF is a slowly progressing lesion, the growth of which is generally limited. Many cases will progress for long periods before patients seek treatment because of the lack of symptoms associated with the lesion. A slowly growing pink soft-tissue nodule in the anterior maxilla of an adolescent should raise suspicion of a POF. Discussion of the differential diagnosis should be done tactfully to prevent unnecessary distress to the patient and family. Zhang and others [16] noted that cancer was included in the differential diagnosis in only 2% of cases. In the current case, the family experienced distress related to the suggestion of squamous cell carcinoma before referral for treatment and definitive diagnosis. Treatment consists of surgical excision, including the periosteum and scaling of adjacent teeth. Close postoperative followup is required because of the growth potential of incompletely removed lesions and the 8%–20% recurrence rate.

References

[1] R. Martin-Granizo, L. A. S. Cuellar, and F. Falahat, "Cemento-ossifying fibroma of the upper gingivae," *Otolaryngology*, vol. 122, no. 5, p. 775, 2000.

[2] C. A. Waldron, "Fibro-osseous lesions of the jaws," *Journal of Oral and Maxillofacial Surgery*, vol. 51, no. 8, pp. 828–835, 1993.

[3] J. C. De Vi Cente Rodriguez, S. G. Mendez, J. S. Zuazua, and B. Rubiales, "Tumors no odontogenicos de los maxilares: classification clinically diagnostic," *Medicina Oral*, vol. 12, pp. 83–93, 1997.

[4] J. N. Kenney, G. E. Kaugars, and L. M. Abbey, "Comparison between the peripheral ossifying fibroma and peripheral odontogenic fibroma," *Journal of Oral and Maxillofacial Surgery*, vol. 47, no. 4, pp. 378–382, 1989.

[5] J. D. Walters, J. K. Will, R. D. Hatfield, D. A. Cacchillo, and D. A. Raabe, "Excision and repair of the peripheral ossifying fibroma: a report of 3 cases," *Journal of Periodontology*, vol. 72, no. 7, pp. 939–944, 2001.

[6] D. A. Orkin and V. D. Amaidas, "Ossifying fibrous epulis. an abbreviated case report," *Oral Surgery, Oral Medicine, Oral Pathology*, vol. 57, no. 2, pp. 147–148, 1984.

[7] Z. E. S. Cuisia and R. B. Brannon, "Peripheral ossifying fibroma—a clinical evaluation of 134 pediatric cases," *Pediatric Dentistry*, vol. 23, no. 3, pp. 245–248, 2001.

[8] S. Das and A. K. Das, "A review of pediatric oral biopsies from a surgical pathology service in a dental school," *Pediatric Dentistry*, vol. 15, no. 3, pp. 208–211, 1993.

[9] B. W. Neville, D. D. Damm, C. M. Allen et al., *Oral and Maxillofacial Pathology*, W.B. Saunders, Philadelpia, Pa, USA, 1995.

[10] S. K. Kumar, S. Ram, M. G. Jorgensen, C. F. Shuler, and P. P. Sedghizadeh, "Multicentric peripheral ossifying fibroma," *Journal of oral science*, vol. 48, no. 4, pp. 239–243, 2006.

[11] L. R. Eversole, A. S. Leider, and K. Nelson, "Ossifying fibroma: a clinicopathologic study of sixty-four cases," *Oral Surgery Oral Medicine and Oral Pathology*, vol. 60, no. 5, pp. 505–511, 1985.

[12] Y. Endo, K. Uzawa, Y. Mochida et al., "Differential distribution of glycosaminoglycans in human cementifying fibroma and fibro-osseous lesions," *Oral Diseases*, vol. 9, no. 2, pp. 73–76, 2003.

[13] R. E. Marx and D. Stern, *Oral And Maxillofacial Pathology: A RationAle for Diagnosis and treatment*, Quintessence Publishing, Ill, USA, 2003.

[14] F. Kendrick and W. F. Waggoner, "Managing a peripheral ossifying fibroma," *Journal of Dentistry for Children*, vol. 63, no. 2, pp. 135–138, 1996.

[15] R. A. Mesquita, S. C. Orsini, M. Sousa, and N. S. De Araújo, "Proliferative activity in peripheral ossifying fibroma and ossifying fibroma," *Journal of Oral Pathology and Medicine*, vol. 27, no. 2, pp. 64–67, 1998.

[16] T. Aoba, C. Yoshioka, Y. Ogawa, and T. Yagi, "A study of the mineral phase of cementifying fibroma," *Journal of Oral Pathology*, vol. 7, no. 3, pp. 156–161, 1978.

[17] L. R. Eversole and S. Rovin, "Reactive lesions of the gingiva," *Journal of oral pathology*, vol. 1, no. 1, pp. 30–38, 1972.

[18] D. G. Gardner, "The peripheral odontogenic fibroma: an attempt at clarification," *Oral Surgery Oral Medicine and Oral Pathology*, vol. 54, no. 1, pp. 40–48, 1982.

[19] A. Buchner and L. S. Hansen, "The histomorphologic spectrum of peripheral ossifying fibroma," *Oral Surgery Oral Medicine and Oral Pathology*, vol. 63, no. 4, pp. 452–461, 1987.

[20] J. N. Kenney, G. E. Kaugars, and L. M. Abbey, "Comparison between the peripheral ossifying fibroma and peripheral odontogenic fibroma," *Journal of Oral and Maxillofacial Surgery*, vol. 47, no. 4, pp. 378–382, 1989.

[21] L. Feller, A. Buskin, and E. J. Raubenheimer, "Cemento-ossifying fibroma: case report and review of the literature," *Journal of the International Academy of Periodontology*, vol. 6, no. 4, pp. 131–135, 2004.

21

Oral Findings of Rothmund-Thomson Syndrome

Emin Murat Canger,[1] Peruze Çelenk,[2] İnci Devrim,[3] and Aysun Avşar[4]

[1] *Department of Oral and Maxillofacial Radiology, Faculty of Dentistry, Erciyes University, Melikgazi, 38039 Kayseri, Turkey*
[2] *Department of Oral and Maxillofacial Radiology, Faculty of Dentistry, Ondokuz Mayis University, 55139 Samsun, Turkey*
[3] *Department of Periodontology, Faculty of Dentistry, Ondokuz Mayis University, 55139 Samsun, Turkey*
[4] *Department of Pediatric Dentistry, Faculty of Dentistry, Ondokuz Mayis University, 55139 Samsun, Turkey*

Correspondence should be addressed to Emin Murat Canger; emcanger@erciyes.edu.tr

Academic Editors: R. V. Lo Vasco, S. Pezelj-Ribaric, M. W. Roberts, and N. H. Rohleder

Rothmund-Thomson syndrome (RTS) is an extremely rare genetic condition exhibiting some dermatological, craniofacial, ophthalmological, and central nervous system abnormalities. It has an autosomal, recessive inheritance and its signs begin at childhood. Essential dermatological alteration is poikilodermatosis. A large head with an frontal bossing and broad low nasal bridge has been described in patients with RTS. Bilateral juvenile cataract is a characteristic finding of patients with RTS. Most of the patients have been markedly short and the growth retardation has been proportionate. Mental retardation is a rare condition. An 11-year-old girl who had been previously diagnosed with RTS was consulted with a chief complaint of delaying in tooth eruption. Intraoral examination revealed median rhomboid glossitis in addition to hyperkeratotic tongue. This report aimed to not only present intraoral findings of RTS, but also to demonstrate the lingual findings of a patient with RTS.

1. Introduction

Rothmund-Thomson syndrome (RTS) is an autosomal recessive dermatosis which comes into existence in infancy with a characteristic facial rush (poikilodermatous) [1–4]. RTS was first introduced by Rothmund in 1863. The form of RTS with a genetic trait, showing hypogonadism and without cataracts, was introduced in 1923 by Thomson as "Poikiloderma congenitale." Those two similar syndromes were first mentioned as Rothmund-Thomson by Taylor in 1957 [1–4].

The diagnostic hallmark and heterogeneous clinical features include short stature, sparse scalp hair, sparse or absent eyelashes and/or eyebrows, juvenile cataracts, skeletal abnormalities, radial ray defects, and premature aging. RTS is extremely rare; although its exact prevalence is unknown, to date about 300 cases have been reported [1–4]. It is also suggested that RTS has a genetic trait [1, 4].

The first signs of RTS are of dermatological origin. The main dermatological alteration is poikilodermatosis, which is patch-like pigmentation which usually develops between the age of 3 and 6 months as erythema, with swelling and blistering on the face [1–4].

Ocular signs are accepted as minor signs specific to the Rothmund-type subset of RTS. Juvenile cataracts appearing bilaterally are a characteristic finding of the patient with RTS. They start rapidly and vision disappears within weeks. Other ocular findings are congenital glaucoma, corneal atrophy, colobomah atrophy in the iris and retina, microphthalmia, and photophobia [1–6].

Hypogonadism is evident in about 25% of patients with RTS. Additionally, the majority of female patients present with a menstrual disorder [1].

This case presented alterations in the tongue as well as the known intraoral findings typical of RTS.

2. Case Report

An 11-year-old girl attended our department with the chief complaint of delayed eruption of her teeth. From her history, it was learned that deciduous teeth extraction had been performed, and no artificial replacement had occurred.

Her medical history revealed that she was born prematurely. The patient's family members were normal; no

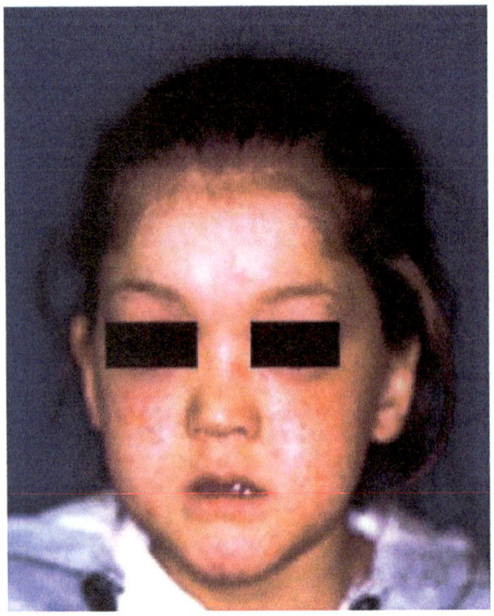

Figure 1: Telangiectatic appearance of the face of patient.

consanguinity or blood incompatibility was reported. In addition, her sister was normal. She had a developmental retardation and was 1-2 years behind her chronological age. Her pediatricians had diagnosed RTS when the patient was 2 years old. At the date of attendance, she was suffering from splenomegaly and lacrimal obliteration.

Our patient had pronounced difficulty in walking and speaking. Extraoral examination revealed exophthalmia and xerophthalmia. Telangiectasia of the face and compressed nose were found (Figure 1). Dermatological findings included macular lesions on the forearm and the front part of the chest, as well as hyperkeratotic depigmented areas on the palms and foot (Figures 2(a), 2(b), and 2(c)).

Intraoral examination disclosed hyperemic and edematous gingiva with hyperplasic papilla. There was evident oligodontia; only the teeth charted below were present in the patient's mouth (Figure 3(a)):

6 3 1	1 3 6
6 2 1	1 2 6

There were widespread carious lesions in all present teeth and coronal destruction due to caries in all permanent first molars (Figures 3(b) and 3(c)).

The following radiograms were obtained: panoramic full mouth and periapical, lateral, cephalometric hand and wrist. Radiographic examination of the hand and wrist radiograms revealed that the bone age of the patient was consistent with the age of 8. The panoramic and full mouth periapical radiograms revealed neither impacted teeth nor germs of teeth. The alveolar bone, periodontal membranes, and lamina dura of the present teeth were radiographically normal (Figure 4).

In addition to the findings described above, median rhomboid glossitis and hyperkeratosis were evident on the patient's tongue (Figure 5).

The patient was originally referred to the periodontology department seeking therapy for gingivitis and later to pediatric dentistry for restorative procedures and construction of a space retainer. Periodontal and restorative treatments were completed and oral hygiene controls are in progress.

3. Discussion

In the Rothmund type of RTS, there are juvenile cataracts; in the Thomson type of RTS, this finding is absent [1]. In our case, although lacrimal obliteration was present as an ophthalmological finding, the cataracts were absent, so the patient can be accepted as a member of the Thomson type of RTS.

It is unclear whether RTS has a sex predilection. Although the patient in our case was female and some research has suggested that RTS is more prevalent in women, other researches found male predominance, so sex predominance has not yet been proven. Further, although certain gene mutations may exist within defined populations, no ethnic predominance has yet been described [1, 2].

Growth delay and the resulting short stature are among the major clinical signs of RTS. Patients are proportionally small; hands and feet are also smaller than normal. Furthermore, bilateral absence of metacarpal and phalanx in the thumbs, deformity of the radius and ulna, and agenesis of the radius are present. Kyphoscoliosis has also been reported. Additionally, osteoporosis, cystic areas resembling fibrous dysplasia, and osteogenesis imperfecta may also be seen [1, 6]. Our patient was proportionally small.

In approximately 50% of RTS cases, hair, eyebrows, and eyelashes are scarce [1–6]. Patients with RTS have a large head with a frontal bossing and a saddle nose. Microcephaly and a triangular face may also be seen [1, 2, 4].

Mental retardation is a rare condition which is seen in approximately 10% of RTS patients. According to some researchers, cases with advanced growth retardation, skeletal anomalies, and ectodermal dysplasia, but without cataracts, constitute a subgroup of the syndrome, and mental retardation is seen prevalently in this subgroup [1, 4–6]. Since cooperation was easily obtained from our patient and her education level was consistent with her coequals, mental retardation was not thought to be present in this case.

Anomalies of teeth were first described by Rothmund in his original article. Overall incidence of dental anomalies has been estimated at between 27% and 59% of cases. Intraoral findings of RTS are listed as microdontia, rudimentary, or hypoplastic teeth, multiple crown malformations, short and conical teeth, increase in prevalence of caries, malocclusion, hypodontia/oligodontia or hyperdontia, ectopic eruption, and delay in eruption. Bifid uvula also has been reported [1, 3, 5, 7]. Our case presented oligodontia. The crowns and roots of teeth were normal. Additionally, widespread and advanced carious lesions were present on both permanent first molars.

Our patient's gingiva was hyperemic and edematous, with hyperplasic papilla. In studies of the periodontal tissue

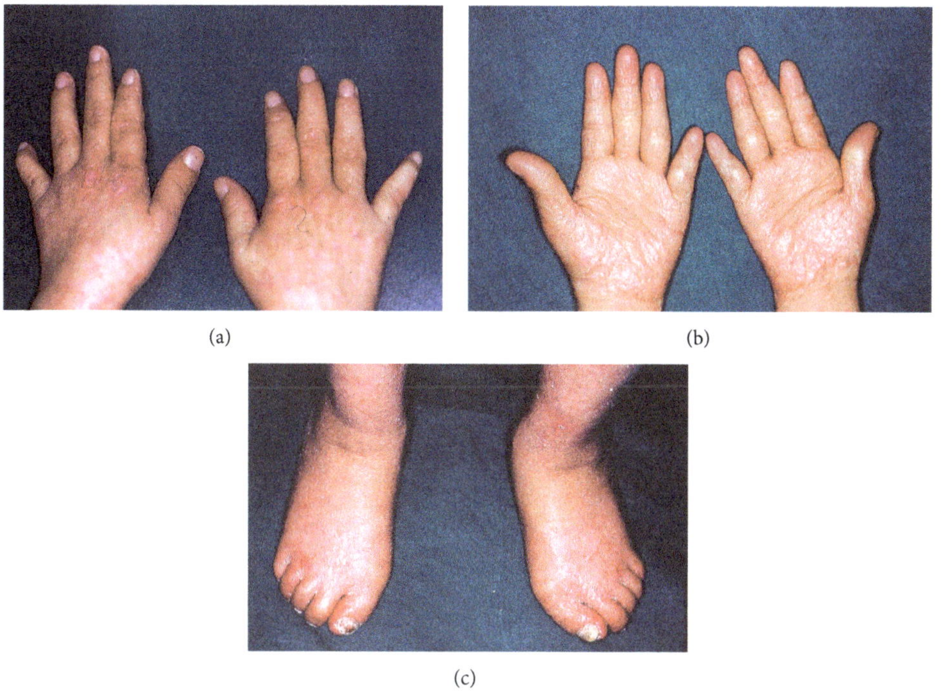

FIGURE 2: (a) The appearance of the outer surface of patient's hand. (b) The hyperkeratotic appearance of the palm. (c) The hyperkeratotic appearance of the foot.

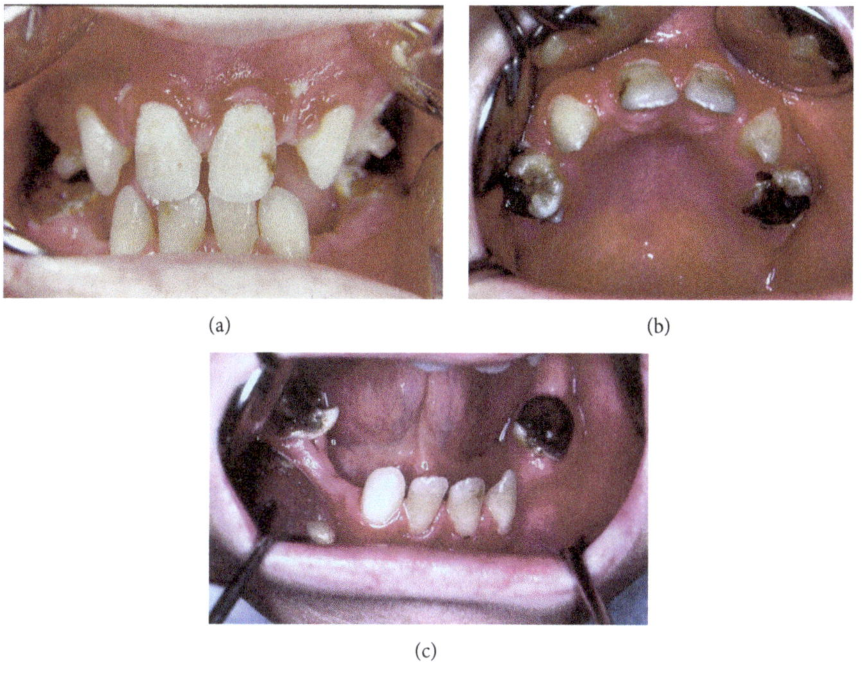

FIGURE 3: (a) The appearance of the edematous gingival and hyperplasic papillae. (b) The appearance of the maxilla reveals that only right and left first molars, canine, and central incisor teeth are present. Also widespread caries are seen on first molars. (c) The appearance of the mandible reveals that only right and left first molars, lateral incisor, and central incisor teeth are present. Also widespread caries are seen on first molars.

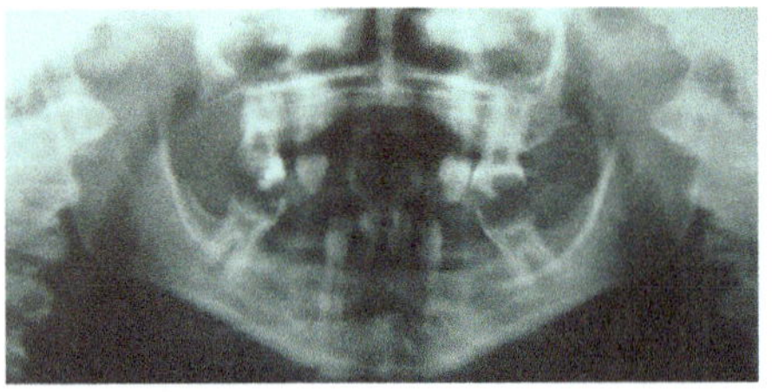

Figure 4: Oligodontia is clearly observed on panoramic radiograph.

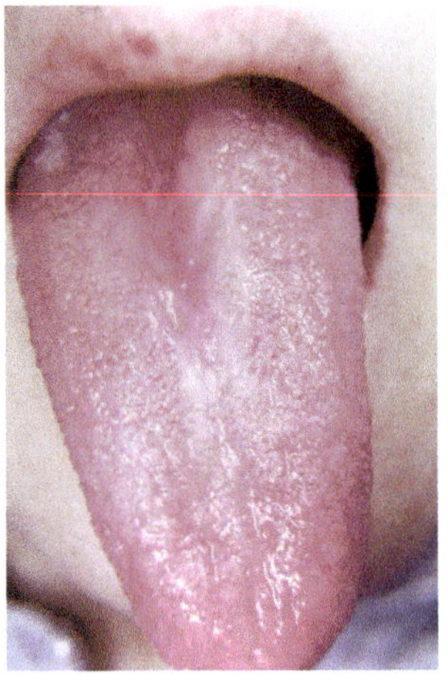

Figure 5: Median rhomboid glossitis on the dorsum of tongue.

destruction in RTS, researchers suggested that the destruction may be related to apoptosis disorders. Apoptosis is a process which removes dysfunctional and undesirable cells from tissues and differs from necrosis. Apoptosis provides a balance between cell proliferation and cell death to achieve growth and proliferation of normal tissues, while exiguous or extreme apoptosis results in death [3].

Cutaneous and noncutaneous malignancies are among the complications of RTS. Osteosarcoma is the most common noncutaneous malignancy, followed by fibrosarcoma, parathyroid adenoma, Hodgkin's sarcoma, and gastric sarcoma. Cutaneous squamous-cell carcinomas have also been reported, as well as noncutaneous squamous-cell carcinoma of the tongue [8].

Median rhomboid glossitis (central papillary atrophy) is a form of erythematous candidiasis which is seen as a well-demarcated erythematous zone in midline, posterior, and dorsal region of the tongue. As its etiology, embryological fault in the fusion of the two lateral processes of the embryological tongue, and covering the central structure from the first and second branchial arches, the tuberculum impar. Generally it is asymptomatic and needs no treatment, but if there is discomfort or irritation, antifungal agents will be administered[9, 10]. Any cases of median rhomboid glossitis in conjunction with RTS couldnot be found. There is only one case of squamous-cell carcinoma of the tongue in a patient of RTS which was written by Marín-Bertolín et al. [8]. Differential diagnosis of RTS is very difficult due to the presence of some identical signs in other syndromes (e.g., Werner, Cockayne, Bloom, and Kindler-Gottner (*Acrogenia*)) and some other poikilodermatosis (e.g., geoderma dysplastica, hereditary sclerosing poikiloderma, dyskeratosis congenita, and xeroderma pigmentosum) [1, 2].

References

[1] R. J. Gorlin, M. M. Cohen, and R. C. M. Hennekam, *Syndromes of the Head and Neck*, Oxford University Press, New York, NY, USA, 4th edition, 2001.

[2] L. Larizza, G. Roversi, and L. Volpi, "Rothmund-thomson syndrome," *Orphanet Journal of Rare Diseases*, vol. 5, no. 1, article 2, 2010.

[3] M. C. Haytaç, H. Öztunç, U.Ö. Mete, and M. Kaya, "Rothmund-Thomson syndrome: a case report," *Oral Surgery, Oral Medicine, Oral Pathology, Oral Radiology, and Endodontics*, vol. 94, pp. 479–484, 2002.

[4] E. Pianigiani, G. De Aloe, A. Andreassi, P. Rubegni, and M. Fimiani, "Rothmund-Thomson syndrome (Thomson-type) and myelodysplasia," *Pediatric Dermatology*, vol. 18, no. 5, pp. 422–425, 2001.

[5] O. Güler, M. Aydın, S. Uğraş, E. Kışlı, and A. Metin, "Rothmund-Thomson syndrome associated with esophageal stenosis: a case report," *Surgery Today*, vol. 28, no. 8, pp. 839–842, 1998.

[6] B. Kerr, G. S. Ashcroft, D. Scott, M. A. Horan, M. W. J. Ferguson, and D. Donnai, "Rothmund-Thomson syndrome: two case reports show heterogeneous cutaneous abnormalities, an association with genetically programmed ageing changes, and increased chromosomal radiosensitivity," *Journal of Medical Genetics*, vol. 33, no. 11, pp. 928–934, 1996.

[7] T. D. Daley, G. P. Wysocki, and R. N. Bohay, "Osteopathia striata, short stature, cataracts, and microdontia: a new syndrome? a case report," *Oral Surgery, Oral Medicine, Oral Pathology, Oral Radiology, and Endodontics*, vol. 81, no. 3, pp. 356–360, 1996.

[8] S. Marín-Bertolín, J. Amorrortu-Velayos, and A. Aliaga Boniche, "Squamous cell carcinoma of the tongue in a patient with Rothmund-Thomson syndrome," *British Journal of Plastic Surgery*, vol. 51, no. 8, pp. 646–648, 1998.

[9] B. D. Neville, D. D. Damm, C. M. Allen, and J. E. Bouquot, *Oral and Maxillofacial Pathology*, Saunders, Philadelphia, Pa, USA, 2nd edition, 2002.

[10] N. Yarom, U. Cantony, and M. Gorsky, "Prevalence of fissured tongue, geographic tongue and median rhomboid glossitis among Israeli adults of different ethnic origins," *Dermatology*, vol. 209, no. 2, pp. 88–94, 2004.

22

Typical Radiographic Findings of Dentin Dysplasia Type 1b with Dental Fluorosis

S. Venkata Suman,[1] Raviraj Jayam,[1] B. Vijay Kumar,[1] Suresh Dirasantchu,[1] K. Venkata Suneel Kumar,[2] and Sameeulla Sk[1]

[1] *Department of Oral Medicine and Radiology, CKS Theja Dental College, Hospital and Research Centre, Tirupati, Andhra Pradesh 517501, India*
[2] *Department of Oral Medicine and Radiology, Narayana Dental College and Hospital, Nellore, Andhra Pradesh 524001, India*

Correspondence should be addressed to S. Venkata Suman; sri_venkat1@yahoo.co.in

Academic Editors: M. A. Chinelatti, J. C. de la Macorra, C. Kitamura, and G. Spagnuolo

Dentin dysplasia is a rare inherited autosomal dominant disorder characterized by rootless teeth. We hereby report a case of dentin dysplasia type 1b with typical radiographic findings: short and blunt roots, pulpal obliteration, horizontal/crescent shaped radiolucencies in pulp chambers, and multiple periapical radiolucencies. However, the present case did not show the autosomal dominant pattern of inheritance and the patient also exhibited concurrent dental fluorosis, transposition of 13 and 14, and multiple cusps in maxillary first molars. Moreover, on careful review of previously documented cases of radiographs of dentin dysplasia, the horizontal/crescent shaped radiolucencies in pulp chambers are a rare finding, which is characteristically seen in the present case.

1. Introduction

Dentin dysplasia (DD) is an autosomal dominant hereditary disturbance in dentin formation, which may present with either mobile teeth or pain associated with spontaneous dental abscesses or cysts. It is a rare anomaly of unknown etiology that affects approximately one patient in every 100,000 [1]. The condition was first described by Ballschmiede, but it was Rushton who termed the condition dentinal dysplasia. This condition is rarely encountered in dental practice. In 1972, Witkop Jr. [2] classified DD into two types: radicular DD as type I and coronal DD as type II. In type I, both the deciduous and permanent dentitions are affected. The crowns of the teeth appear clinically normal in morphology, but defects in dentin formation and pulp obliteration are present. Radiographic examination is important for the identification of DD type I. In the coronal type, the pulps are enlarged and are described as having a "thistle tube" appearance, in permanent dentition. In the deciduous dentition, coronal dentin dysplasia bears a resemblance to dentinogenesis imperfecta type II.

The present case is dentin dysplasia type 1b with typical radiographic findings: short and blunt roots, pulpal obliteration, horizontal/crescent shaped radiolucencies in pulp chambers, and multiple periapical radiolucencies.

Though dentin dysplasia is transmitted as autosomal dominant disorder, the present case did not show the autosomal dominant pattern of inheritance and the patient also exhibited concurrent dental fluorosis, transposition of 13 and 14, and multiple cusps in maxillary first molars. Moreover, on careful review of previously documented cases of radiographs of dentin dysplasia, the horizontal/crescent shaped radiolucencies in pulp chambers are a rare finding, which is characteristically seen in the present case.

2. Case Report

A 16-year-old male patient presented with a chief complaint of partial edentulousness due to early shedding of teeth. Patient did znot give any history of trauma. Extraoral

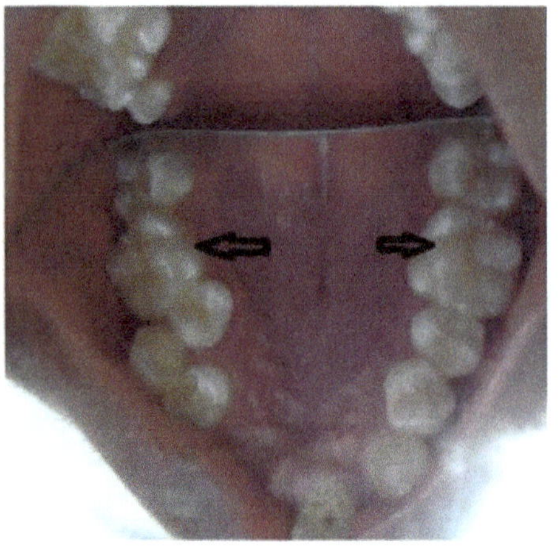

FIGURE 1: Intraoral photograph showing transposition between 13 and 14 and multiple cusps in occlusal surface of the 1st maxillary molars (black arrows).

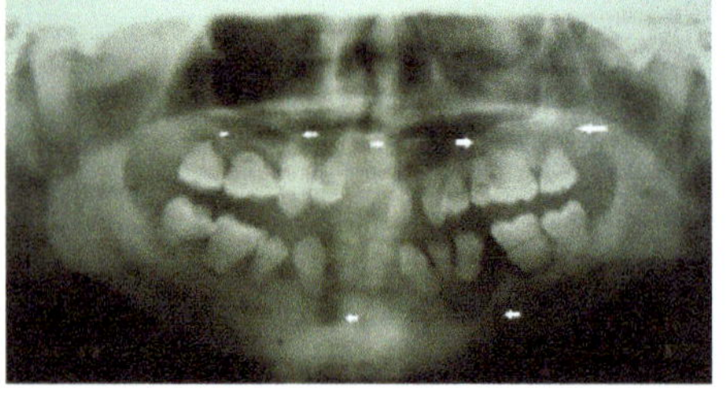

FIGURE 2: Cropped panoramic radiograph showing generalized short and tapered roots, pulpal obliteration, horizontal/crescent shaped pulpal remnants in pulp chambers, and multiple periapical radiolucencies (white arrows).

examination did not reveal any abnormality. On intraoral examination, teeth present were

17 16 15 13 14 22 23 24 25 26 27

47 46 45 43 33 34 35 36 37

The majority of the teeth exhibited grade I mobility except for 35 which had grade II mobility. The crowns of teeth showed brownish yellow discoloration with white chalky areas, corresponding to dental fluorosis. The maxillary first molars showed multiple cusps and there was transposition of 13 and 14 (Figure 1). Patient was subjected to panoramic radiograph and full mouth intraoral periapical radiographs. The radiographs revealed features like generalized short and blunt roots, pulpal obliteration, horizontal/crescent shaped pulpal remnants in pulp chambers, and multiple periapical radiolucencies (Figures 2 and 3(a)–3(d)). With the above radiographic findings, this case was diagnosed as dentin dysplasia type 1b. Patient was treated conservatively by advising dietary and oral hygiene instructions, oral prophylaxis, and removable partial denture fabrication for esthetic purpose.

3. Discussion

Dentin dysplasia is a rare disorder which is thought to arise due to abnormal differentiation or function of the ectomesenchymally derived odontoblasts [1]. Witkop attributed the ectopic dentin formation to the displacement of internal cells of the developing dental organ and proliferation in the dentin papilla [2]. Logan et al. proposed that obliteration of pulpal space could be due to abnormal degeneration and calcification in dental papilla [3].

Dentin dysplasia is inherited as an autosomal dominant trait. However, in this case none of the family members exhibited radiographic features of dentin dysplasia. This indicated that the patient is a first generation sufferer. Such similar incidence was also reported by Toomarian et al. [4].

Carroll et al. [5] subclassified dentin dysplasia into four types. In type 1a, there are no pulp chambers and root formation, and there are frequent periapical radiolucencies; type 1b has a single small horizontally oriented and crescent shaped pulp, and roots are only a few millimeters in length and there are frequent periapical radiolucencies; in type 1c, there are two horizontal or vertical and crescent shaped pulpal remnants surrounded by a central island of dentin and with significant but shortened root length and variable periapical radiolucencies; in type 1d, there are visible pulp chambers and canal with near normal root length and large pulp stones that are located in the coronal portion of the canal and create a localized bulging in the canal, as well as root constriction of the pulp canal apical to the stone and few periapical radiolucencies.

The present case exhibited classical radiographic features of type 1b. Though the previous literature has documented considerable number of cases of dentin dysplasia type 1,

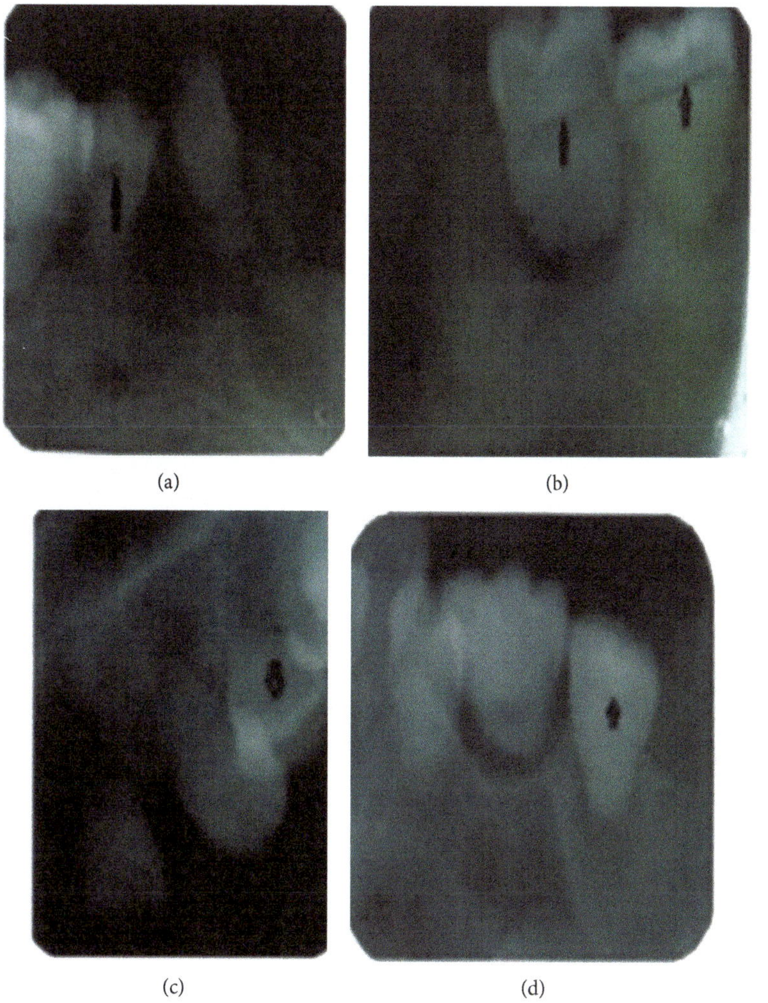

FIGURE 3: Intraoral periapical radiographs showing horizontal/crescent shaped pulpal remnants in pulp chambers (black arrows).

very few of them had successfully demonstrated the horizontal/crescent shaped pulp in their radiographs. Our case clearly demonstrates this feature in addition to other radiographic findings like short roots, pulpal obliterations, and multiple periapical radiolucencies.

The present case also showed other associated clinical findings like dental fluorosis, transposition of 13 and 14, and multiple cusps in maxillary first molars. Dental fluorosis in the present case is attributed to the fact that the patient belonged to the geographical area which is endemic to fluorosis.

Management of dentin dysplasia has always been a challenging task to the dentists. Followup and routine conservative treatment are often advised. Maintenance of periodontal health through adherence to oral hygiene instructions is vital to the survival of mobile teeth. Endodontic treatment is contraindicated in teeth with total obliteration of root canals and pulp chambers [6].

In conclusion, dentin dysplasia is a rare genetic disorder. The present case exhibited characteristic radiographic findings along with other associated clinical findings like dental fluorosis, transposition of 13 and 14, and multiple cusps in maxillary first molars. Also this case did not show the expected pattern of inheritance. Cases of dentin dysplasia have to be treated conservatively to prevent premature exfoliation of teeth.

References

[1] M. Melnick, L. S. Levin, and J. Brady, "Dentin dysplasia type I: a scanning electron microscopic analysis of the primary dentition," *Oral Surgery Oral Medicine and Oral Pathology*, vol. 50, no. 4, pp. 335–340, 1980.

[2] C. J. Witkop Jr., "Hereditary defects of dentin," *Dental Clinics of North America*, vol. 19, no. 1, pp. 25–45, 1975.

[3] J. Logan, H. Becks, S. Silverman Jr., and J. J. Pindborg, "Dentinal dysplasia," *Oral Surgery, Oral Medicine, Oral Pathology*, vol. 15, no. 3, pp. 317–333, 1962.

[4] L. Toomarian, F. Mashhadiabbas, M. Mirkarimi, and L. Mehrdad, "Dentin dysplasia type I: a case report and review of the literature," *Journal of Medical Case Reports*, vol. 4, article 1, 2010.

[5] M. K. O. Carroll, W. K. Duncan, and T. M. Perkins, "Dentin dysplasia: review of the literature and a proposed subclassification based on radiographic findings," *Oral Surgery Oral Medicine and Oral Pathology*, vol. 72, no. 1, pp. 119–125, 1991.

[6] N. E. Steidler, B. G. Radden, and P. C. Reade, "Dentinal dysplasia: a clinicopathological study of eight cases and review of the literature," *British Journal of Oral and Maxillofacial Surgery*, vol. 22, no. 4, pp. 274–286, 1984.

23

Florid Cementoosseous Dysplasia: A Rare Case Report

Mehmet Fatih Şentürk,[1] Recep Kestane,[2] Elif Naz Yakar,[3] and Ahmet Keskin[2]

[1] *Department of Oral and Maxillofacial Surgery, Faculty of Dentistry, University of Süleyman Demirel, East Campus, 32260 Çünür Isparta, Turkey*
[2] *Department of Oral and Maxillofacial Surgery, Faculty of Dentistry, University of Ankara, Ankara, Turkey*
[3] *Department of Dentomaxillofacial Radiology, Faculty of Dentistry, University of Ankara, Ankara, Turkey*

Correspondence should be addressed to Mehmet Fatih Şentürk; fatih.senturk84@gmail.com

Academic Editors: R. A. de Mesquita and C. S. Farah

Florid cementoosseous dysplasia (FCOD) is a rare, benign, fibroosseous, and multifocal dysplastic lesion of the jaw that consists of cellular fibrous connective tissue with bone and cementum-like tissue. FCOD is most commonly found in middle-aged black women, is generally asymptomatic, and is usually detected during radiological examination. FCOD associated with multiple impacted teeth and bone expansion is a very rare phenomenon, and there are only a few familial cases reported in the literature. In this report, a 35-year-old male Turkish patient is presented who was diagnosed with nonfamilial FCOD from clinical, radiological, and histopathological findings. To our knowledge this is the first case of the nonfamilial FCOD with this many impacted teeth and severely expanded bones.

1. Introduction

Florid cementoosseous dysplasia (FCOD) is a benign, fibroosseous, and multifocal dysplastic lesion of the jaw that consists of cellular fibrous connective tissue with bone and cementum-like tissue [1]. FCOD was previously known as gigantiform cementoma, multiple cementoossifying fibroma, sclerosing osteitis, multiple enostosis, and sclerotic cemental masses of the jaws. It was first comprehensively described by Melrose et al. [2]. This lesion is most commonly found in middle-aged black women, although it also may occur in Caucasians and Asians [3, 4]. The etiology of FCOD is unknown, and there is no clear explanation for its gender and racial predilections [5]. Clinically these lesions are often asymptomatic. Symptoms such as dull pain or drainage are almost always associated with exposure of the sclerotic calcified masses in the oral cavity [2, 4, 5]. Radiographically, the lesions appear as multiple sclerotic masses located in two or more quadrants, usually in the tooth-bearing regions. They are often confined within the alveolar bone [6].

A search of the literature showed that only a few cases have been reported concerning the familial form of FCOD associated with multiple impacted teeth. However, no examples were found of the nonfamilial form of FCOD associated with multiple impacted teeth. In this study, a very rare case of nonfamilial FCOD associated with multiple impacted teeth and bone expansion is presented and the current literature regarding this lesion reviewed.

2. Case Presentation

A 35-year-old male patient was referred to the Department of Oral and Maxillofacial Surgery, Faculty of Dentistry, at Ankara University, with severe swelling, notably in the maxilla. The patient had no systemic symptoms. Clinical examination revealed expansion of the bone and partially edentulous areas on both the maxilla and mandible. Several decayed roots were discovered in both jaws, and some of the erupted teeth were malposed due to bone expansion. The overlying gingiva and mucosa were normal with no clinical signs of inflammation; the patient stated that he had never experienced pain in any part of his jaws (Figures 1 and 2). The familial history was taken and some of the family members were examined, but no familial aspects of the disease could be established. Radiological examination revealed multiple,

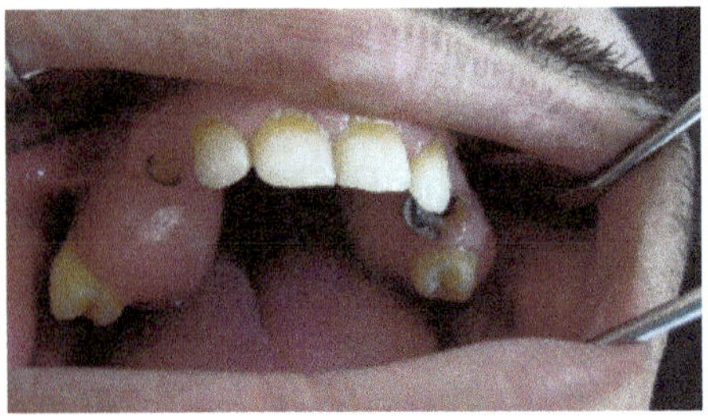

FIGURE 1: Preoperative view of the maxilla with bone expansions intraorally.

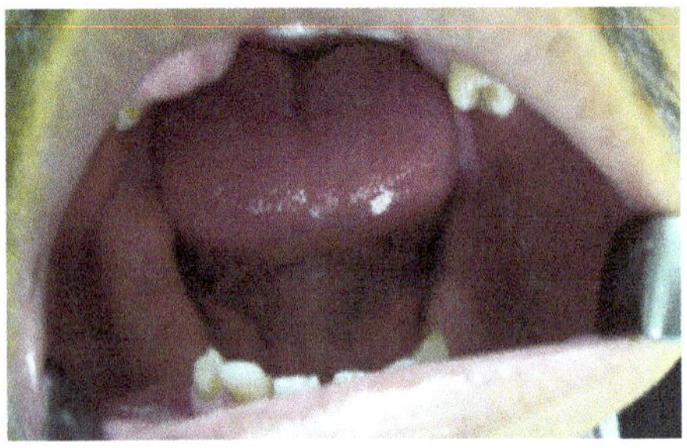

FIGURE 2: Preoperative mandible intraorally.

diffuse, lobular radioopacities throughout the edentulous areas of the maxilla and mandible with multiple impacted teeth. Most of the impacted teeth seemed to be pushed through the periphery of the jaws by the expansile lesions (Figure 3). The serum alkaline phosphatase level was within normal limits, and a scintigraphic bone scan showed no increased osteoblastic activity on the other bony formations (Figure 4). Thus, the differential diagnosis of FCOD was made rather than Paget's disease or Gardner's syndrome. However, the case was extraordinary in many ways and surgery was required to allow prosthetic rehabilitation. A bone biopsy was performed to support the initial diagnosis. Histopathologically, rounded cement bone-like structures, showing irregular lamellation, were seen in fibrous stroma consisting of fibroblastic cells (Figure 5). When clinical, radiological, and histopathological findings were evaluated together, the definitive diagnosis was made of FCOD. Cortical bone expansions were recontoured in two operations under local anesthesia. No impacted teeth were extracted due to their location. The remaining roots and malposed teeth were extracted, and the removed bony segments were sent for histopathological examination (Figure 6). Histopathological findings confirmed the diagnosis of FCOD once again. The postoperative course was uneventful. A partial, removable prosthesis was fabricated 1 month after the surgery. Care was taken to avoid any trauma as a result of the prosthesis. Routine controls were performed every 6 months. The postoperative 1-year course was uneventful (Figures 7, 8, 9, and 10). The patient has been followed up for 16 months with no complication. Followup is continuing.

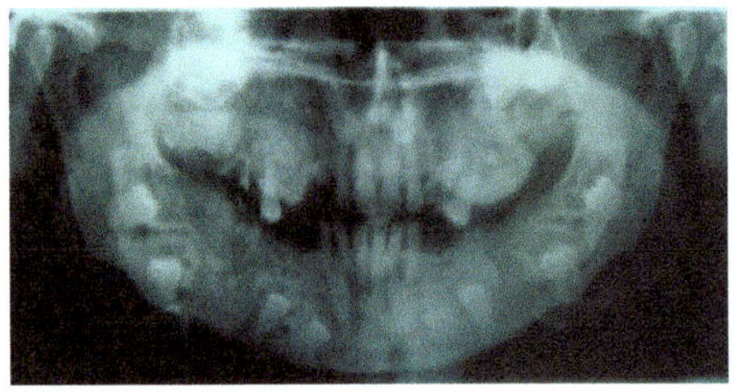

FIGURE 3: Preoperative panoramic radiograph showing multiple impacted teeth and bone expansion.

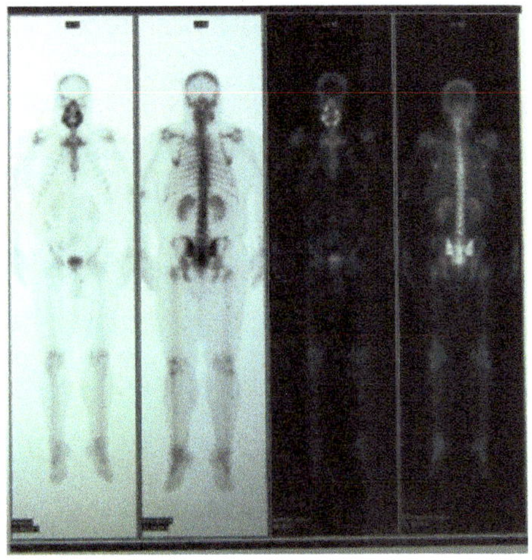

FIGURE 4: Scintigraphic bone scans showing no increased osteoblastic activity on the other bony formations.

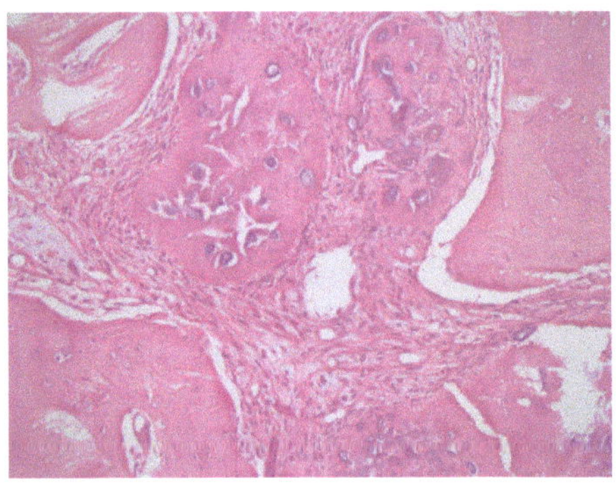

FIGURE 5: Histopathologically rounded cement bone-like structures showing irregular lamellation are seen in fibrous stroma consisting of fibroblastic cells (HEx100).

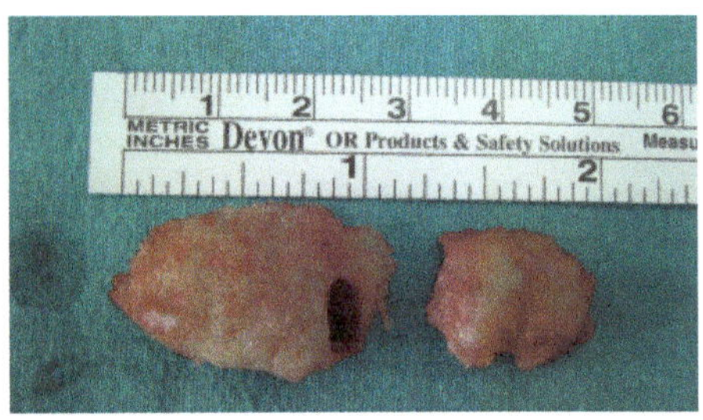

FIGURE 6: Bony segments removed from maxilla.

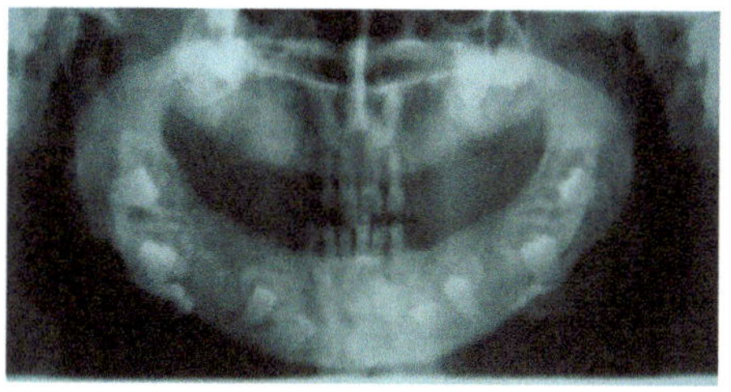

FIGURE 7: Postoperative panoramic radiograph.

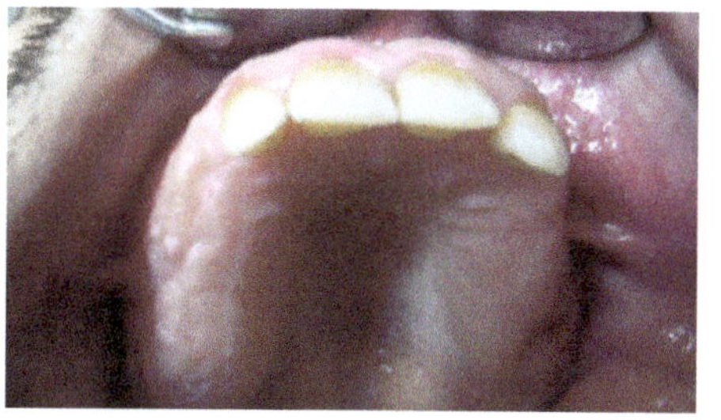

FIGURE 9: Postoperative 1-year view of maxillary arch intraorally.

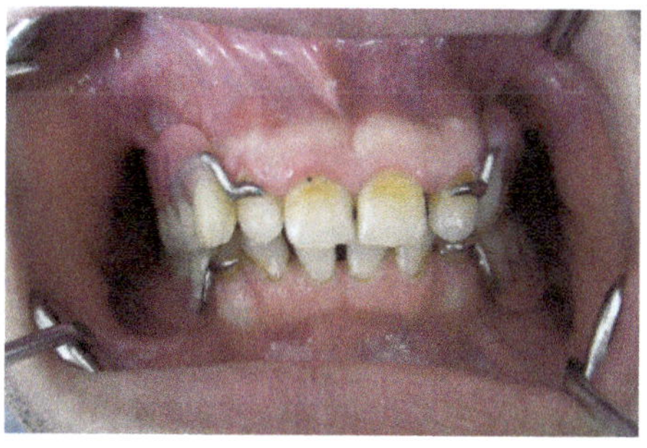

FIGURE 8: Postoperative 1-year view of occlusion with removable partial prosthesis.

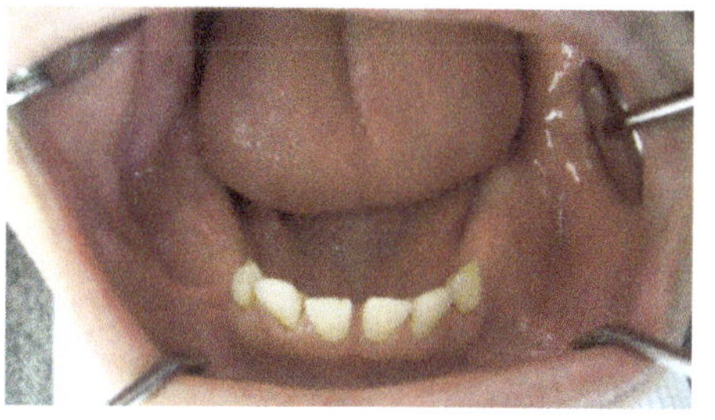

FIGURE 10: Postoperative 1-year view of mandibular arch intraorally.

3. Discussion

FCOD refers to a set of radiolucent-radiopaque periapical and interradicular lesions involving the mandible bilaterally and sometimes the maxilla. It is basically an extended form of periapical cementoosseous dysplasia. These lesions are also asymptomatic dysmorphic bone-cementum complexes. Radiographs show large, radiolucent, mixed, or most often, dense radiopaque masses, limited to the periapical alveolar bone. They do not involve the inferior border, except through direct focal extension, and do not occur in the rami [7]. The present case was a severe form of FCOD, involving all four quadrants, including the angle and the basal bone in some areas of the mandible.

FCOD typically occurs in middle-aged black women [8]. Melrose et al. [2] reported a study with 34 cases of similar lesions, of which 32 were black women (in a predominantly Caucasian population) with a mean age of 42. The present case of a 35-year-old Turkish man may represent the first of such a rare combination of features being reported in the English and Turkish language literature.

FCOD should be differentiated from Paget's disease, chronic diffuse osteomyelitis, and Gardner's syndrome. FCOD has no other skeletal changes, skin tumors, or dental anomalies. Thus FCOD can be differentiated from Gardner's syndrome. Paget's disease is polyostotic and shows raised alkaline phosphatase level which is not a consistent feature of FCOD. Chronic diffuse sclerosing osteomyelitis is not confined to tooth-bearing areas. It is a primary inflammatory condition of the mandible, with cyclic episodes of unilateral pain and swelling. The affected lesion of the mandible exhibits a diffuse opacity with poorly defined borders [9].

FCODs are most often painless and detected through routine radiographs [10, 11]. Their presence is not usually associated with expansion, but rare cases may show mild expansion [7]. FCOD affecting multiple family members appears to be quite uncommon. There are only a few reports in which the hereditary nature of the lesion could be demonstrated [12–15]. Unlike the sporadic cases, the familial form is characterized by more expansile lesions, which may recur after surgery, and it tends to occur in younger subjects. In all of the familial cases reported, FCOD appears to be inherited as an autosomal dominant trait with variable phenotypic expression [12, 14–16]. Toffanin et al. [17] reported a case of FCOD affecting multiple family members. Some of the affected subjects had multiple impacted teeth, and one also had marked expansion of the symphyseal region. That patient underwent resection and reconstruction of the mandibular body with a free osteomyocutaneous fibula graft. In the present case, no familial aspects of the disease could be established. The case was also painless, but it showed several impacted teeth and marked expansion in both jaws. The nonfamilial form of FCOD very rarely shows such a combination.

Multiple impacted teeth are a rare phenomenon in cases diagnosed as FCOD. A search of the literature showed only two reports of FCOD associated with multiple impacted teeth. Toffanin et al. [17] reported 4 cases of FCOD with multiple impacted teeth; 12 were the highest number of impacted teeth among those cases. Srivastava et al. [18] also reported a case of FCOD associated with multiple impacted teeth. Seventeen impacted teeth were recorded in this case. In both of these reports, the FCOD was familial in nature. However, in our case 15 impacted teeth were seen, and there were no familial aspects. To our knowledge, our case has the maximum number of impacted teeth among nonfamilial FCOD cases reported thus far.

Normally, the diagnosis of FCOD in the jaws is made through the clinical and radiographic features [19]. In the asymptomatic patient, it is probably wise to keep the patient under observation without surgical intervention. A biopsy is not required to confirm the diagnosis as this is usually established radiographically. It is not normally justified to surgically remove these lesions, as the surgery involved can be extensive. Instead, followup and recontouring are recommended when cortical expansion occurs [20]. Whenever surgical treatment is planned, the lack of vascularity of the lesion and increased risk of osteomyelitis should be considered. The affected area undergoes changes from normal vascular bone into an avascular cementum-like lesion. Furthermore, complete removal of necrotic tissue may result in a large discontinuity defect [21]. However, in lesions causing pain and disturbance, surgery and the risks it entails might be necessary for adequate treatment. However, recontouring should be the treatment of choice where there is only cortical expansion and mucosal perforation due to the cementoosseous lesions [22]. Our case had cortical expansion in all four quadrants making prosthetic rehabilitation impossible. As a result we decided to perform recontouring surgery to obtain adequate interocclusal space for prosthesis. We performed a bone biopsy conservatively to confirm the initial diagnosis of FCOD. Histologic examination supported our clinical and radiological diagnosis. Subsequently, we performed surgery in all four quadrants in two sessions under local anesthesia.

In conclusion, bone expansion and multiple impacted teeth are very rarely seen in nonfamilial forms of FCOD. If the lesions and impacted teeth are asymptomatic, it is wise to avoid surgical intervention. However, if the expansion makes prosthetic rehabilitation impossible in edentulous jaws, recontouring surgery may be the best choice to obtain sufficient space for prosthesis.

References

[1] T. Wakasa, N. Kawai, H. Aiga, and K. Kishi, "Management of florid cemento-osseous dysplasia of the mandible producing solitary bone cyst: report of a case," *Journal of Oral and Maxillofacial Surgery*, vol. 60, no. 7, pp. 832–835, 2002.

[2] R. J. Melrose, A. M. Abrams, and B. G. Mills, "Florid osseous dysplasia. A clinical pathologic study of thirty four cases," *Oral Surgery Oral Medicine and Oral Pathology*, vol. 41, no. 1, pp. 62–82, 1976.

[3] M. Miyake and S. Nagahata, "Florid cemento-osseous dysplasia report of a case," *International Journal of Oral and Maxillofacial Surgery*, vol. 28, no. 1, pp. 56–57, 1999.

[4] C. A. Waldron, "Fibro-osseous lesions of the jaws," *Journal of Oral and Maxillofacial Surgery*, vol. 43, no. 4, pp. 249–262, 1985.

[5] I. Beylouni, P. Farge, J. F. Mazoyer, and J. L. Coudert, "Florid cemento-osseous dysplasia: report of a case documented with computed tomography and 3D imaging," *Oral Surgery, Oral Medicine, Oral Pathology, Oral Radiology, and Endodontics*, vol. 85, no. 6, pp. 707–711, 1998.

[6] D. D. Damm and J. E. Fantasia, "Multifocal mixed radiolucencies. Florid cemento-osseous dysplasia," *General Dentistry*, vol. 49, no. 5, pp. 461–538, 2001.

[7] R. E. Marx and D. Stern, *Oral and Maxillofacial Pathology: A Rationale for Diagnosis and Treatment*, Quintessence, London, UK, 2004.

[8] S.-T. Ong and C.-H. Siar, "Florid cemento-osseous dysplasia in a young Chinese man. Case report," *Australian Dental Journal*, vol. 42, no. 6, pp. 404–408, 1997.

[9] J. H. Kim, B. C. Song, S. H. Kim, and Y. S. Park, "Clinical, radiographic and histological findings of florid cemento-osseous dysplasia: a case report," *Imaging Science in Dentistry*, vol. 41, pp. 139–142, 2011.

[10] G. Minhas, T. Hodge, and D. S. Gill, "Orthodontic treatment and cemento-osseous dysplasia: a case report," *Journal of Orthodontics*, vol. 35, no. 2, pp. 90–95, 2008.

[11] N. A. Said-al-Naief and E. Surwillo, "Florid osseous dysplasia of the mandible: report of a case," *Compendium of Continuing Education in Dentistry*, vol. 20, no. 11, pp. 1017–1022, 1999.

[12] S. K. Young, N. R. Markowitz, S. Sullivan, T. W. Seale, and R. Hirschi, "Familial gigantiform cementoma: classification and presentation of a large pedigree," *Oral Surgery Oral Medicine and Oral Pathology*, vol. 68, no. 6, pp. 740–747, 1989.

[13] H. O. Sedano, R. Kuba, and R. J. Gorlin, "Autosomal dominant cemental dysplasia," *Oral Surgery Oral Medicine and Oral Pathology*, vol. 54, no. 6, pp. 642–646, 1982.

[14] H. Coleman, M. Altini, J. Kieser, and M. Nissenbaum, "Familial florid cemento-osseous dysplasia–a case report and review of the literature," *The Journal of the Dental Association of South Africa*, vol. 51, no. 12, pp. 766–770, 1996.

[15] A. E. Musella and L. J. Slater, "Familial florid osseous dysplasia: a case report," *Journal of Oral and Maxillofacial Surgery*, vol. 47, no. 6, pp. 636–640, 1989.

[16] J. S. Cannon, E. E. Keller, and D. C. Dahlin, "Gigantiform cementoma: report of two cases (mother and son)," *Journal of Oral Surgery*, vol. 38, no. 1, pp. 65–70, 1980.

[17] A. Toffanin, R. Benetti, and R. Manconi, "Familial florid cemento-osseous dysplasia: a case report," *Journal of Oral and Maxillofacial Surgery*, vol. 58, no. 12, pp. 1440–1446, 2000.

[18] A. Srivastava, R. Agarwal, R. Soni, A. Sachan, G. C. Shivakumar, and T. P. Chaturvedi, "Familial florid cemento-osseous dysplasia: a rare manifestation in an Indian family," *Case Reports in Dentistry*, vol. 2012, Article ID 574125, 5 pages, 2012.

[19] D. J. D. S. Sarmento, B. V. de Brito Monteiro, A. M. C. de Medeiros, and E. J. D. da Silveira, "Severe florid cemento-osseous dysplasia: a case report treated conservatively and literature review," *Oral and Maxillofacial Surgery*, vol. 17, no. 1, pp. 43–46, 2013.

[20] W. Jerjes, B. Banu, B. Swinson, and C. Hopper, "Florid cemento-osseous dysplasia in a young Indian woman. A case report," *British Dental Journal*, vol. 198, no. 8, pp. 477–478, 2005.

[21] S. Bencharit, D. Schardt-Sacco, J. R. Zuniga, and G. E. Minsley, "Surgical and prosthodontic rehabilitation for a patient with aggressive florid cemento-osseous dysplasia: a clinical report," *Journal of Prosthetic Dentistry*, vol. 90, no. 3, pp. 220–224, 2003.

[22] S. Kayaaltı Özarslan, H. H. Yılmaz, M. Ç. Aksoy, and T. Baykul, "Florid cemento-osseous dysplasia: a case report," *Journal of Dental Faculty of Atatürk University*, vol. 4, supplement, pp. 128–132, 2011.

24

Hereditary Gingival Fibromatosis: A Review and a Report of a Rare Case

Hossein Aghili and Mahdjoube Goldani Moghadam

Department of Orthodontics, Faculty of Dentistry, Shahid Sadoughi University of Medical Sciences, Yazd 89195/165, Iran

Correspondence should be addressed to Mahdjoube Goldani Moghadam; mahdjoube.gm@gmail.com

Academic Editors: L. Junquera and A. Markopoulos

Hereditary gingival fibromatosis (HGF) is a rare condition which manifests itself by an enlarged gingival tissue covering teeth to various extents. The condition may occur isolated or as part of a syndrome. This paper presents a case of 9-year-old female patient suffering from HGF with chief complaint of mouth protrusion. Cephalometric findings showed severe mandibular deficiency and vertical maxillary excess. Patient exhibited perioral muscle contraction on mouth closing. After discussing the treatment possibilities with the patient and her parents, the decision was made to wait until growth potential decreases (following the adolescent growth spurt) and to correct the problem with orthognathic surgery.

1. Introduction

Hereditary gingival fibromatosis (HGF) is a rare condition with the prevalence of one per 175000 population and equal distribution in sexes [1]. The onset of disease is concurrent with the eruption of permanent teeth [2]. The excessive growth of gingival tissue may cause displacement of teeth, overretention of primary teeth, and spacing [2]. Both autosomal dominant and autosomal recessive modes of inheritance have been reported [3–5]. The gingival enlargement may occur alone or in combination of other symptoms as part of a syndrome. Examples of syndromic GF are Zimmerman-Laband syndrome (GF, hypoplastic distal phalanges, hepatosplenomegaly, epilepsy, hypertrichosis, and mental retardation), Jones syndrome (GF and progressive neural deafness), Klippel-Trenaunay syndrome (GF, hemihypertrophy, Nevus flammeus, hemangioma, hypertlorism, and macrocephaly), Ramon syndrome (GF, hypertrichosis, mental retardation, epilepsy, rheumatoid arthritis, and diabetes mellitus), Rutherfurd syndrome (GF, unerupted teeth, corneal dystrophy, and mental retardation), and Cross syndrome (GF, nanophthalmos, microcornea, and severe mental retardation) [6]. A case of nonsyndromic HGF with skeletal jaw discrepancy is presented in this paper.

2. Case Presentation

A 9-year-old female patient visited the department of orthodontics complaining of mouth protrusion (Figure 1) and enlargement of gingival tissues. The patient and her parents noticed gingival enlargement when she was seven years old with gradual spacing of teeth. At the time they visited a general dental practitioner who suggested quadrant wise gingivectomy. Patient's dental records represented that maxillary and mandibular quadrant wise gingivectomies with reverse bevel incision had been performed 1 year ago under local anesthesia, but the enlargement has recurred to the significant degree. Patient's medical history was noncontributory and revealed no significant medication. Upon interviewing it was disclosed that the patient's father, sister, and paternal grandfather had a history of similar gingival enlargement. Her intelligence was normal and clinical examination failed to reveal any sign of associated syndromes. A general physician was consulted who confirmed that the condition was an isolated occurrence.

Intraoral examination showed normal development of the dentition. Excessive overjet and protrusion of upper teeth were observed (Figure 2). The patient showed muscle tension on mouth closing, lip strain and lip incompetency at rest

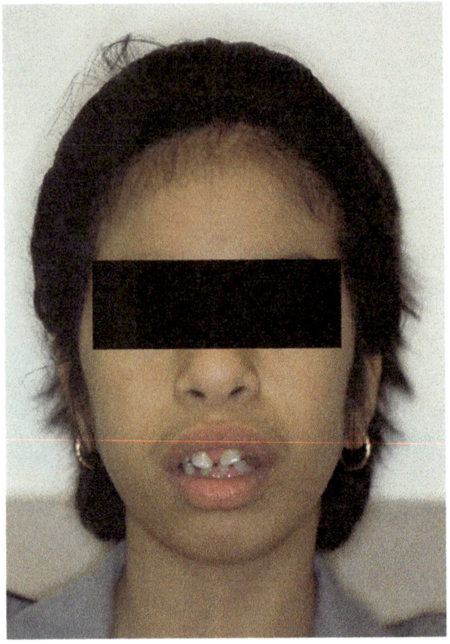

FIGURE 1: Frontal view of the patient showing lip incompetency and mouth protrusion.

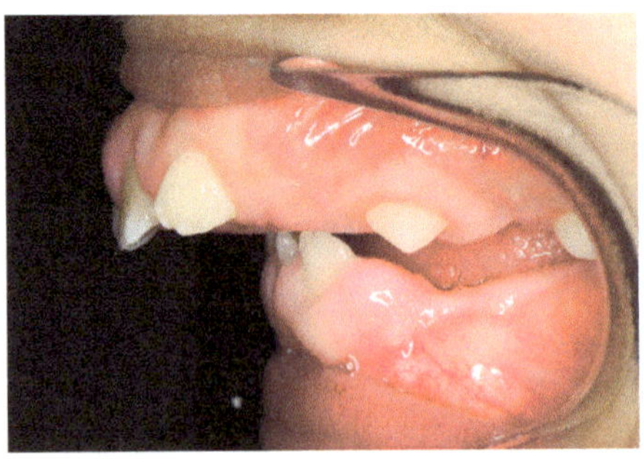

FIGURE 2: Excessive overjet.

(Figures 3 and 4). The enlarged gingival tissues were normal in color and firm in palpation, and the most affected sites were anterior regions of jaws especially in upper anterior palatal mucosa (Figures 5 and 6).

Panoramic radiograph showed normal development of the dentition (Figure 7). Permanent teeth were all present (except for maxillary right first and left second premolars) and in their normal developmental stages. In lateral cephalogram of the patient severe mandibular deficiency and vertical maxillary excess were obvious. Upper anterior teeth were protruded and mandibular plane angle was large (vertical growth pattern) (Figure 8).

Since the dentition showed normal development and the eruption of permanent teeth was not affected by the condition, repeated gingivectomies were not included in the treatment plan. Treatment options were discussed with the patient and her parents, including growth modification (functional appliance combined with high pull headgear) before adolescent growth spurt or orthognathic surgery well

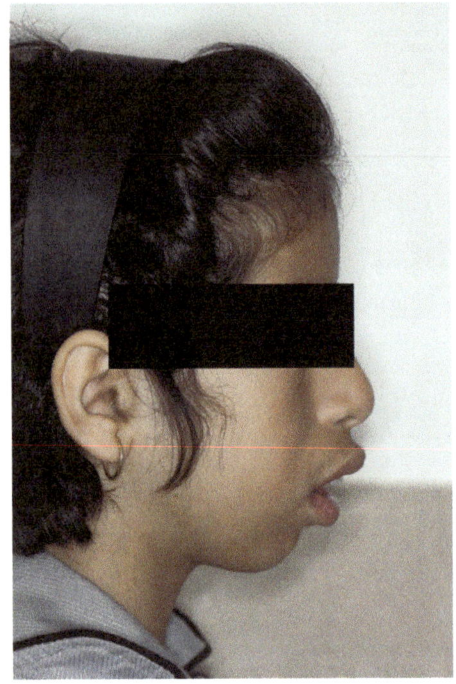

FIGURE 3: Profile view of the patient showing lip incompetency at rest.

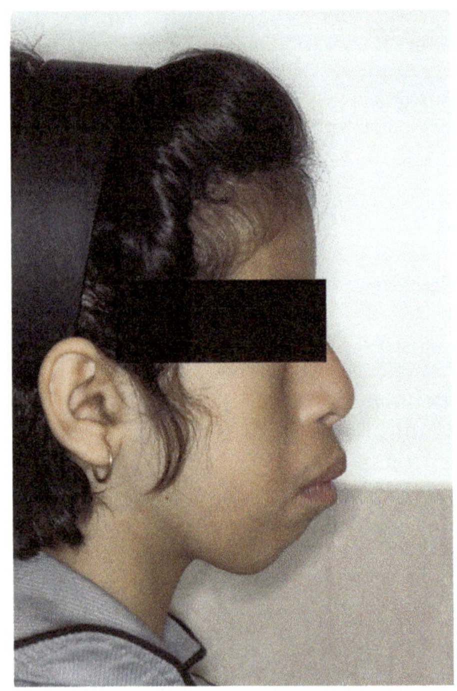

FIGURE 4: Profile view of the patient showing lip strain.

after patient's growth spurt at puberty. It was explained for the parents that the long face growth pattern is hard to modify and the treatment must continue over many years which needs excellent cooperation [7]. It also was explained that in a trial on a sample of at least moderately severe Class II patients, the number of patients who needed orthognathic surgery

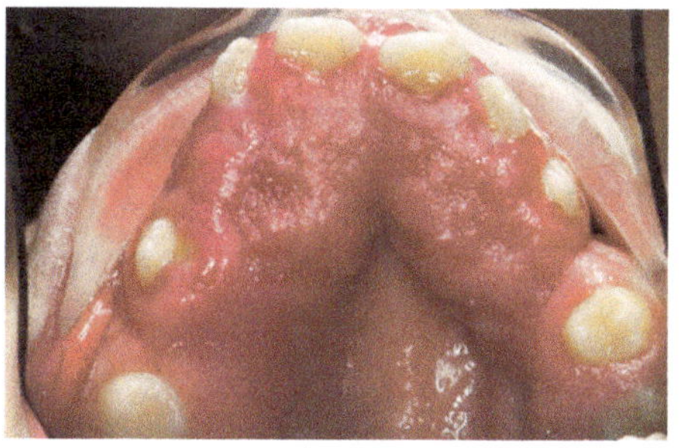

FIGURE 5: Upper occlusal view.

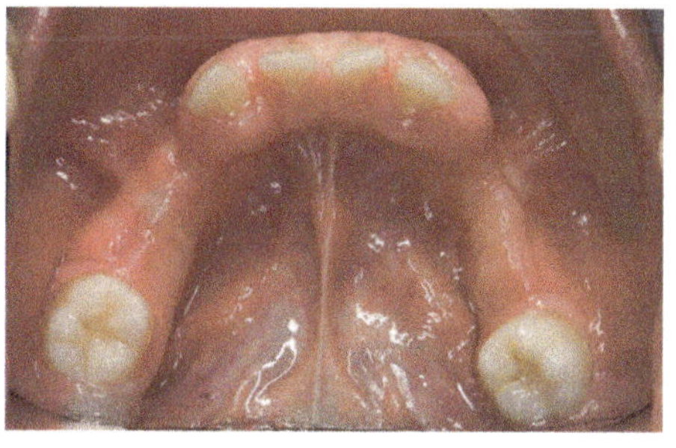

FIGURE 6: Lower occlusal view.

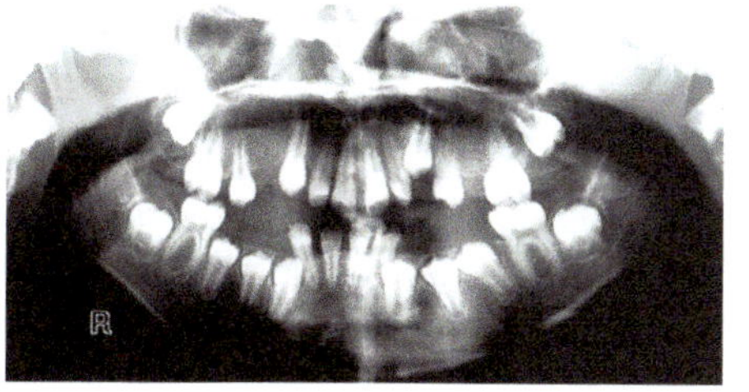

FIGURE 7: Panoramic radiograph showing normal development of permanent teeth and missing of maxillary right first and left second premolars.

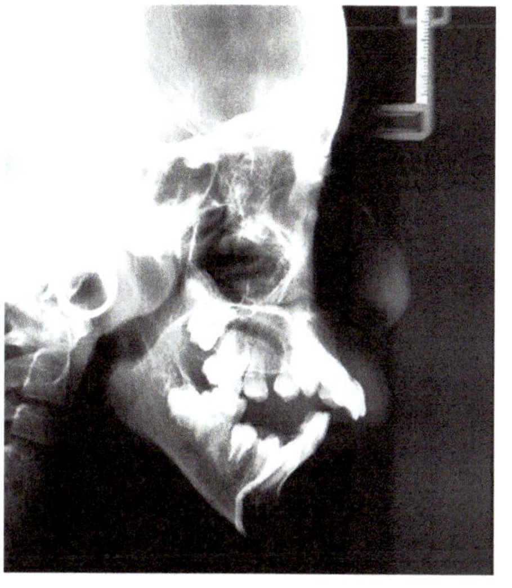

FIGURE 8: Lateral cephalogram showing mandibular deficiency and vertical growth pattern.

later in life showed insignificant difference between treated children (with growth modification) and control group (no treatment). Regarding the severity of the problem and their unwillingness to attempt growth modification, the decision was made to wait until slowing down the growth (after adolescent growth spurt) and correcting the jaw discrepancy through bimaxillary orthognathic surgery for mandibular advancement and the impact of the posterior maxilla. Until then periodic monitoring of the patient to become assure of normal eruption of permanent teeth was planned. To improve the patient psychological state, it was suggested to temporarily eliminate upper teeth spacing and protrusion by means of a 2 × 4 appliance along with resective periodontal surgery in upper anterior region (vestibular and palatal) which her parents refused.

3. Discussion

The mode of genetic transmission in this patient was consistent with an autosomal dominant inheritance since both sexes and successive generations were affected (the patient, her sister, father and paternal grandfather). As stated earlier both autosomal dominant and recessive modes of transmission of HGF have been reported [3–5]. Recently, four genetically separated loci on chromosome 2p (GINGF and GINGF3), chromosome 5q (GINGF2), and chromosome 11p (GINGF4) have been determined in association with HGF [6, 8–10].

Differential diagnosis of gingival enlargements includes enlargement associated with hormonal changes (such as in pregnancy), drug-induced gingival overgrowth, or enlargements due to genetic disorders [11]. Inflammations, tumors, and cysts can also present themselves as gingival enlargements [1]. Enlargement can be further categorized as localized and generalized depending on the extent of involvement [12]. In the present case the diagnosis of HGF was given based on the family history and clinical examination. The enlargement in our patient was particularly prominent in the anterior palate and mandibular anterior region. HGF generally has two forms based on the extent of involved tissue, including nodular (localized, mostly seen in the maxillary tuberosity and molar area) and symmetric (generalized, which is more common and both arches are equally affected) forms [13]. The affected gingival tissue is pink, usually shows exaggerated stippling, and is firm and fibrous on palpation which helps to differentiate the condition from drug-induced gingival enlargements in those where the tissue is often movable [13]. Inflamed gingival tissue due to plaque accumulation may become red. Free and attached gingival tissues are both involved, but extension beyond the mucogingival junction is not observed [13].

The histological findings are nonspecific and include acanthotic and hyperkeratotic epithelium with elongated rete ridges deeply extended to a relative avascular connective tissue with densely arranged collagen bundles and numerous fibroblasts [1, 14]. Two types of fibroblasts are present in HGF:

inactive fibroblast with little cytoplasm and highly active fibroblast with fully developed cytoplasmic organelles [15]. Activation of certain fibroblasts by physical trauma, such as tooth eruption, can be a possible explanation for simultaneity of HGF development with tooth eruption [16].

As stated earlier HGF can be an isolated or syndrome-associated condition. The association of the entity with growth hormone deficiency secondary to lack of growth hormone releasing factor secretion has also been reported [17]. The presented patient seemed to be a case of nonsyndromic HGF which the isolated nature of the condition was further confirmed by a physician.

The side effects of gingival enlargement in HGF include speech problems, painful mastication, spacing and diastema, malocclusion, and overretention of primary teeth [18]. In our patient, gingival enlargement had led to spacing especially between upper anterior teeth. In order to address patients' esthetic and functional needs usually surgical excision of the enlarged tissue is necessary. Since the enlargement recurs to a various extent, repeated gingivectomies are needed for restoring the gingival contours. In the patient presented, deferring orthodontic treatment until growth potential decreases and correcting the problem through combined orthodontic and orthognathic procedures were planned. Gingivectomy had little to do in improving the patient's condition. Regarding the higher rate of recurrence in children and teenagers compared to adults [18], we found it better to delay surgical intervention (gingivectomy) until commencement of the presurgical orthodontic phase and planned periodic visits to monitor eruption of remained permanent teeth. Early treatment with growth modification was rejected by the parents.

4. Conclusion

This paper presents diagnosis and treatment plan of a patient with HGF and severe skeletal malocclusion. Regarding the rarity of the condition only few case reports addressing the orthodontic management of the condition exist. The case presented in this paper differs from previous reports since she needed combined orthodontic and orthognathic treatment because of severe skeletal discrepancies of the jaws. After precise evaluation of risks, costs, and benefits associated with different treatment possibilities and discussing them with the patient and her parents, orthognathic surgery at appropriate time was planned.

Conflict of Interests

The authors declared no conflict of interests.

References

[1] J. Kather, M. A. C. Salgado, U. F. L. Salgado, J. R. Cortelli, and D. Pallos, "Clinical and histomorphometric characteristics of three different families with hereditary gingival fibromatosis," *Oral Surgery, Oral Medicine, Oral Pathology, Oral Radiology and Endodontology*, vol. 105, no. 3, pp. 348–352, 2008.

[2] G. H. Breen, R. Addante, and C. C. Black, "Early onset of hereditary gingival fibromatosis in a 28-month-old," *Pediatric Dentistry*, vol. 31, no. 4, pp. 286–288, 2009.

[3] L. Bozzo, O. P. de Almeida, C. Scully, and M. J. Aldred, "Hereditary gingival fibromatosis. Report of an extensive four-generation pedigree," *Oral Surgery, Oral Medicine, Oral Pathology*, vol. 78, no. 4, pp. 452–454, 1994.

[4] R. J. Jorgenson and M. E. Cocker, "Variation in the inheritance and expression of gingival fibromatosis," *Journal of Periodontology*, vol. 45, no. 7, pp. 472–477, 1974.

[5] S. L. Singer, J. Goldblatt, L. A. Hallam, and J. C. Winters, "Hereditary gingival fibromatosis with a recessive mode of inheritance. Case reports," *Australian Dental Journal*, vol. 38, no. 6, pp. 427–432, 1993.

[6] L. Häkkinen and A. Csiszar, "Hereditary gingival fibromatosis: characteristics and novel putative pathogenic mechanisms," *Journal of Dental Research*, vol. 86, no. 1, pp. 25–34, 2007.

[7] W. R. Proffit, R. P. White Jr., and D. M. Sarver, *Contemporary Treatment of Dentofacial Deformity*, Mosby, St. Louis, Mo, USA, 2003.

[8] T. C. Hart, D. Pallos, D. W. Bowden, J. Bolyard, M. J. Pettenati, and J. R. Cortelli, "Genetic linkage of hereditary gingival fibromatosis to chromosome 2p21," *The American Journal of Human Genetics*, vol. 62, no. 4, pp. 876–883, 1998.

[9] S. Xiao, L. Bu, L. Zhu et al., "A new locus for hereditary gingival fibromatosis (GINGF2) maps to 5q13-q22," *Genomics*, vol. 74, no. 2, pp. 180–185, 2001.

[10] X. Ye, L. Shi, Y. Cheng et al., "A novel locus for autosomal dominant hereditary gingival fibromatosis, GINGF3, maps to chromosome 2p22.3-p23.3," *Clinical Genetics*, vol. 68, no. 3, pp. 239–244, 2005.

[11] G. C. Armitage, "Development of a classification system for periodontal diseases and conditions," *Annals of Periodontology*, vol. 4, no. 1, pp. 1–6, 1999.

[12] F. Carranza, "Gingival enlargement," in *Periodontology*, F. Carranza, Ed., pp. 125–149, WB Saunders, Philadelphia, Pa, USA, 7th edition, 1990.

[13] J. Katz, M. Guelmann, and S. Barak, "Hereditary gingival fibromatosis with distinct dental, skeletal and developmental abnormalities," *Pediatric Dentistry*, vol. 24, no. 3, pp. 253–256, 2002.

[14] A. Doufexi, M. Mina, and E. Ioannidou, "Gingival overgrowth in children: epidemiology, pathogenesis, and complications. A literature review," *Journal of Periodontology*, vol. 76, no. 1, pp. 3–10, 2005.

[15] Y. Collan, H. Ranta, and T. Vartio, "Histochemical and biochemical study of hereditary fibrous hyperplasia of the gingiva," *Scandinavian Journal of Dental Research*, vol. 90, no. 1, pp. 20–28, 1982.

[16] K. Shirasuna, M. Okura, K. Watatani, Y. Hayashido, M. Saka, and T. Matsuya, "Abnormal cellular property of fibroblasts from congenital gingival fibromatosis," *Journal of Oral Pathology*, vol. 17, no. 8, pp. 381–385, 1988.

[17] K. Oikarinen, T. Salo, M. L. Kaar, P. Lahtela, and M. Altonen, "Hereditary gingival fibromatosis associated with growth hormone deficiency," *The British Journal of Oral and Maxillofacial Surgery*, vol. 28, no. 5, pp. 335–339, 1990.

[18] L. P. Bittencourt, V. Campos, L. F. M. Moliterno, D. P. B. Ribeiro, and R. K. Sampaio, "Hereditary gingival fibromatosis: review of the literature and a case report," *Quintessence International*, vol. 31, no. 6, pp. 415–418, 2000.

25

Severe Osteolysis of the Mandibular Angle and Total Condylolysis in Progressive Systemic Sclerosis

Amin Rahpeyma,[1] Seyed Hosein Hoseini Zarch,[2] and Saeedeh Khajehahmadi[3]

[1] *Oral and Maxillofacial Surgery, Oral and Maxillofacial Diseases Research Center, Faculty of Dentistry, Mashhad University of Medical Sciences, Vakilabad Boulevard, Mashhad, Iran*
[2] *Oral and Maxillofacial Radiology, Dental Research Center, Faculty of Dentistry, Mashhad University of Medical Sciences, Vakilabad Boulevard, Mashhad, Iran*
[3] *Oral and Maxillofacial Pathology, Dental Research Center, Faculty of Dentistry, Mashhad University of Medical Sciences, Vakilabad Boulevard, P.O. Box 91735-984, Mashhad, Iran*

Correspondence should be addressed to Saeedeh Khajehahmadi; saeedeh.ahmady@yahoo.com

Academic Editors: M. H. K. Motamedi and S. R. Watt-Smith

Progressive systemic sclerosis is an autoimmune disease characterized by gradual deposition of abnormal collagen which causes fibrous changes of the skin and visceral organs such as lung, heart, and kidney, which lead to serious complication. Microangiopathy and firm skin cause extrinsic pressure and obliteration of the vessels that lead to ischemia and destruction of the underlying bone. Salivary gland fibrosis causes xerostomia that increases risk of dental caries. Therefore, oral hygiene instruction (OHI) and preventive dentistry are recommended for these patients. We present a 36-year-old female that suffers from systemic sclerosis with total lysis of the mandibular condyle.

1. Introduction

Scleroderma or progressive systemic sclerosis (PSS) was first reported in 1752 by Curzio of Naples [1]. PSS, also known as scleroderma, is a connective tissue disorder characterized by fibrosis of the skin and visceral organs [2]. The cause of PSS is immunologically mediated pathogenesis. PSS occurs predominately in the adult but it can also be seen in childhood, with females affected three to four times as often as males [3]. The most common manifestations is microstomia that causes a limitation of opening the mouth in two-thirds of the cases. In addition, salivary gland fibrosis causes xerostomia; therefore, these patients are more prone to dental decay.

In some patients, as loss of attachment gingival occurs, multiple area of gingival recession may be present. In scleroderma patients, preventive care is of foremost importance. Meticulous oral hygiene must be established and maintained. Occasionally slight bilateral erosion of mandibular condyle causes anterior open bite. Bone resorption is caused by the increased pressure associated with the deposition of collagen.

Bone resorption has been reported in maxillofacial region, which occurs in masticatory muscle attachments [4]. On radiographic appearance a characteristic resorption of the ramus and condyle may be observed.

We reported a case of total osteolysis of the mandibular condyle in a 36-year-old female patient with oral manifestations of the disease.

2. Case Report

A 36-year-old female suffering from PSS with 9-year history of disease was referred to oral and maxillofacial surgery for extraction of her decayed posterior teeth.

The patient had reduced maximal interincisal opening (MIO = 12 mm), mask-like face, perioral deep rhytides, pinched nose, facial telangiectasia, and atrophic ulcerated finger tips (sclerodactyly). Pain accompanying bone resorption is present in her fingers (painful digital ischemia).

In medical history, there was pulmonary fibrosis. Limitation in mouth opening, malformed fingers, dry mouth,

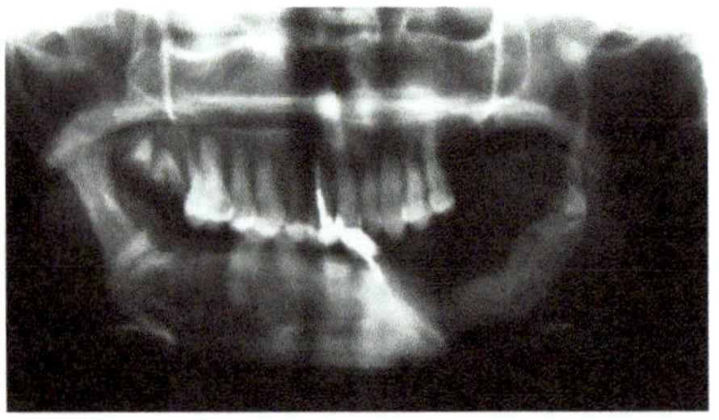

FIGURE 1: Dental panoramic tomogram relieved extensive bone resorption of bilateral mandibular angles and total left condylolysis.

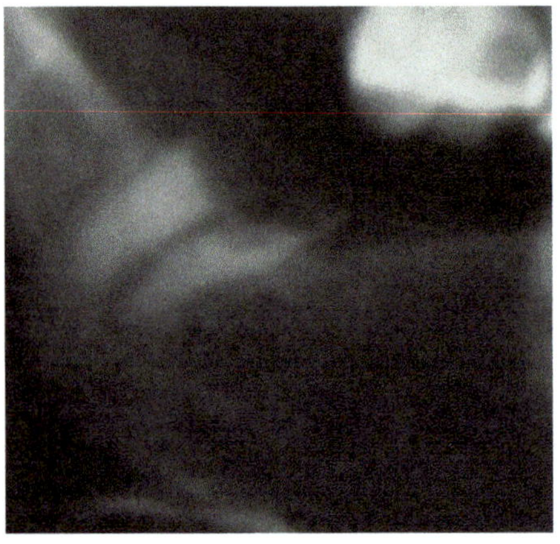

FIGURE 2: Resorption of the right mandibular angle and decayed remnant root tooth.

tight tongue, and reduced movement of the cheeks created problems in oral hygiene maintenance; hence molar teeth were severely decayed. Root canal therapy (RCT) of teeth number 9 and number 22 with pin composite buildup was observed (Figure 1). Decayed remained roots were present in posterior quadrants (Figure 2). Dental treatment such as posterior teeth restorations, fixed or removable prosthesis, was difficult to do in this patient because of restricted mouth opening.

Dental panoramic view relieved extensive bone resorption of bilateral mandibular angles and total left condylolysis (Figure 3). Left coronoid process was thinned and elongated which extended up to zygomatic arch. Contralateral coronoid process length was normal. There was a 1.5 cm vertical length difference between right and left coronoid processes. Patient has no history of jaw trauma or surgery.

Under local anesthesia, decayed roots were removed. Limitation in mouth opening and severe bone resorption made dental procedures difficult. Great caution is required to avoid iatrogenic jaw fracture.

3. Discussion

Scleroderma or PSS is an autoimmune disease characterized by gradual deposition of collagen in reticular dermis, gastrointestinal tract, heart, lung, and other organs [2]. most cases of PSS most commonly occur during the third to fifth decades of life [2]. PSS has a low prevalence (130 per million) [3] and it occurs about three times more common in women.

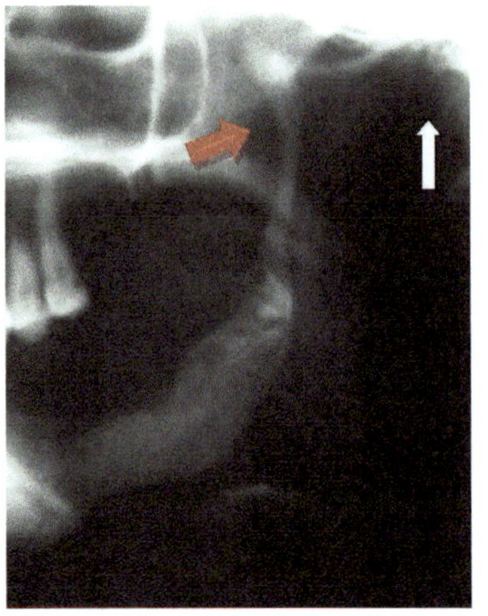

FIGURE 3: Empty glenoid fossa (white arrow), thin elongated coronoid process (red arrow), and left angle bone resorption.

Bone resorption is an uncommon occurrence but recognized complication of long standing PSS [5]. Posterior inferior ramal bone resorption of the jaws was first described in 1959 by Taversa [6]. It is hypothesized that pressure from overlying skin and atrophic muscles with ischemia from small vessels angiopathy has role in bone resorption pathogenesis [7]. In maxillofacial regions resorption occurs in attachment area of masticatory muscles including masseter, temporal, lateral pterygoid, and anterior belly of digastrics muscle. Bone resorption in other skeletal bones such as terminal phalanges, distal radius, ulna, cervical spine, zygomatic arch, and the ribs has been reported [8].

Mandibular bone resorption usually happens in mandibular angle area and is more likely to happen bilaterally [8–10].

Pervious reported cases of bilateral mandibular condylolysis in scleroderma patients had open bite except the case of Caplan [11–13]. Despite extensive resorption of the condyle, the present case had no open bite or alteration in jaw relationship.

Pain, preauricular tenderness, occlusal disturbance, TMJ sounds, and reduction of ramus height are common clinical features, but in our case despite huge bone resorption, there were no pain and tenderness. Dental radiographic manifestations of the scleroderma patient include PDL widening, root resorption, and decayed posterior teeth [14] similar to our case. Patients with PSS exhibit an increased prevalence of external root resorption [5].

Root canal therapies of the teeth with external root resorption require special consideration.

Fibrosis of the salivary glands leads to xerostomia [15]. Because of dry mouth, these patients have a greater risk for dental caries and periodontal disease and in this case we should consider concurrent secondary sjogren syndrome. In addition, there is an increased prevalence of oral candidacies in patients with xerostomia because of reduction in saliva production.

In the present case, dry mouth was an important clinical feature; thus preventive dentistry is too important in scleroderma patients.

Also diffuse widening of the periodontal ligament space is often present in dental radiograph.

In our case, despite complete left mandibular condylolysis and bilateral angle resorption, there were appropriate jaw relations.

Perimandibular connective tissue (PMCT) adaptation and presence of mandibular canines help in stabilization of three dimensional spatial positions of jaws.

Limited mouth opening and reduced movement of the cheek and tongue made dental practice very difficult. Dental treatment including removable partial dentures, traditional fixed prosthodontics, or implant is difficult [5]. In order to reduce dental problems, programmed preventive dentistry and regular followup of the scleroderma patients are recommended.

Deposition of abnormal collagen in the tongue causes a firm and hypomobile tongue [5]. The oral chief compliant in scleroderma patients is xerostomia, which causes difficulty in speaking. Some patients who complain of dry mouth may appear to have adequate salivary flow and oral moistness.

4. Conclusion

Because of the increased potential for dental caries in scleroderma patient, programmed preventive dentistry and regular followup are recommended.

Reduced maximal interincisal opening and severe bone resorption made dental procedures difficult. Great caution is required for avoiding iatrogenic jaw fracture in severely resorbed mandibular bone.

Conflict of Interests

The authors declare that they have no conflict of interests.

References

[1] W. P. Naylor, "Oral management of the scleroderma patient," *The Journal of the American Dental Association*, vol. 105, no. 5, pp. 814–817, 1982.

[2] M. M. Rubin and R. J. Sanfilippo, "Resorption of the mandibular angle in progressive systemic sclerosis: case report," *Journal of Oral and Maxillofacial Surgery*, vol. 50, no. 1, pp. 75–77, 1992.

[3] M. A. Z. de Figueiredo, J. A. P. de Figueiredo, and S. Porter, "Root resorption associated with mandibular bone erosion in a patient with scleroderma," *Journal of Endodontics*, vol. 34, no. 1, pp. 102–103, 2008.

[4] H. Çankaya and Y. Kabasakal, "Mandibular resorption due to progressive systemic sclerosis: a case report," *Journal of Oral and Maxillofacial Surgery*, vol. 59, no. 5, pp. 565–567, 2001.

[5] C. Cazal, A. P. V. Sobral, R. F. S. N. Neves, F. W. V. Freire Filho, Á. B. Cardoso, and M. M. F. da Silveira, "Oral complaints in progressive systemic sclerosis: two cases report," *Medicina Oral, Patologia Oral y Cirugia Bucal*, vol. 13, no. 2, pp. 114–118, 2008.

[6] S. C. White, N. W. Frey, D. D. Blaschke et al., "Oral radiographic changes in patients with progressive systemic sclerosis (scleroderma)," *The Journal of the American Dental Association*, vol. 94, no. 6, pp. 1178–1182, 1977.

[7] W. P. Naylor, "Oral management of the scleroderma patient," *The Journal of the American Dental Association*, vol. 105, no. 5, pp. 814–817, 1982.

[8] R. E. Wood and P. Lee, "Analysis of the oral manifestations of systemic sclerosis (scleroderma)," *Oral Surgery Oral Medicine and Oral Pathology*, vol. 65, no. 2, pp. 172–178, 1988.

[9] M. M. Rubin and R. J. Sanfilippo, "Resorption of the mandibular angle in progressive systemic sclerosis: case report," *Journal of Oral and Maxillofacial Surgery*, vol. 50, no. 1, pp. 75–77, 1992.

[10] F. E. Hopper and A. D. Giles, "Orofacial changes in systemic sclerosis. Report of a case of resorption of mandibular angles and zygomatic arches," *British Journal of Oral Surgery*, vol. 20, no. 2, pp. 129–134, 1982.

[11] R. G. Jagger, E. G. Absi, H. G. Jeremiah, and A. W. Sugar, "Bilateral mandibular condylysis in a patient with systemic sclerosis," *Dentomaxillofacial Radiology*, vol. 35, no. 6, pp. 461–463, 2006.

[12] P. E. Haers and H. F. Sailer, "Mandibular resorption due to systemic sclerosis. Case report of surgical correction of a secondary open bite deformity," *International Journal of Oral and Maxillofacial Surgery*, vol. 24, no. 4, pp. 261–267, 1995.

[13] H. I. Caplan and R. A. Benny, "Total osteolysis of the mandibular condyle in progressive systemic sclerosis," *Oral Surgery Oral Medicine and Oral Pathology*, vol. 46, no. 3, pp. 362–366, 1978.

[14] E. Alpöz, H. Cankara, and P. Güneri, "Facial subcutaneous calcinosis and mandibular resorbtion in systemic sclerosis: a case report," *Dentomaxillofacial Radiology*, vol. 36, pp. 172–174, 2007.

[15] G. Nagy, J. Kovács, M. Zeher, and L. Czirják, "Analysis of the oral manifestations of systemic sclerosis," *Oral Surgery, Oral Medicine, Oral Pathology and Oral Radiology*, vol. 77, pp. 141–146, 1994.

26

Rehabilitation of Posterior Maxilla with Zygomatic and Dental Implant after Tumor Resection: A Case Report

Faysal Ugurlu, Coskun Yıldız, B. C. Sener, and Atilla Sertgoz

Department of Oral and Maxillofacial Surgery, Dentistry Faculty, Marmara University, 34365 Istanbul, Turkey

Correspondence should be addressed to Faysal Ugurlu; faysalugurlu@hotmail.com

Academic Editors: R. S. Brown, D. Cogulu, and R. A. de Mesquita

Zygomatic implants have been used for dental rehabilitation in patients with insufficient bone in the posterior upper jaw, due to, for example, tumor resection, trauma, or atrophy. Zygomatic implants are an alternative to complex free or vascularized bone grafting and distraction osteogenesis. A 42-year-old male patient with a severe defect in the right posterior maxilla, starting from the first canine region, which had occurred after tumor resection 3 years earlier, was referred to our department. One zygomatic implant (Brenemark System, Nobel Biocare, Goteborg, Sweden) to the zygoma and one dental implant to the canine region were placed. After a 5-month osseointegration period, a fixed denture was fabricated and adapted to the implants. Although the surgical and prosthetic procedures for zygoma implants are not easy, the final outcomes can be successful with appropriate planning.

1. Introduction

Maxillary posterior defects that occur after tumor resection or trauma are challenging to reconstruct and rehabilitate. The aim of rehabilitation is not only to provide a cosmetically acceptable appearance, but also to restore oral functions, such as deglutition, mastication, and phonation. To provide better function, an implant-supported prosthesis can be fabricated. However, implant placement in the zygoma and pterygoid bone is difficult due to the variable anatomy and varying degrees of atrophy possible in the maxillofacial region [1, 2]. The surgery is not without risk because the drill path is close to critical anatomical structures, such as the maxillary sinus, the nasal cavity, and the eyes [2, 3]. A small angular error may result in significant positional errors at the end of the tool trajectory. Furthermore, the limited intraoperative visibility, especially given the anatomical intricacies of the curved zygomatic bone, makes this kind of surgery a demanding procedure.

In recent years, preoperative 3D planning of implant treatment that takes into account both the quality and quantity of the jawbone and prosthodontic considerations has had a major influence on final implant treatment outcome. In particular, before zygoma implant placement, 3D imaging and planning should be performed to ensure the safety of surgery and rehabilitation. This case study describes the clinical management of prosthetic rehabilitation of a patient who underwent zygoma implant placement.

2. Case Report

A 42-year-old male patient was referred to our department with functional and esthetic issues. His anamnesis revealed that tumor resection had been performed to his right posterior maxilla 3 years earlier. His clinical examination revealed a severe defect in the right posterior maxilla, starting from the canine region (Figure 1). To be able to make an implant-supported fixed prosthesis, a zygoma implant was planned for the posterior maxilla, due to the huge bone defect in that area, and one dental implant was planned (Figures 2 and 3). The patient was evaluated preoperatively with respect to jaw size, bone volume, bone density, jaw relationships, intermaxillary distance, occlusal relation, and condition of the opposing dentition. Preoperative analysis of the anatomical conditions and possible maxillary pathology was evaluated using panoramic radiographs and a cone-beam CT scan.

The operation was performed under intravenous sedation. A crestal incision was made and a mucoperiosteal flap

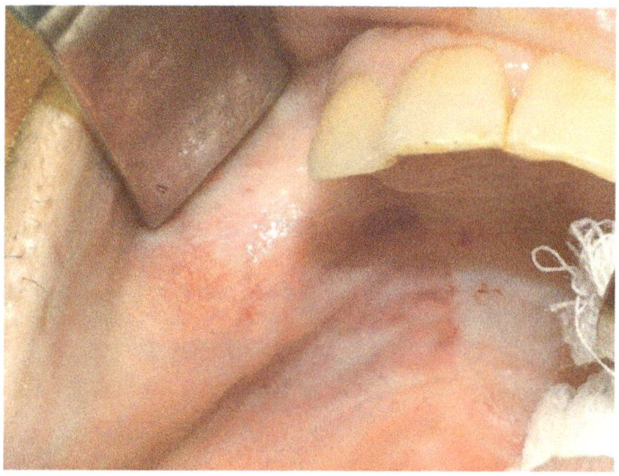

FIGURE 1: Preoperative intraoral view.

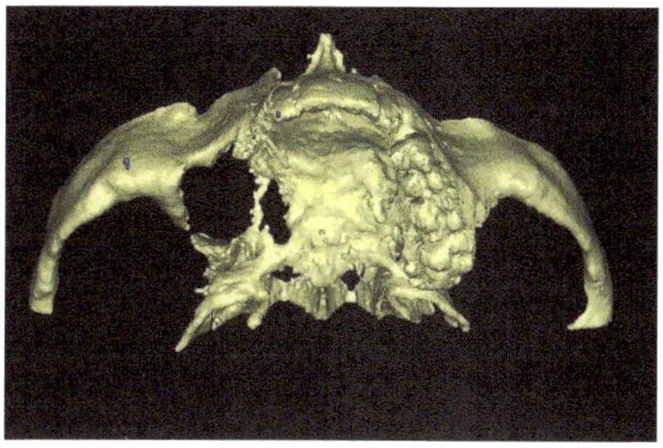

FIGURE 2: 3D view of defect.

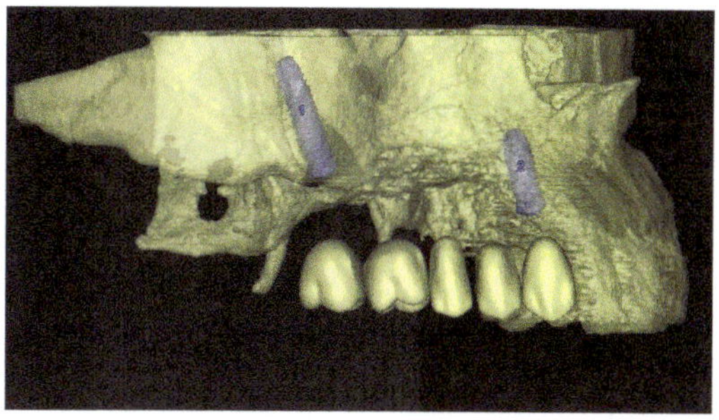

FIGURE 3: Preoperative simulation of implant planning.

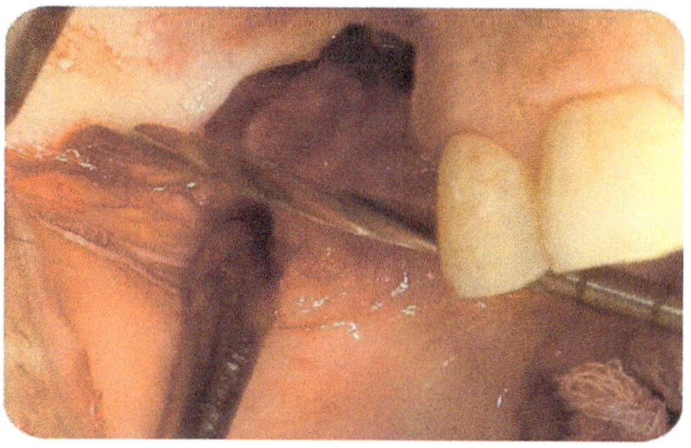

FIGURE 4: Intraoperative view of zygoma after flap elevation.

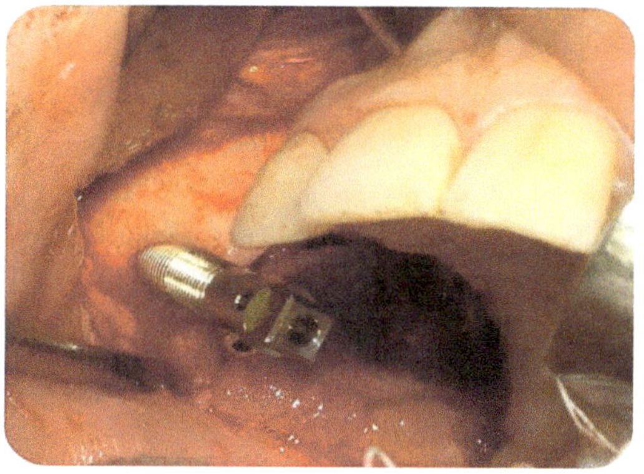

FIGURE 5: Implant placement of zygomatic implant.

was elevated up to the zygomatic buttress (Figure 4). The zygoma implant was drilled and placed to the posterior; one dental implant was placed in the premolar region (Figure 5). The soft tissues were readapted and sutured back into position with silk sutures. An antibiotic (clindamycin, 600 mg/day) was prescribed for 10 days postoperatively. The remaining sutures were removed after 10 days.

Permanent prosthetic rehabilitation was initiated 5 months after implant placement (Figure 6). Metal impression copings were screwed onto the implants after removal of the healing screws. An impression was taken using an open-tray technique. Metal-supported porcelain restorations were constructed using conventional methods (Figures 7 and 8).

The patient was followed up at 5 years after the prosthetic rehabilitation. The last clinical and radiographic assessments were uneventful, and the patient's satisfaction with the esthetic result was excellent (Figures 9 and 10).

3. Discussion

Reconstruction of posterior maxillary defects is a challenge. Many procedures, such as onlay grafts [4], free or microvascular bone grafts [5, 6], transport distraction osteogenesis [7], and apposition grafts with or without a Le Fort I osteotomy [8] are well documented and have success rates of 60–90%. However, these often involve invasive and lengthy surgeries, long treatment time, and some morbidity. Microvascular bone grafts are complex and risky operations. In addition, these conventional techniques cause donor site morbidity during harvesting of soft tissues and bone grafts [4]. Furthermore, free bone grafts are commonly associated with unpredictable resorption during healing [4, 5, 9].

Zygomatic implants, an alternative to these techniques, have survival rates of 98–100% [10]. Although no randomized clinical trial that compared sinus grafts or onlay grafts and zygomatic implants has been reported, the survival rates suggest that zygomatic implants should be considered an alternative to bone grafting and applied in routine rehabilitation of the totally edentulous patient with high resorption of the maxilla and severe defects in the posterior maxilla after tumor resection. However, the placement of zygoma implants is not without risk, due to the anatomically complex operation site. Implant-guided surgery is a suitable method

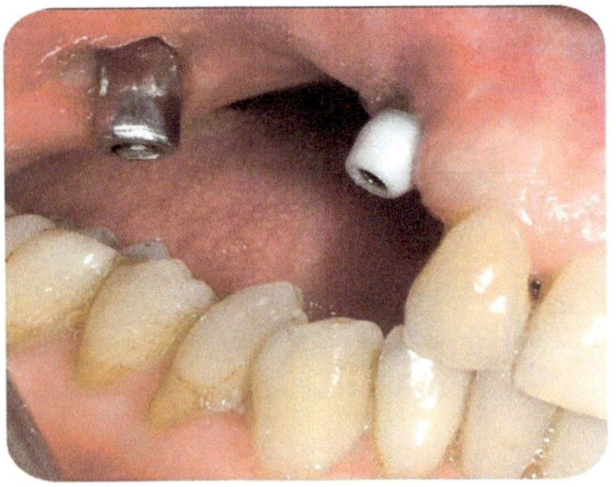

FIGURE 6: Intraoral view during osteointegration period.

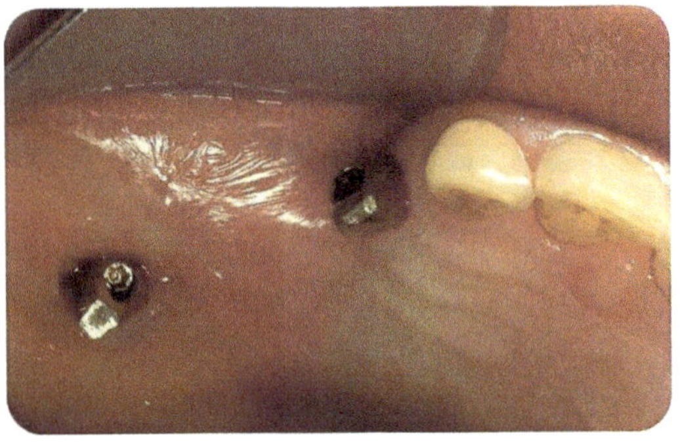

FIGURE 7: Intraoral view after implant abutments.

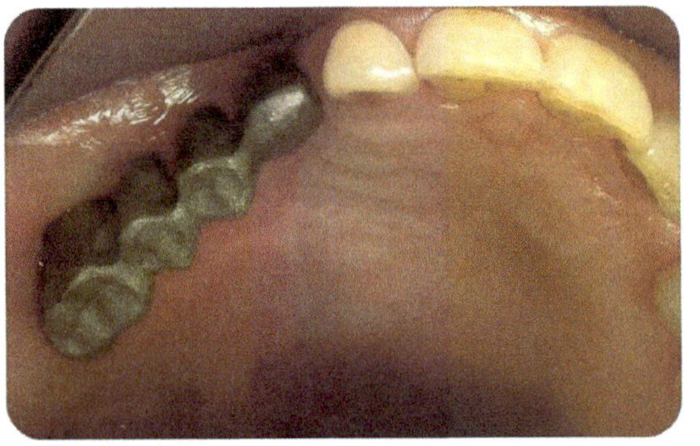

FIGURE 8: Fabricated Metal base of bridge.

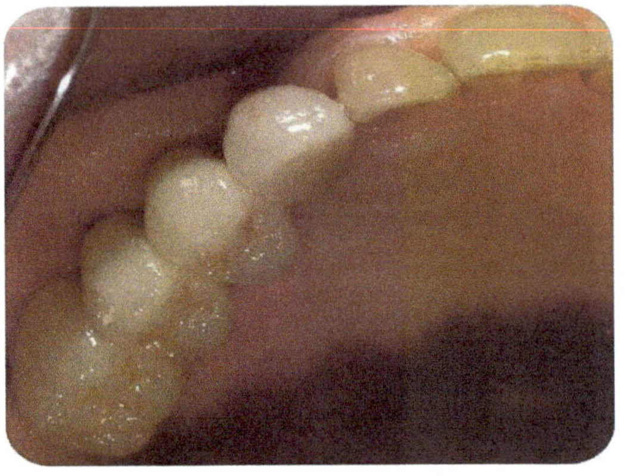

FIGURE 9: Metal supported porcelain bridge.

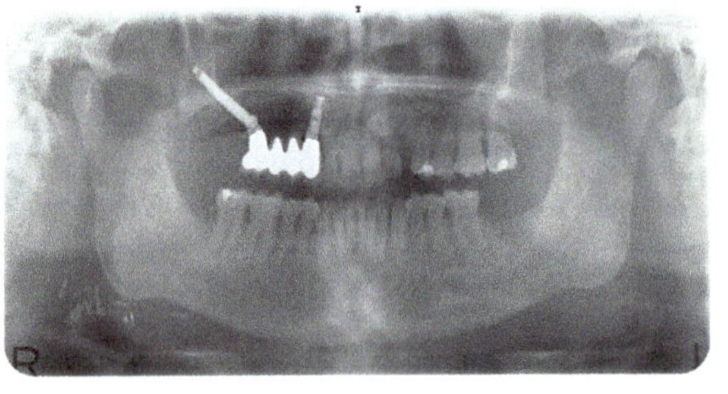

FIGURE 10: Radiographic view after 1 year follow-up.

for minimizing the risks and improving the precision of the surgery. This method enables the transfer of the preoperative plan accurately to the operating theatre.

The drill guides dictate the location, angle, and depth of insertion of the implant, so as to provide a link between the planning and the actual surgery by transferring the simulated plan accurately to the patient [11, 12]. Another possibility to establish the relationship between the operation site and the computer-generated additional information is the use of tracking technology, which continually registers the position of the patient and surgical tools by means of special sensors ("computer-aided navigation") [13]. This navigation technology has now been tested and demonstrated by many research groups and clinicians for use in many applications [11–13]. However, these methods are expensive to use.

With a thick cortical layer, the zygoma bone offers a solid and extended anchorage that can support the masticatory forces applied at the occlusal level. The amount of bone volume in the zygoma has been reported in several studies. These concluded that the high volume of bone and the possibility of tricortical anchorage increased both the success and survival rate of zygomatic implants [14, 15].

The greatest advantage of zygomatic implants is elimination of donor site morbidity and infection in the graft material. Also, treatment time is decreased significantly by avoiding the need for bone healing after grafting. Also, their use reduces the number of surgical operations required and so also the associated hospital costs [16].

Despite their advantages, zygomatic implants also have many complications and problems after implantation. Soft tissue inflammation around the abutments has been reported in some studies of zygomatic implants [17]. The depth of the palatal mucosa at the level of the posterior implant is normally 5 mm, consisting of parakeratinized epithelium that is not comparable with the normal pocket [18]. Lack of soft tissue with the bone defect can lead to gingival problems around the implant during or after osseointegration, as in our case. To overcome this, oral hygiene levels must be high. With good oral hygiene and close follow-up (every 3 months) no inflammation was recorded around the zygoma implant in the present case.

Sinusitis has been reported by a number of authors [19, 20]. The incidence was 14–30%. In some cases, patients with an oroantral fistula may develop suppuration with or without sinusitis. Treatment involves the administration of antibiotics and/or repositioning soft tissue, without removal of the stable zygomatic implant. Causes of sinusitis include perforation of the sinus membrane and leakage at the level of the maxilla due to a hole in the zygomatic implant, leading to migration of bacteria from the mouth to the sinus [16]. In the present case, no sinusitis or oroantral fistula occurred.

The zygomatic implant-supported prosthesis requires special care due to the biomechanical forces that affect the long-term stability of an implant-supported restoration. Use of a stiff prosthesis is necessary because flexing of the materials can cause deformation and deviation, resulting in loss of implant or loosening of the junction between the prosthesis and fixation. The success rates of implants in the zygomatic bone vary from 95% to 97% with 12–124 months of follow-up observation [21, 22], and the patient satisfaction rate is 80% 1 year after installation of the prosthesis [23].

4. Conclusions

Zygoma implants are a unique alternative for rehabilitation of the posterior maxilla after tumor resection or trauma. Due to both the anatomical intricacies of the zygomatic bone and the implant length, the placement of zygoma implants still represents a challenge to prosthodontists. To minimize the risks of surgery, 3D reconstruction, preoperative planning, registration, surgical implant guidance, and a motion tracking algorithm should be used.

References

[1] L. Vrielinck, C. Politis, S. Schepers, M. Pauwels, and I. Naert, "Image-based planning and clinical validation of zygoma and pterygoid implant placement in patients with severe bone atrophy using customized drill guides. Preliminary results from a prospective clinical follow-up study," *International Journal of Oral and Maxillofacial Surgery*, vol. 32, no. 1, pp. 7–14, 2003.

[2] Y. Uchida, M. Goto, T. Katsuki, and T. Akiyoshi, "Measurement of the maxilla and zygoma as an aid in installing zygomatic implants," *Journal of Oral and Maxillofacial Surgery*, vol. 59, no. 10, pp. 1193–1198, 2001.

[3] S. M. Parel, P. I. Brånemark, L. O. Ohrnell, and B. Svensson, "Remote implant anchorage for the rehabilitation of maxillary defects," *Journal of Prosthetic Dentistry*, vol. 86, no. 4, pp. 377–381, 2001.

[4] J. Clavero and S. Lundgren, "Ramus or chin grafts for maxillary sinus inlay and local onlay augmentation: comparison of donor site morbidity and complications," *Clinical Implant Dentistry and Related Research*, vol. 5, no. 3, pp. 154–160, 2003.

[5] M. J. Yaremchuk, "Vascularized bone grafts for maxillofacial reconstruction," *Clinics in Plastic Surgery*, vol. 16, pp. 29–39, 1989.

[6] M. Sjöström, L. Sennerby, H. Nilson, and S. Lundgren, "Reconstruction of the atrophic edentulous maxilla with free iliac crest grafts and implants: a 3-year report of a prospective clinical study," *Clinical Implant Dentistry and Related Research*, vol. 9, no. 1, pp. 46–59, 2007.

[7] L. K. Cheung, Q. Zhang, Z. G. Zhang, and M. C. M. Wong, "Reconstruction of maxillectomy defect by transport distraction osteogenesis," *International Journal of Oral and Maxillofacial Surgery*, vol. 32, no. 5, pp. 515–522, 2003.

[8] E. Nyström, H. Nilson, J. Gunne, and S. Lundgren, "Reconstruction of the atrophic maxilla with interpositional bone grafting/Le Fort I osteotomy and endosteal implants: a 11-16 year follow-up," *International Journal of Oral and Maxillofacial Surgery*, vol. 38, no. 1, pp. 1–6, 2009.

[9] R. G. Triplett and S. R. Schow, "Autologous bone grafts and endosseous implants: complementary techniques," *Journal of Oral and Maxillofacial Surgery*, vol. 54, no. 4, pp. 486–494, 1996.

[10] M. Del Fabbro, T. Testori, L. Francetti, and R. Weinstein, "Systematic review of survival rates for implants placed in the grafted maxillary sinus," *International Journal of Periodontics and Restorative Dentistry*, vol. 24, no. 6, pp. 565–577, 2004.

[11] L. Vrielinck, C. Politis, S. Schepers, M. Pauwels, and I. Naert, "Image-based planning and clinical validation of zygoma and pterygoid implant placement in patients with severe bone atrophy using customized drill guides. Preliminary results from a prospective clinical follow-up study," *International Journal of Oral and Maxillofacial Surgery*, vol. 32, no. 1, pp. 7–14, 2003.

[12] K. Lal, G. S. White, D. N. Morea, and R. F. Wright, "Use of stereolithographic templates for surgical and prosthodontic implant planning and placement. Part I. The concept," *Journal of Prosthodontics*, vol. 15, no. 1, pp. 51–58, 2006.

[13] R. Ewers, K. Schicho, G. Undt et al., "Basic research and 12 years of clinical experience in computer-assisted navigation technology: a review," *International Journal of Oral and Maxillofacial Surgery*, vol. 34, no. 1, pp. 1–8, 2005.

[14] L. R. Duarte, H. N. Filho, C. E. Francischone, L. G. Peredo, and P. I. Brånemark, "The establishment of a protocol for the total rehabilitation of atrophic maxillae employing four zygomatic fixtures in an immediate loading system—a 30-month clinical and radiographic follow-up," *Clinical Implant Dentistry and Related Research*, vol. 9, no. 4, pp. 186–196, 2007.

[15] P. Maló, M. de Araujo Nobre, and I. Lopes, "A new approach to rehabilitate the severely atrophic maxilla using extramaxillary anchored implants in immediate function: a pilot study," *Journal of Prosthetic Dentistry*, vol. 100, no. 5, pp. 354–366, 2008.

[16] M. Stiévenart and C. Malevez, "Rehabilitation of totally atrophied maxilla by means of four zygomatic implants and fixed prosthesis: a 6-40-month follow-up," *International Journal of Oral and Maxillofacial Surgery*, vol. 39, pp. 358–363, 2010.

[17] B. Al-Nawas, J. Wegener, C. Bender, and W. Wagner, "Critical soft tissue parameters of the zygomatic implant," *Journal of Clinical Periodontology*, vol. 31, no. 7, pp. 497–500, 2004.

[18] M. Stiévenart and C. Malevez, "Rehabilitation of totally atrophied maxilla by means of four zygomatic implants and fixed prosthesis: a 6-40-month follow-up," *International Journal of Oral and Maxillofacial Surgery*, vol. 39, pp. 358–363, 2010.

[19] J. P. Becktor, S. Isaksson, P. Abrahamsson, and L. Sennerby, "Evaluation of 31 zygomatic implants and 74 regular dental implants used in 16 patients for prosthetic reconstruction of the atrophic maxilla with cross-arch fixed bridges," *Clinical Implant Dentistry and Related Research*, vol. 7, no. 3, pp. 159–165, 2005.

[20] C. Malevez, M. Abarca, F. Durdu, and P. Daelemans, "Clinical outcome of 103 consecutive zygomatic implants: a 6-48 months follow-up study," *Clinical Oral Implants Research*, vol. 15, no. 1, pp. 18–22, 2004.

[21] J. P. Urgell, V. R. Gutiérrez, and C. G. Escoda, "Rehabilitation of atrophic maxilla: a review of 101 zygomatic implants," *Medicina*

Oral, Patologia Oral y Cirugia Bucal, vol. 13, no. 6, Article ID 10489698, pp. E363–E370, 2008.

[22] C. A. Landes, "Zygoma implant-supported midfacial prosthetic rehabilitation: a 4-year follow-up study including assessment of quality of life," *Clinical Oral Implants Research*, vol. 16, no. 3, pp. 313–325, 2005.

[23] M. Peñarrocha, C. Carrillo, A. Boronat, and E. Martí, "Level of satisfaction in patients with maxillary full-arch fixed prostheses: zygomatic versus conventional implants," *International Journal of Oral and Maxillofacial Implants*, vol. 22, no. 5, pp. 769–773, 2007.

27

Coverage of Gingival Fenestration Using Modified Pouch and Tunnel Technique: A Novel Approach

Sunil Pendor,[1] Vidya Baliga,[1] A. Muthukumaraswamy,[2] Prasad V. Dhadse,[1] Kiran Kumar Ganji,[1] and Kaustubh Thakare[1]

[1] *Department of Periodontics, Sharad Pawar Dental College and Hospital, Sawangi (M), Wardha, Maharashtra 442004, India*
[2] *Department of Periodontics, Tamilnadu Government Dental College and Hospital, Chennai, Tamilnadu 600003, India*

Correspondence should be addressed to Vidya Baliga; baligavs@gmail.com

Academic Editors: S. Anil and M. De Bruyne

Gingival fenestration defects are a rare phenomenon. Gingival fenestration means the exposure of the tooth due to loss of the overlying bone and gingiva. Though treatment of mucosal fenestration occurring in association with chronic periapical inflammation has been reported previously, the occurrence and treatment of gingival fenestration have not been documented in great detail. This report describes the occurrence of a gingival fenestration that developed secondarily to a gutka chewing habit. Treatment of the fenestration along with coverage of an adjacent recession defect in a single-step procedure using a pouch and tunnel technique is described.

1. Introduction

Gingival fenestrations are of uncertain etiology and have rarely been reported in the dental literature [1]. Gingival fenestration defects may create problems regarding plaque control, root hypersensitivity, and esthetics.

Gingival recession may be caused by periodontal disease, improper oral hygiene, frenal pull, bone dehiscence, improper restorations, tooth malposition, viral infections of the gingiva, and oral habits [2]. Recession defects are treated to resolve a variety of patient-centered concerns including, but not limited to, root sensitivity, increased potential for root caries, difficulty in plaque control, and esthetics [3]. Furthermore, it must be remembered that exposed roots are prone to abrasion and erosion.

Several innovations, modifications, and variations have been developed for surgical root coverage since Grupe and Warren [4] first described the laterally positioned flap. However, greater predictability of results became achievable only with the introduction of bilaminar connective tissue grafting techniques [5]. Raetzke in 1985 [6] described a bilaminar technique for isolated recession defects, creating an envelope or pouch around the recession area to receive connective tissue graft. Zabalegui and others [7] treated multiple gingival recessions by creating a tunnel under the areas of gingival recession to receive the connective tissue graft thus avoiding dissecting the intermediate papilla and improving blood supply to the flap. Highly successful root coverage was reported with these two techniques [6, 7].

Gutka is chiefly a mixture of powdered tobacco, areca nut (fruit of *Areca catechu*), and slaked lime (aqueous calcium hydroxide), usage of which is seen mainly in the Indian subcontinent and also enjoyed by immigrant communities settled in Europe and the United States [8]. Habitual gutka use has been associated with the occurrence of several oral mucosal disorders, including oral submucous fibrosis (OSF), oral cancer, and periodontal disease [9, 10].

The following case describes a rare situation of occurrence of a gingival fenestration in a gutka chewer. Treatment of the fenestration, as well as simultaneous root coverage of a class I recession defect on the adjacent tooth, creating a pouch and subjacent tunnel is described. A conservative incision technique for the preparation of the tunnel was used.

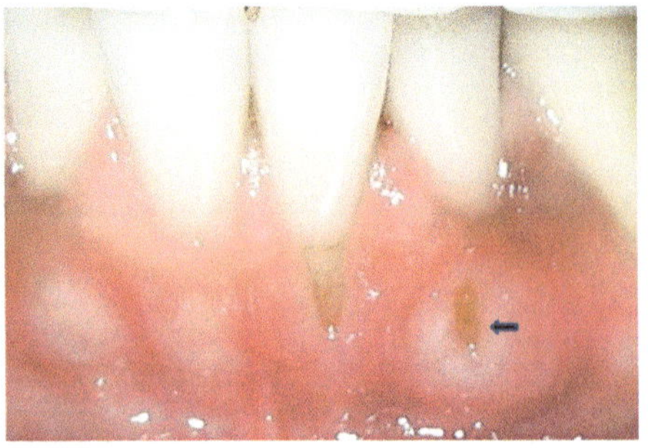

FIGURE 1: Intraoral photograph showing Miller's class I recession in the mandibular left central incisor and the fenestration defect (arrow).

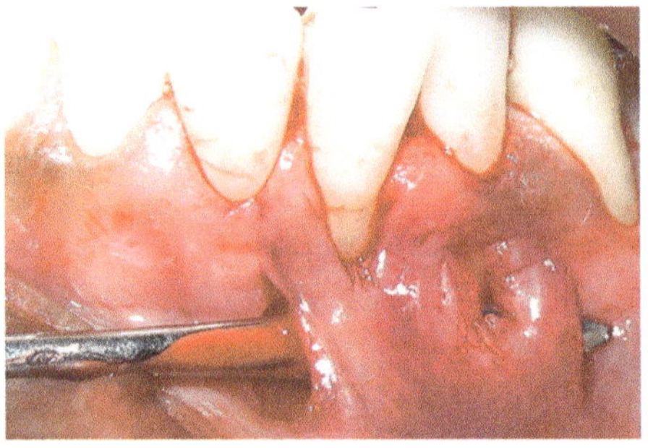

FIGURE 2: Partial thickness tunnel connecting two vertical incisions for fenestration coverage.

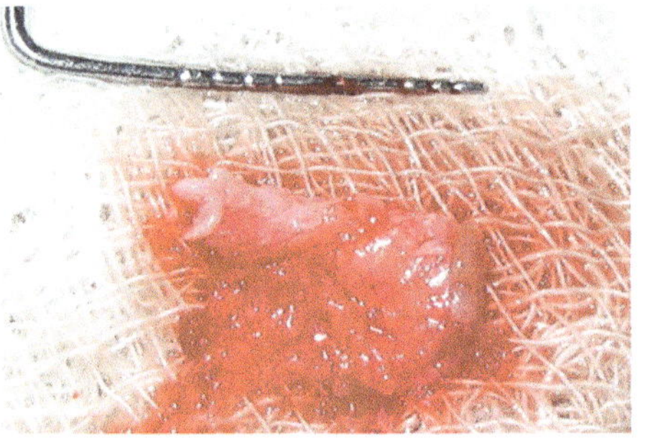

FIGURE 3: Harvested connective tissue graft.

2. Case Report

A 27-year-old male reported to the authors' department with a complaint of hypersensitivity and burning sensation in the lower left front region since one month. History of two years of gutka chewing with placement of the gutka quid in the lower labial vestibule was reported. On examination, a portion of the root of mandibular left lateral incisor was visible through a gingival and alveolar bone fenestration on the labial surface (Figure 1). The fenestration was oval in shape, measuring approximately 4 × 2 mm in diameter. The area was free of pus and calculus, and the surrounding gingiva appeared whitish in color. All probing depth measurements around the tooth were within the normal limit, and the fenestrated area could not be probed through the gingival sulcus. The adjacent central incisor showed the presence of a Miller's class I recession [11] (Figure 1).

The patient was counselled regarding the harmful effects of gutka chewing and was referred to a tobacco-cessation center. Professional prophylaxis was performed 1 month after cessation of the habit. Informed consent was obtained from the patient.

The surgery was initiated after administration of a local anesthetic agent (Xicaine, ICPA, Mumbai, India). A sulcular incision was given with a number 15C blade and a supraperiosteal pouch was created apically and laterally to the recession extending 3 to 5 mm in all directions. Two conservative submarginal vertical releasing incisions extending beyond the mucogingival junction were made on the mesial line angle of the right central incisor and distal line angle of the lateral incisor. A partial thickness tunnel was prepared extending horizontally, connecting the two vertical incisions (Figure 2). The tunnel was connected to the pouch, and the apical extension was carried beyond the mucogingival junction to facilitate the placement of the connective tissue graft.

Connective tissue graft of adequate dimensions (Figure 3) as measured with a template was procured from the palate (site: mesial aspect of the maxillary left first premolar to the distal aspect of the first molar) by the "trap door" approach [12] and the palatal donor site was sutured using a 4-0 nonresorbable, silk suture.

The harvested connective tissue graft was positioned in the prepared pouch by sliding it through the vertical incision area (Figure 4) and securing it to the adjacent interdental papillae using 5-0 absorbable suture (Vicryl, Ethicon, Johnson and Johnson, USA) and independent sling sutures. With the help of elevators the graft was further slid through the tunnel to cover the fenestration (Figure 5) and securing it to the adjacent flap using 5-0 Vicryl sutures. The vertical incisions were closed with interrupted sutures (Figure 6).

The patient was discharged after placement of a periodontal dressing (PerioCare, Pulpdent Corporation, Watertown, MA, USA). He was advised to refrain from mechanical cleansing of the surgical site, which could disturb initial healing, and instructed to rinse with 0.2% chlorhexidine gluconate solution (Hexidine, ICPA Health Care Products Ltd., Mumbai, India) twice a day for one minute. An analgesic was prescribed for the relief from any postsurgical pain.

Healing was uneventful. The sutures placed in the palate were removed after 1 week. The sutures placed on the buccal aspect and the periodontal pack was removed after 15 days. At the 1-month, 2-month, 3-month, and 6-month (Figure 7) postsurgical appointments, progressive adaptation of the edges of the graft to the surrounding tissues and increased morphologic and chromatic mimicking were observed. Six months after surgery, sulcular probing depth was less than 2 mm at the recession site, and no bleeding on probing was present. The gingival margin at the centre of labial surface was 0.5 mm short of the CEJ, but a recession depth reduction of 2.5 mm was seen (Prior to the surgery recession depth was 3 mm; after 6 months the residual recession at the site was 0.5 mm). The position of the mucogingival junction remained the same, but the amount of keratinized gingival

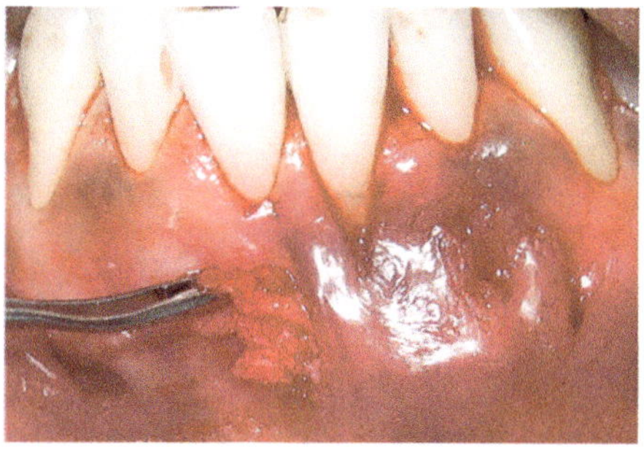

FIGURE 4: Placement of the connective tissue graft in the prepared tunnel.

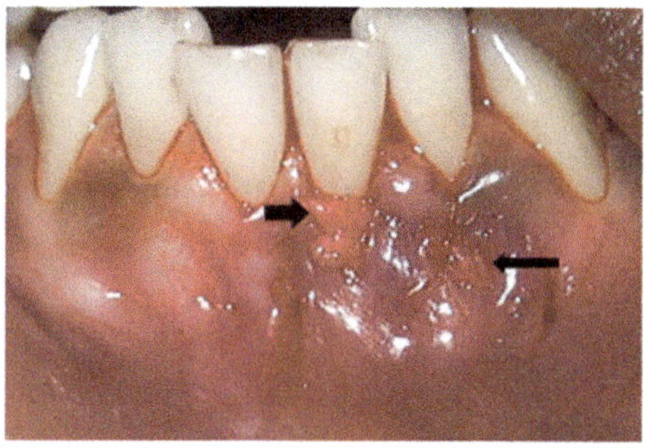

FIGURE 5: Extending the graft coronally into the prepared pouch (short and thick arrow-shows the graft placed in the prepared pouch); note coverage of the fenestration defect (long arrow) also.

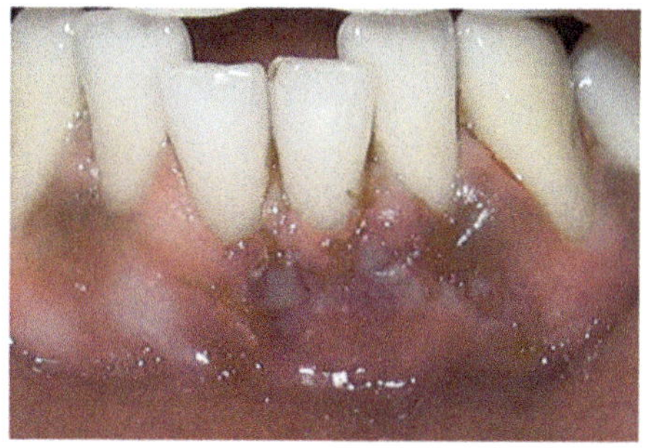

FIGURE 6: The graft was sutured by independent sling sutures and secured to the adjacent papillae by interrupted sutures in the recession area. Graft covering the fenestration defect was secured to the adjacent flap with interrupted sutures.

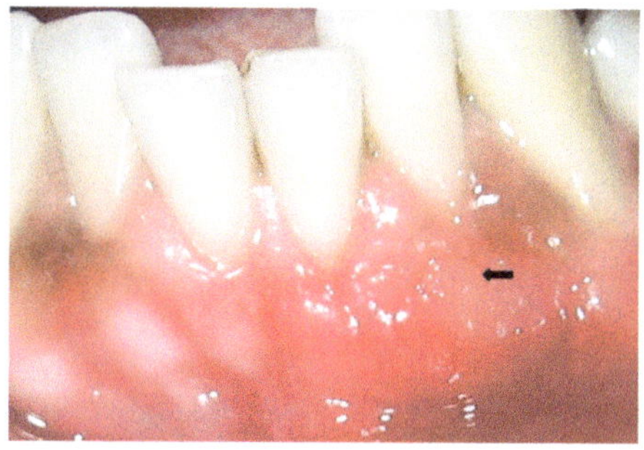

FIGURE 7: At 6-month followup the fenestration was completely covered and adequate root coverage of the recessed tooth was achieved.

on the left central incisor increased by 2.5 mm (1.0 mm before surgery, 3.5 mm after surgery). Though an indentation was seen at the fenestration area, complete coverage of the defect was completely seen. The patient was placed in maintenance program consisting of prophylaxis and motivation.

3. Discussion

Bilateral fenestration of the labial gingival tissue of the permanent mandibular central incisors has been reported in a developing child, which resulted in an apical positioning of the gingival margin even after maintenance of good oral hygiene over a 2-year period [2]. No etiologic factors were identified other than labial positioning of the teeth and the changes in gingival contour were noted as a part of the continuous process of remodeling.

Isolated gingival fenestration has also been reported to occur in association with cervical enamel projections (CEPs) [1]. The attachment between epithelium and enamel as a junction has been described to be composed of hemidesmosomes and a basal lamina [18, 19] thought to constitute an area of lessened resistance to plaque-associated inflammatory degradation [20].

Mucosal fenestrations have been reported previously [16, 17], and the probable etiological factors reported were extreme buccal inclination of root tips with very thin or nonexistent buccal cortical plate combining with chronic periapical inflammation [16, 17]. The various fenestration defects and the treatment modalities employed are summarized in Table 1.

Gutka contains fine grains of areca nut, which, besides causing mechanical injury to oral tissues, also allows ground tobacco to adhere to the traumatized mucosa, leading to morphologic changes and membrane damage [21]. In the present case the tooth with fenestration defect was free of periapical inflammation as indicated by radiographic and clinical examination. Oral hygiene performance was found to be adequate. Hence, it can be said that mechanical injury caused by gutka chewing may have led to the development of gingival fenestration. In addition, exposure of the tooth favored further deposition of plaque as well as subjecting it to constant mechanical injury caused by continued gutka chewing that prevented reformation of the mucosal covering. Mechanical injury combined with a labially aligned tooth may be the probable etiologic factors for occurrence of recession.

Cessation of the gutka chewing habit may help to reduce the severity of the condition and may also prevent its progression; however, the defect caused required surgical intervention. Due to the presence of two adjacent defects, which would otherwise require two separate procedures for root coverage, were treated using a single-step procedure thus reducing patient morbidity.

Table 1: Reported cases with fenestration and various treatment modalities employed.

Fenestration type	Region	Etiologic factors	Treatment
Gingival [2]	Mandibular centrals	Labial placement was considered part of development process	Observation—2-year period
Gingival [1]	Maxillary central incisor	Cervical enamel projections	Flap elevation with odontoplasty
Mucosal [13]	Maxillary central incisor	Chronic periapical inflammation	Re-root planing + chlorhexidine mouth rinsing
Mucosal [14]	Maxillary first molar	Chronic periapical inflammation, buccally inclined root tip	Full thickness mucoperiosteal flap with primary closure
Mucosal [15]	Mandibular incisor	Chronic periapical inflammation	Full thickness rectangular flap with healing by secondary intention
Mucosal [16]	Maxillary premolar	Buccally inclined root, chronic periapical inflammation	Laterally positioned flap
Mucosal [17]	Maxillary premolar	Chronic periapical inflammation	Connective tissue graft

One of the prerequisites for complete recuperation of the periodontal tissues is the maintenance of adequate vascularization in the flaps and grafts, which is an advantage offered by bilaminar techniques. Also, the presence of releasing incisions interrupts the superficial and intramural vascularization [5]. In the case discussed since the fenestration was located submarginally, the coronoapical extension of the releasing incisions was kept to the minimum necessary to facilitate access without involving the gingival margin and the papilla thereby improving the blood supply to the graft and further reducing patient morbidity.

Complete root coverage has been clinically defined on the basis of the following criteria [5]: (1) the marginal tissue reaches the level of the cementoenamel junction (CEJ); (2) clinical attachment is present; (3) sulcus depth is 2 mm or less; and (4) bleeding on probing is absent. Though primary coverage could not be attained in a small area, midlabially, one cannot rule out the possibility of secondary coverage that occurs by creeping attachment [22].

4. Conclusion

This case report shows the advantages in terms of predictability of coverage and esthetics when care is taken to ensure proper access through minimal releasing incisions. We believe that this technique is valuable when a single-step procedure is required to cover adjacent recession as well as a gingival fenestration defect. Given the widespread incidence of marginal tissue recession and associated esthetic concern of patients, the single-stage pouch and tunnel surgical technique may be beneficial in meeting the esthetic and functional demands of patients and also contribute to increased treatment acceptance and overall patient satisfaction.

Contribution

S. Pendor was responsible for concept and is the guarantor. V. Baliga was responsible for design, definition of intellectual content, literature search, data acquisition, statistical analysis, and paper preparation and revision. A. Muthukumaraswamy performed clinical studies. P. V. Dhadse acquired data and edited the paper. K. K. Ganji acquired and analyzed data. K. Thakare acquired and analyzed data and edited the paper.

References

[1] B. G. Askenas, H. R. Fry, and J. W. Davis, "Cervical enamel projection with gingival fenestration in a maxillary central incisor: report of a case," *Quintessence International*, vol. 23, no. 2, pp. 103–107, 1992.

[2] L. A. M. Santos-Pinto, N. Sue Seale, A. K. Reddy, and R. C. L. Cordeiro, "Fenestration gingival defect in erupting permanent mandibular incisors: a case report," *Quintessence International*, vol. 29, no. 4, pp. 239–242, 1998.

[3] M. K. McGuire and M. Nunn, "Evaluation of human recession defects treated with coronally advanced flaps and either enamel matrix derivative or connective tissue. Part 1: comparison of clinical parameters," *Journal of Periodontology*, vol. 74, no. 8, pp. 1110–1125, 2003.

[4] H. Grupe and R. Warren, "Repair of gingival defects by a sliding flap operation," *Journal of Periodontology*, vol. 27, no. 2, pp. 92–95, 1956.

[5] G. Santarelli, R. Ciancaglini, F. Campanari, C. Dinoi, and S. Ferraris, "Connective tissue grafting employing the tunnel technique: a case report of complete root coverage in the anterior maxilla," *International Journal of Periodontics and Restorative Dentistry*, vol. 21, no. 1, pp. 77–83, 2001.

[6] P. B. Raetzke, "Covering localized areas of root exposure employing the "envelope" technique," *Journal of Periodontology*, vol. 56, no. 7, pp. 397–402, 1985.

[7] I. Zabalegui, A. Sicilia, J. Cambra, J. Gil, and M. Sanz, "Treatment of multiple adjacent gingival recessions with the tunnel subepithelial connective tissue graft: a clinical report," *International Journal of Periodontics and Restorative Dentistry*, vol. 19, no. 2, pp. 199–206, 1999.

[8] F. Javed, M. Chotai, A. Mehmood, and K. Almas, "Oral mucosal disorders associated with habitual gutka usage: a review," *Oral Surgery, Oral Medicine, Oral Pathology, Oral Radiology and Endodontology*, vol. 109, no. 6, pp. 857–864, 2010.

[9] F. Javed, M. Altamash, B. Klinge, and P. Engström, "Periodontal conditions and oral symptoms in gutka-chewers with and without type 2 diabetes," *Acta Odontologica Scandinavica*, vol. 66, no. 5, pp. 268–273, 2008.

[10] P. R. Murti, R. B. Bhonsle, J. J. Pindborg, D. K. Daftary, P. C. Gupta, and F. S. Mehta, "Malignant transformation rate in oral submucous fibrosis over a 17-year period," *Community Dentistry and Oral Epidemiology*, vol. 13, no. 6, pp. 340–341, 1985.

[11] P. D. Miller Jr., "A classification of marginal tissue recession," *The International Journal of Periodontics and Restorative Dentistry*, vol. 5, no. 2, pp. 8–13, 1985.

[12] J. L. Wennström and G. P. Pini Prato, "Mucogingival therapy-periodontal plastic surgery," in *Clinical Periodontology and Implant Dentistry*, J. Lindhe, T. Karring, and N. P. Lang, Eds., p. 955, Blackwell Munksgaard, Oxford, UK, 5th edition, 2008.

[13] Z.-P. Yang, "Treatment of labial fenestration of maxillary central incisor," *Endodontics and Dental Traumatology*, vol. 12, no. 2, pp. 104–108, 1996.

[14] W. L. Sawes and I. E. Barnes, "The surgical treatment of fenestrated buccal roots of an upper molar-a case report," *International Endodontic Journal*, vol. 16, no. 2, pp. 82–86, 1983.

[15] A. Rawlinson, "Treatment of a labial fenestration of a lower incisor tooth apex," *British Dental Journal*, vol. 156, no. 12, pp. 448–449, 1984.

[16] Y. Ju, A. H. Tsai, Y. Wu, and W. Pan, "Surgical intervention of mucosal fenestration in a maxillary premolar: a case report," *Quintessence International*, vol. 35, no. 2, pp. 125–128, 2004.

[17] G. Chen, C. T. Fang, and C. Tong, "The management of mucosal fenestration: a report of two cases," *International Endodontic Journal*, vol. 42, no. 2, pp. 156–164, 2009.

[18] I. B. Stern, "Electron microscopic observatons of oral epithelium. I. Basal cells and the basement membrane," *Periodontics*, vol. 3, no. 5, pp. 224–238, 1965.

[19] H. Ito, S. Enomoto, and K. Kobayashi, "Electron microscopic study of the human epithelial attachment," *The Bulletin of Tokyo Medical and Dental University*, vol. 14, no. 2, pp. 267–277, 1967.

[20] A. R. Goldstein, "Enamel pearls as contributing factor in periodontal breakdown," *The Journal of the American Dental Association*, vol. 99, no. 2, pp. 210–211, 1979.

[21] G. Parmar, P. Sangwan, P. Vashi, P. Kulkarni, and S. Kumar, "Effect of chewing a mixture of areca nut and tobacco on periodontal tissues and oral hygiene status," *Journal of Oral Science*, vol. 50, no. 1, pp. 57–62, 2008.

[22] J. Matter and G. Cimasoni, "Creeping attachment after free gingival grafts," *Journal of Periodontology*, vol. 47, no. 10, pp. 574–579, 1976.

28

Microabrasion: An Effective Method for Improvement of Esthetics in Dentistry

Biji Balan,[1] Chengappa Madanda Uthaiah,[2] Sreejesh Narayanan,[3] and Priyadarshini Mookalamada Monnappa[4]

[1] *Department of Conservative Dentistry and Endodontics, Kannur Dental College, Anjarakandy, Kannur, Kerala 670612, India*
[2] *Department of Prosthodontics, Kannur Dental College, Anjarakandy, Kannur, Kerala 670612, India*
[3] *District HQ Hospital, Kannur, Kerala 670017, India*
[4] *Kannur Medical College, Anjarakandy, Kannur, Kerala 670612, India*

Correspondence should be addressed to Biji Balan; docbiji@gmail.com

Academic Editors: C. Evans and A. Milosevic

Enamel microabrasion can eliminate enamel irregularities and discoloration defects, thus improving the appearance of teeth. This paper presents the latest treatment protocol of enamel microabrasion to remove stains on the enamel surface. It has been verified that teeth submitted to microabrasion acquire a yellowish colour because of the thinness of the remaining enamel, revealing the colour of dentinal tissue to a greater degree. Enamel microabrasion is a technique that can be used to correct discoloured enamel. Enamel microabrasion was developed in the mid-1980s as a method of eliminating enamel discolouration defects and improving the appearance of teeth. Several years after the method was developed, much has been learned about this technique, long-term results of treatment, and microscopic changes to the enamel surface that have distinguishable clinical implications. In addition, certain patients can benefit from enamel microabrasion to yield attractive cosmetic results. The aim of this study was to report the clinical case of a male patient of 25 years with moderate fluorosis, whose smile was re-established by the use of an enamel microabrasion technique, with 18% hydrochloric acid and pumice slurry shown to be a safe and efficient method for removing fluorosis stains.

1. Introduction

It is well documented that fluoride can have both beneficial and detrimental effects on the dentition ever since Mc Kay and G. V. Black published the effect of fluoride on dentition in 1916 [1]. The beneficial effects of fluoride on dental caries are due primarily to the topical effect of fluoride after the teeth have erupted in the oral cavity. In contrast, detrimental effects are due to systemic absorption during tooth development resulting in dental fluorosis that is one of the most common types of enamel demineralisation [1]. Initially, it involves subsurface hypomineralization and/or porosity of the enamel but may extend through the whole thickness as the severity increases [2]. The discoloration may range from yellow to dark brown [3]. Enamel discoloration especially in the anterior teeth may raise esthetic concerns in patients. Conservative non-restorative methods such as microabrasion technique have been used in the treatment of demineralization defects and discolorations of teeth [4]. This technique which involves mild acid etching in combination with rotary application of an abrasive medium [5] was first described by Dr. Walter Kane (Colorado Springs, 1916). By rubbing six maxillary anterior teeth with hydrochloric acid (HCl) under the flame of an alcohol torch, he found favourable results in the treatment of enamel fluorosis without any destruction or damage of enamel. However, for more than 60 years, most clinicians avoided applying this technique, because of fear of damage or destruction of the enamel [6, 7]. In 1984, McCloskey introduced the use of acid combined with pumice [7] which was named "microabrasion" by Croll two years later [8]. Considering its high incidence, the dentist must be able to diagnose fluorosis properly and treat it efficiently.

If the stains are present in the outer layers of enamel, they can be easily removed, leaving a smooth, glassy enamel

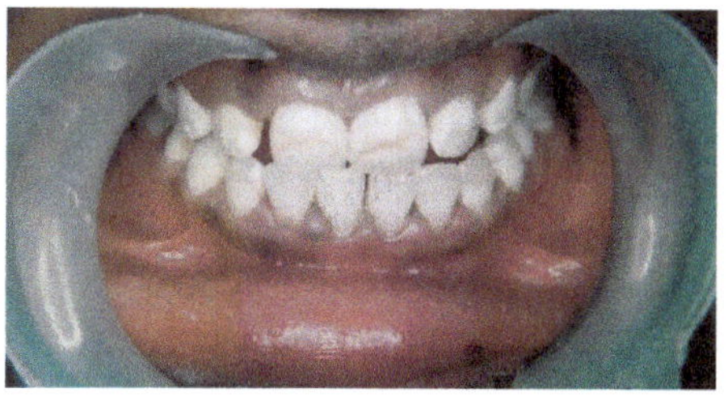

FIGURE 1: Preoperative.

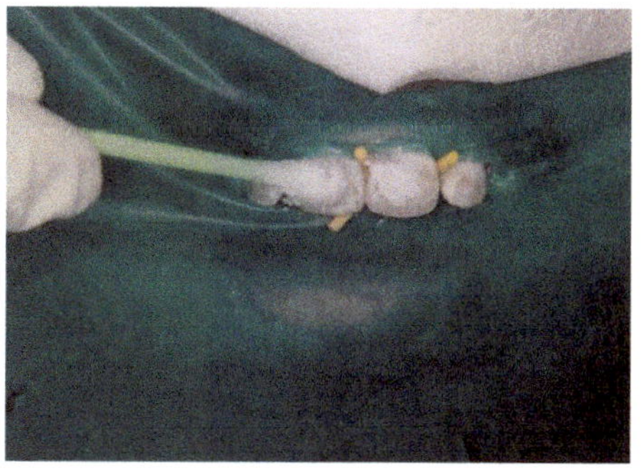

FIGURE 2: Application of HCL and pumice slurry on teeth.

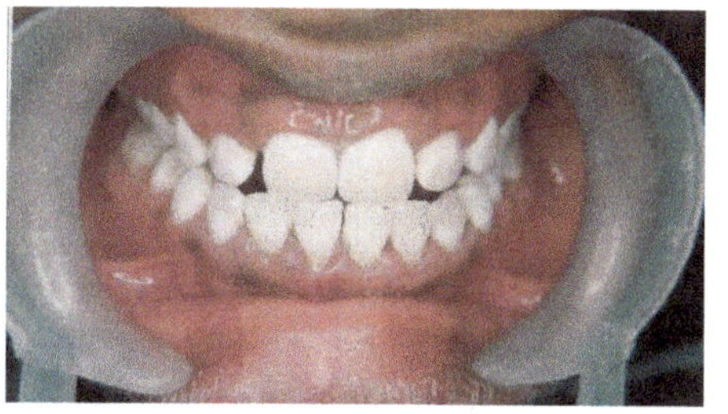

FIGURE 3: Postoperative.

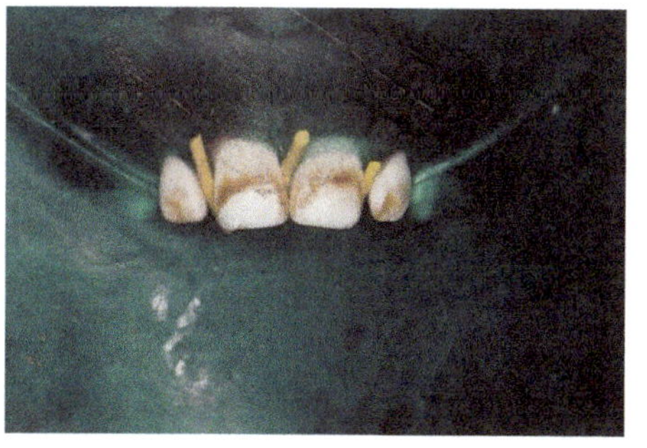

FIGURE 4: Preoperative. Isolation done using rubber dam.

surface as the finished result. This surface is seen to be more caries resistant than the original surface. This paper deals with a case report of how effectively mild to moderate stains that are removed using microabrasion technique.

2. Case Report-1

A twenty-five year-old-male patient came to the dental clinics for routine dental care. His chief complaint was to remove and/or minimize the noticeable brown/yellow staining of his teeth. He wanted the least invasive and most cost-effective treatment to change his smile. A review of his medical history and past dental history revealed no contraindications to dental treatment. In consideration of his age, the patient was not interested in treatment options that involved significant removal of tooth structure, such as porcelain or composite resin veneers. From the appearance of his teeth, a diagnosis of mild fluorosis staining determined by using Dean's Fluorosis Index (Table 1) was sent on the anterior teeth in the aesthetic zone, with the most significant staining occurring on the maxillary anterior teeth, with light brown streaks in the middle third of the facial surfaces (Figure 1).

A treatment plan was presented to the patient that would fulfill his request for minimally invasive treatment which proposed microabrasion of the superficial enamel. Upon completion of treatment, the tooth shade would be evaluated.

The teeth was isolated with a rubber dam to protect the gums from coming into contact with the acid (18% HCl). The pumice-acid slurry is then applied to the tooth or teeth to the facial surfaces of the maxillary teeth using cotton (Figure 2) and rubbed either manually or with a very slow speed rubber cup. Using a right angle latch type slow-speed handpiece running the motor at 1,000 rpm, a hybrid bristle brush-cup was used to rub the pumice acid slurry for three separate applications of 30 to 40 seconds each. Between each application, the slurry was rinsed and dried from the tooth surfaces. This procedure was repeated three times. At the completion of the microabrasion technique, the enamel surfaces were polished with a cup-shaped porcelain polishing rubber abrasive to smooth and polish the enamel surface. After a few layers of enamel are removed, the slurry was rinsed with water and the result was evaluated. This process is repeated until the stain is gone or the process must be stopped for other reasons (enamel getting too thin or tooth getting sensitive). After the process was complete, fluoride gel was placed on the teeth in order to reduce postoperative sensitivity. The entire process takes less than an hour and is permanent. The rubber dam was removed and the patient viewed the result of treatment (Figure 3). He was pleased with the result from the immediate removal of the dark staining on his maxillary anterior teeth.

3. Case Report-2

A thirty-year-old male came to the dental hospital with chief complaint of dark brown staining of the anterior teeth. He also wanted a least invasive, cost-effective treatment to enhance his esthetics. From the appearance of his teeth, diagnosis of moderate flourosis staining was determined by Dean's Fluorosis Index (Table 1). The most significant staining occurring on the maxillary anterior teeth contained dark brown streaks in the middle third of the facial surfaces (Figure 4). The same procedure for the microabrasion was repeated as was done in Section 2. After the procedure was completed, fluoride gel application was placed on the teeth to reduce the postoperative sensitivity.

TABLE 1

Normal	The enamel represents the usual translucent semivitriform type of structure. The surface is smooth, glossy, and usually of a pale creamy white colour.
Questionable	The enamel discloses slight aberrations from the translucency of normal enamel, ranging from a few white flecks to occasional white spots. This classification is utilized in those instances where a definite diagnosis of the mildest form of fluorosis is not warranted and a classification of "normal" is not justified.
Very mild	Small, opaque, paper-white areas scattered irregularly over the tooth but not involving as much as 25% of the tooth surface. Frequently included in this classification are teeth showing no more than about one to 2 mm of white opacity at the tip of the summit of the cusps of the bicuspids or second molars.
Mild	The white opaque areas in the enamel of the teeth are more extensive but do not involve as much as 50% of the tooth.
Moderate	All enamel surfaces of the teeth are affected, and the surfaces subject to attrition show wear. Brown stain is frequently a disfiguring feature
Severe	Includes teeth formerly classified as "moderately severe and severe." All enamel surfaces are affected and hypoplasia is so marked that the general form of the tooth may be affected. The major diagnostic sign of this classification is discrete or confluent pitting. Brown stains are widespread and teeth often present a corroded-like appearance.

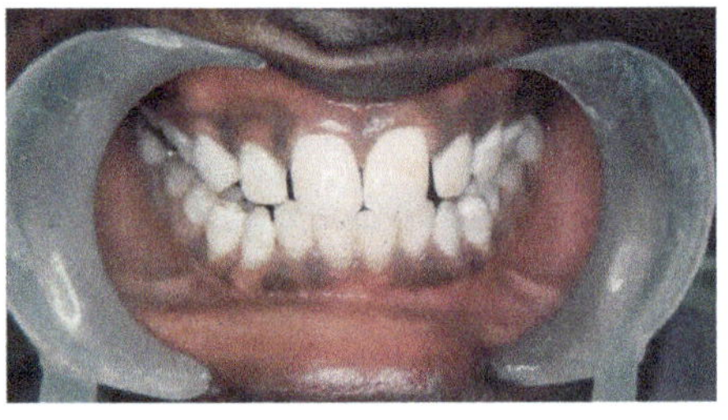

FIGURE 5: Postoperative.

The rubber dam was removed for the evaluation of the result by the patient (Figure 5). The patient was quite satisfied with the results. In the above mentioned cases, patients were asked not to smoke, eat, or drink anything that could possibly stain the teeth for 24–48 hours after the treatment.

4. Discussion

Dental fluorosis is defined as hypomineralisation of enamel resulting from excessive intake of fluoride during tooth development. It is characterized by diffuse opacities on the enamel surface. These are differentiated from other conditions by the characteristic bilaterally symmetric distribution of the enamel defects. The degree to which the enamel is affected is dependent upon the duration, timing, and intensity of the fluoride concentration. In its mild form, most commonly the teeth present with small white streaks and the enamel appear mottled. As the severity of the condition increases, black and brown stains develop. The enamel microabrasion technique is an excellent method to remove intrinsic enamel stains of any etiology and colour, as well as to correct superficial irregularities on the buccal aspect of enamel, caused by either amelogenesis imperfecta or defects acquired after removal of orthodontic appliance [9]. These alterations, however, should have a hard texture and may affect the superficial layers of dental enamel. Because it is very difficult to determine the real depth of intrinsic stains or surface irregularities, the application of the microabrasion technique on intrinsic stains, regardless of their dimensions and depths, should always be considered before trying a restorative procedure [10]. Recurrence of staining on the teeth was not seen in these cases after two months on their recall visits. Maintenance of oral hygiene and caries prevention methods was advised to the patients.

Tooth discoloration due to fluorosis is an aesthetic problem for certain patients. While there is a range of restorative interventions that can be used to change the appearance of fluorosed teeth, the goal of minimally invasive treatment for mild-moderate fluorosis is the one that should be evaluated first. For the case presented in this article, a minimally invasive treatment option of microabrasion is the best choice.

5. Conclusion

The current evidence demonstrates that when a diagnosis of fluorosis has been made, the majority of cases are very mild or mild and do not require restorative treatment. For mild fluorosis discoloration and for moderate/severe fluorosis, treatment to change the aesthetic appearance of the teeth can be accomplished with minimally invasive treatment using microabrasion or in case of moderate-severe condition, combinations of microabrasion with bleaching can be done to provide the patient with an aesthetically acceptable results. For more severe fluorosis with dark discolorations and surface pitting, adhesive restorative dentistry may be necessary to fulfill a patient's aesthetic desires.

References

[1] F. S. McKay and G. V. Black, "An investigation of mottled teeth: an endemic developmental imperfection of the enamel of the teeth, heretofore unknown in the literature of dentistry," *Dental Cosmos*, vol. 58, pp. 477–484, 1916.

[2] A. C. B. Bezerra, S. C. Leal, S. A. M. Otero, D. B. L. Gravina, V. R. N. Cruvinel, and O. A. De Toledo, "Enamel opacities removal using two different acids: an *in vivo* comparison," *Journal of Clinical Pediatric Dentistry*, vol. 29, no. 2, pp. 147–150, 2005.

[3] B. W. Nevil, D. D. Dann, C. M. Allen, and J. Bouquot, Eds., *Oral and Maxillofacial Pathology*, Saunders; Elsevier, Philadelphia, Pa, USA, 2009.

[4] C. D. Lynch and R. J. McConnell, "The use of microabrasion to remove discolored enamel: a clinical report," *Journal of Prosthetic Dentistry*, vol. 90, no. 5, pp. 417–419, 2003.

[5] T. P. Croll, "A case of enamel color modification: 60-year results," *Quintessence International*, vol. 18, no. 7, pp. 493–495, 1987.

[6] T. P. Croll and R. R. Cavanaugh, "Enamel color modification by controlled hydrochloric acid-pumice abrasion. I. technique and examples," *Quintessence International*, vol. 17, no. 2, pp. 81–87, 1986.

[7] R. J. McCloskey, "A technique for removal of fluorosis stains," *The Journal of the American Dental Association*, vol. 109, no. 1, pp. 63–64, 1984.

[8] T. P. Croll, "Enamel microabrasion: the technique," *Quintessence International*, vol. 20, no. 6, pp. 395–400, 1989.

[9] R. H. Sundfeld, V. Rahal, T. P. Croll, R. S. De Aalexandre, and A. L. F. Briso, "Enamel microabrasion followed by dental bleaching for patients after orthodontic treatment—case reports," *Journal of Esthetic and Restorative Dentistry*, vol. 19, no. 2, pp. 71–77, 2007.

[10] R. H. Sundfeld, T. P. Croll, A. L. F. Briso, R. S. De Alexandre, and D. S. Neto, "Considerations about enamel microabrasion after 18 years," *American Journal of Dentistry*, vol. 20, no. 2, pp. 67–72, 2007.

Circummandibular Wiring of Symphysis Fracture in a Five-Year-Old Child

Krishna Priya Vellore,[1] Srinivas Gadipelly,[2] Brahmananda Dutta,[1] Vijay Bhaskar Reddy,[2] Sri Ram,[1] and Arun Parsa[1]

[1] *Department of Pedodontics and Preventive Dentistry, MNR Dental College and Hospital, Andhra Pradesh, Sangareddy 502001, India*
[2] *Department of Oral and Maxillofacial Surgery, MNR Dental College and Hospital, Andhra Pradesh, Sangareddy 502001, India*

Correspondence should be addressed to Krishna Priya Vellore; krishnapriyavllr@gmail.com

Academic Editors: M. B. D. Gaviao and M. A. Polack

The treatment of pediatric maxillofacial fractures is unique due to the psychological, physiological, developmental, and anatomical characteristics of children. *Method.* This case report describes the management of symphysis fracture of mandible in a 5-year-old boy. The fracture was treated by acrylic splint with circummandibular wiring. *Results.* The splint was removed after 3 weeks. The patient had no complaints, and radiograph revealed a healed fracture. *Conclusion.* The clinical outcome in the present case indicates the management of mandibular fractures in pediatric patients using acrylic splint with circummandibular wiring.

1. Introduction

Mandibular fractures are the most common (56%) facial skeletal injury in hospitalized pediatric trauma patients [1, 2]. Boys are affected twice as frequently as girls [2, 3]. Dentoalveolar injuries are more frequent facial injury (60%) in children (especially under the age of 5) but rarely require hospitalization. In pediatric patients symphysis and parasymphysis fractures account for 15%–20% and body fracture rare [4]. The treatment choice of fractures in the pediatric mandible depends on the age and the state of tooth development.

Major injuries affecting the face are associated with hyperactivity of the child, fall, road traffic accidents (RTA), assault, and child abuses which are the most frequent risks of facial bone fractures in children [5].

Majority of the body and symphysis fractures in children are undisplaced because of elasticity of mandible and embedded tooth buds that holds the fragments together "like glue" [6, 7]. If displaced, closed reduction and immobilization are performed.

The following paper will review the triage, evaluation, and management of facial trauma in children. It highlights the role of acrylic splint with the use of circummandibular wiring technique in the management of symphysis fracture in a 5-year-old child.

2. Case Report

A 5-year-old male child reported to the Outpatient Department of Pedodontics and Preventive Dentistry, MNR Dental College and Hospital, Sangareddy, India, with a history of fall from steps. The patient was conscious, not well oriented with dressings in the lower jaw and no history of convulsions, vomiting, and bleeding from ear and nose. Haematological parameters such as blood count, CT, and BT were normal at the time of examination.

3. Clinical and Radiological Examination

Extraoral examination revealed the presence of a swelling in the anterior region of mandible. There was limited mouth opening because of pain and possible muscle spasm. On intraoral examination, bleeding was evident within the mouth. All primary teeth were present. A clinically minimally displaced fracture of the mandible in the area between two mandibular primary central incisors was noted. This

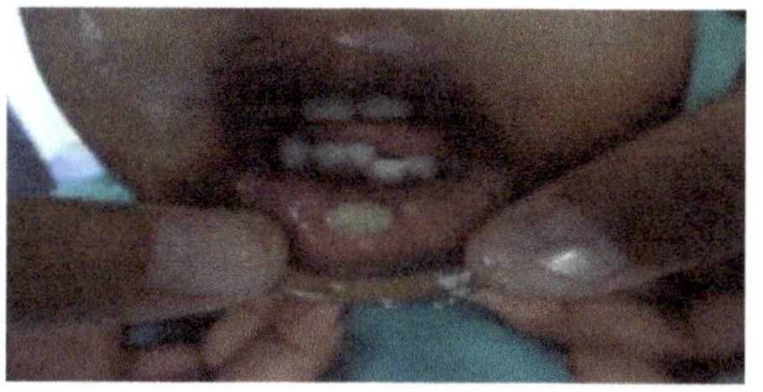

FIGURE 1: Preoperative photograph showing symphysis fracture.

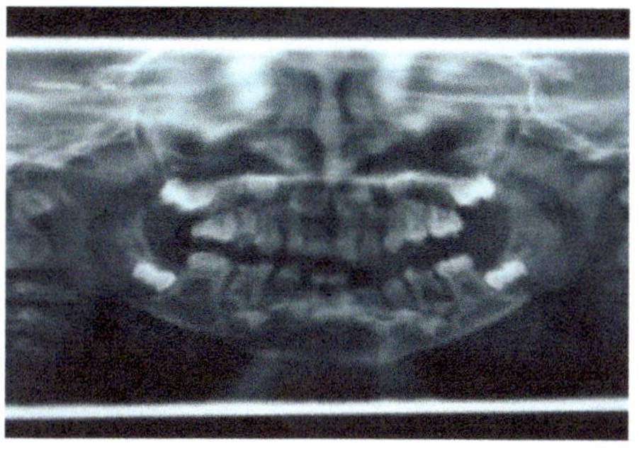

FIGURE 2: Preoperative OPG.

resulted in an altered occlusion and a midline diastema in the fractured area. The examination also revealed a subluxation of the upper right primary incisor which was not treated as followup is required and a deep laceration on the chin (Figure 1).

In the radiographs, mandibular symphysis fractures were evident between lower central incisors (Figures 2 and 9). Impressions of both jaws were taken with alginate impression material before mandibular reduction (Figure 3). An acrylic cap splint was then constructed on the model of the patient's arches after reducing the fracture on the models (Figure 4).

4. Management

Under general anaesthesia, the dislocated segments were reduced by bidigital pressure with the guidance of the surgical splint (Figure 5). A small stab incision was placed at the inferior border of the mandible in the right side. A William velsey Fry awl was introduced through the stab incision. The bone awl was guided along the body of the mandible and taken out lingually. Next the wire was tied in and the awl was gently guided along the lower border of the mandible and passed into the buccal sulcus (Figure 6).

The wire was held together and ironing was done to adapt the wire in close approximation to the bone. This also prevents soft tissue injury and an unesthetic scar. The acrylic cap splint was then stabilized on the right side by winding the wire in a clockwise direction. The same procedure was followed on the left side. Care was taken to avoid pulling the wire through the mandible since the child was young and at this stage the mandibular cortex is thin and relatively less dense. The external wound on the chin was thoroughly debrided and primary closure was done in two layers.

OPG radiograph was taken postoperatively to check if the wires were properly secured to bone (Figure 7). Postoperative antibiotic treatment was started for 1 week. Soft diet, avoidance of physical activities, and antibacterial mouth rinse were prescribed. Postoperative monitoring was performed on a weekly basis and was favourable in both healing and function. No signs of complications were observed during the healing period (Figures 8 and 10). The interdental wiring and acrylic splint were removed after 3 weeks.

5. Discussion

Fractures of the mandible comprise the most common facial skeletal injury among hospitalised pediatric trauma patients. They are the second most common facial skeletal injury, behind nasal fractures in the general pediatric population [8–11]. Boys outnumber girls in the incidence of mandible fractures by a ratio of two in one, with falls, blunt trauma, and motor vehicle accidents cited as the most common causes [10–12]. The areas of pediatric mandible that are most frequently fractured are in condyles, subcondylar, and angle regions (80%), and the symphysis/parasymphyseal area (15% to 20%) fractures of the body of the mandible are rare in pediatric population [10].

Factors to be considered in the definitive treatment of the dentoalveolar injury include (1) age and cooperation of the patient; (2) duration between trauma and treatment; (3) location or extent of the injury; (4) injury to primary or permanent dentition; (5) stages of root development; (6) presence of fracture of supporting bone; and (7) periodontal health of remaining teeth [13]. Among the commonly used treatment options, acrylic cap splints are ideal. They avail support not only from the adjacent teeth but also from bone. They are easy to fabricate and are economical. Routinely, they

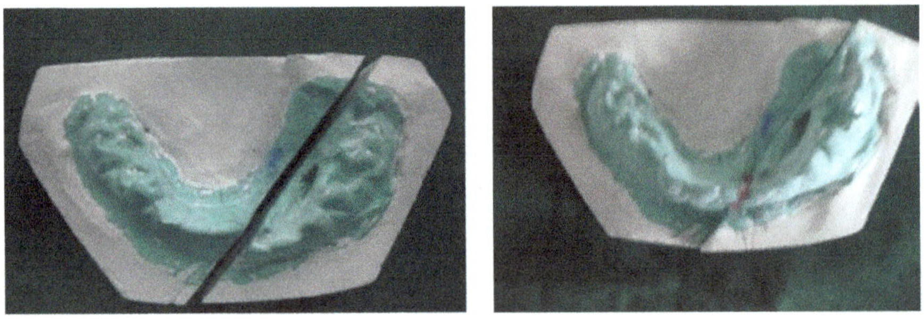

(a) (b)

Figure 3: Preoperative model setup.

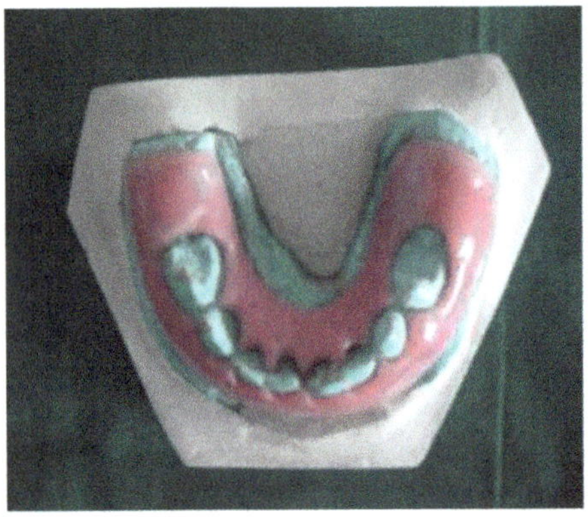

Figure 4: Prefabricated surgical splint on the model.

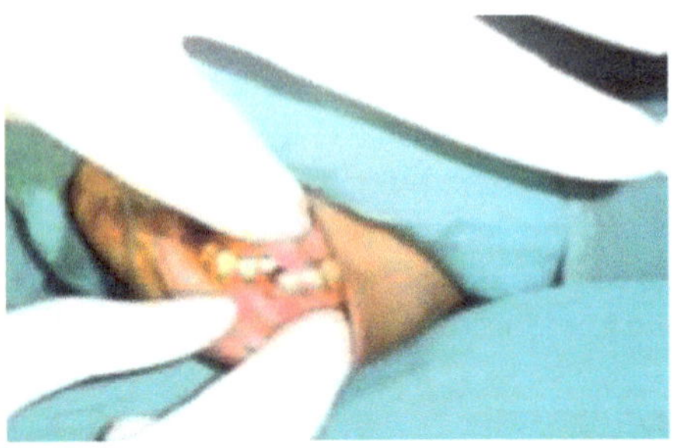

Figure 5: Intraoperative reduction of the segments.

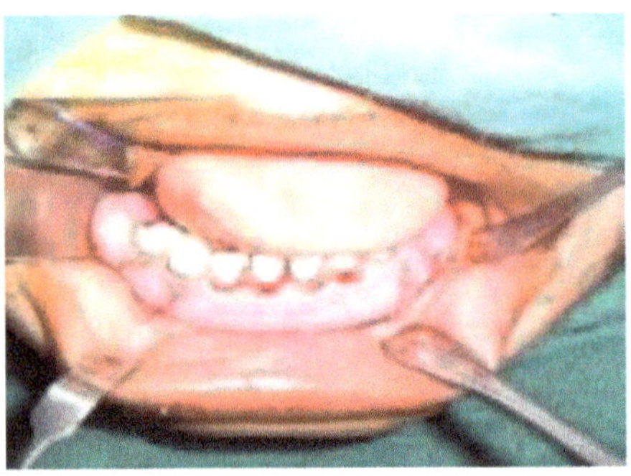

Figure 6: Intraoperative photograph showing splint in position, secured with circummandibular wires.

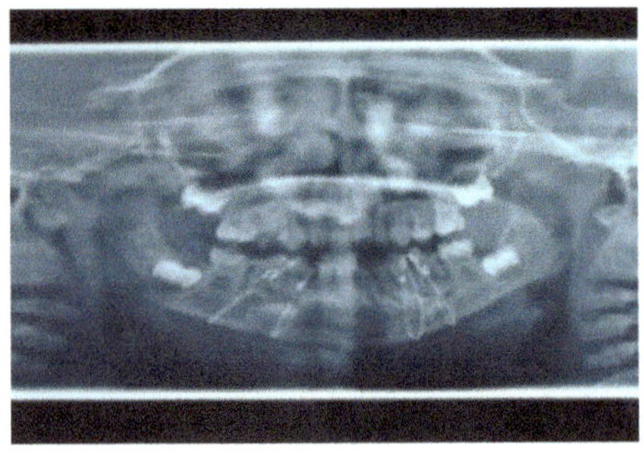

Figure 7: Intraoperative OPG with circummandibular wiring.

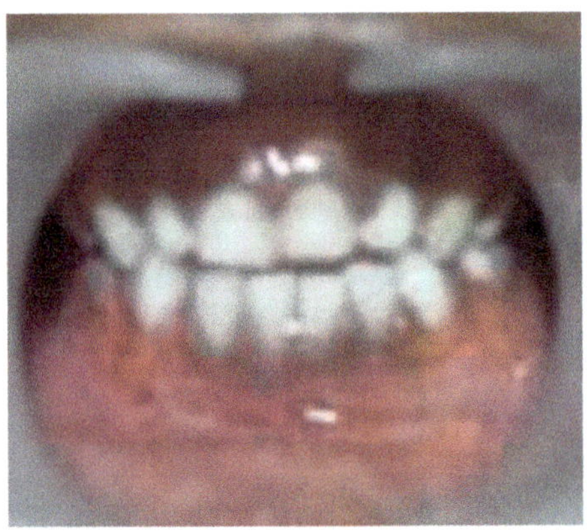

Figure 8. Postoperative followup.

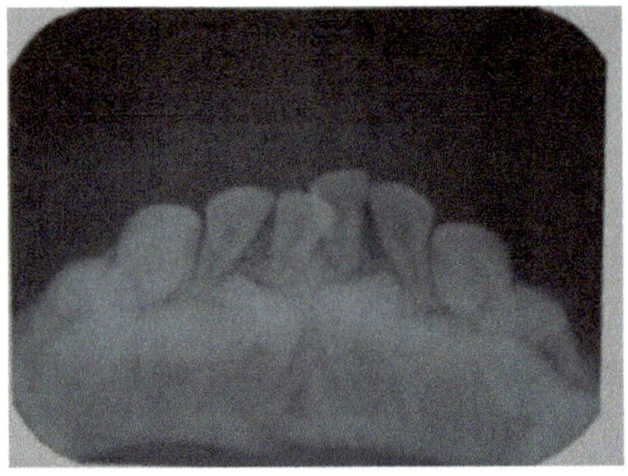

Figure 9: Preoperative IOPA of 73–83 region showing displaced 71 and 81.

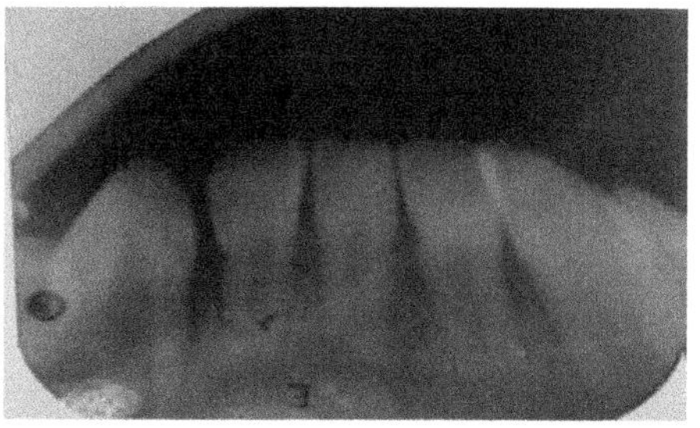

FIGURE 10: Postoperative IOPA of 73–83 region after 3 weeks with well-aligned 71 and 81.

are used in stabilising mandibular fractures, as they can be stabilised by the use of circum-mandibular wire.

6. Conclusion

"Facial fracture in children is a common type of injury suffered by pediatric patients. Causes and patterns of facial fractures vary with age. Knowledge of the association of dental injuries and maxillofacial fractures is a basic tool for their prevention. The majority of these fractures can be managed conservatively. The results of the fracture treatment presented here verified the usefulness of open cap splint in cases of mandibular body, parasymphysis, symphysis fracture."

References

[1] T. B. Dodson, "Mandibular fractures in children," *OMS Knowledge Update*, vol. 1, part II, pp. 95–107, 1995.

[2] S. Iida and T. Matsuya, "Paediatric maxillofacial fractures: their aetiological characters and fracture patterns," *Journal of Cranio-Maxillofacial Surgery*, vol. 30, no. 4, pp. 237–241, 2002.

[3] J. C. Posnick, M. Wells, G. E. Pron, and B. Alpert, "Pediatric facial fractures: evolving patterns of treatment," *Journal of Oral and Maxillofacial Surgery*, vol. 51, no. 8, pp. 836–845, 1993.

[4] A. B. Bataineh, "Etiology and incidence of maxillofacial fractures in the north of Jordan," *Oral Surgery, Oral Medicine, Oral Pathology, Oral Radiology, and Endodontics*, vol. 86, no. 1, pp. 31–35, 1998.

[5] R. Lalloo, "Risk factors for major injuries to the face and teeth," *Dental Traumatology*, vol. 19, no. 1, pp. 12–14, 2003.

[6] J. B. Mulliken, L. B. Kaban, and J. E. Murray, "Management of facial fractures in children," *Clinics in Plastic Surgery*, vol. 4, no. 4, pp. 491–502, 1977.

[7] M. A. Fortunato, A. F. Fielding, and L. H. Guernsey, "Facial bone fractures in children," *Oral Surgery Oral Medicine and Oral Pathology*, vol. 53, no. 3, pp. 225–230, 1982.

[8] K. C. Yerit, S. Hainich, G. Enislidis et al., "Biodegradable fixation of mandibular fractures in children: stability and early results," *Oral Surgery, Oral Medicine, Oral Pathology, Oral Radiology and Endodontology*, vol. 100, no. 1, pp. 17–24, 2005.

[9] R. H. Haug, L. L. Cunningham, and M. T. Brandt, "Plates, screws, and children: their relationship in craniomaxillofacial trauma," *Journal of Long-Term Effects of Medical Implants*, vol. 13, no. 4, pp. 271–287, 2003.

[10] A. Baumann, M. J. Troulis, and L. B. Kaban, "Facial trauma II. Dentoalveolar injuries and mandibular fractures," in *Pediatric Oral and Maxillofacial Surgery*, pp. 445–461, Saunders, Philadelphia, Pa, USA, 2004.

[11] R. W. T. Myall, K. H. Dawson, and M. A. Egbert, "Maxillofacial injuries in children," in *Oral and Maxillofacial Surgery*, R. J. Fonseca, Ed., vol. 3, pp. 423–426, WB Saunders, Philadelphia, Pa, USA, 2000.

[12] J. C. Posnick, B. J. Costello, and P. S. Tiwana, "pediatric craniomaxillofacial fracture management," in *Peterson's Principles of Oral and Maxillofacial Surgery*, vol. 1, pp. 528–532, BC Decker, Hamilton, Canada, 2nd edition, 2004.

[13] G. H. Blakey III, R. L. Ruiz, and T. A. Tuarey, "Management of facial fractures in growing patient," in *Oral and Maxillofacial Trauma and Endodontics*, R. J. Fonseca and R. V. Walker, Eds., vol. 2, pp. 1003–1041, WB Saunders, Philadelphia, Pa, USA, 1997.

30

Modified and Grafted Coronectomy: A New Technique and a Case Report with Two-Year Followup

Michael Leizerovitz and Olga Leizerovitz

UCLA School of Dentistry, 10833 Le Conte Avenue, Los Angeles, CA 90095-1668, USA

Correspondence should be addressed to Michael Leizerovitz; travel.surgery@hotmail.com

Academic Editors: N. Brezniak, M. De Bruyne, and K. H. Zawawi

Purpose. A standard coronectomy (intentional partial odontectomy) is recommended for mandibular third molar (MTM) extraction cases with a high risk of inferior alveolar nerve injury (IANI). However, complications such as inadvertent intraoperative root removal, post-op root migration, second molar (MSM) periodontal defects and others do exist. This report presents a new technique, the Modified and Grafted Coronectomy (MGC), describes the measures to prevent or minimize the known drawbacks of the standard coronectomy, and reviews the literature for comparison with three other IANI-prevention techniques. *Materials and Methods.* MGC was performed on two MTMs with nerve involvement and severe periodontal pockets on the distal of MSM. Modifications were: stabilizing the root stump to prevent intraoperative movement, creation of a large intrabony space for bone graft material, and grafting for periodontal healing while minimizing the possibility of post-op root migration. *Results.* Excellent overall periodontal improvement, with probing depths reduced to 3-4 mm. Panoramic radiograph displayed remarkable bone regeneration. No residual root migration was evident at the two year follow up. *Conclusion.* MGC may be a good alternative, especially in cases with periodontal defects on the distal of MSM. It may also help to minimize inadvertent intraoperative root removal and postoperative root migration.

1. Introduction

The removal of impacted mandibular third molar (MTM) in close proximity to the mandibular canal has proven to be problematic. One of the more severe risks is inferior alveolar nerve injury (IANI). The prevalence of this type of nerve injury in the twenty-four prospective studies reviewed varies between a minimum of 0% [1, 2] and a maximum of 8.4% [3]. The need to prevent these kinds of injuries is especially important since current treatment modalities of neurosensory deficit management (four surgical and two nonsurgical [4]) show only limited improvement in sensation. According to studies, complete recovery is uncommon with all types of available treatments [4, 5].

Coronectomy is the oldest and the best researched of the IANI-risk reducing procedures [6–19]. First described in 1984 [14], it has been extensively reviewed in multiple articles and retrospective studies, has been examined in eight prospective trials (Table 1), and has been now listed as a standard treatment option for surgical management of third molars by AAOMS ParCare 2012 in USA [20]. Despite those facts, coronectomy has not yet been accepted by the majority of the oral surgery community.

In the regular coronectomy, the aspect of the third molar root/s in the closest proximity to the inferior alveolar nerve (IAN) is intentionally retained. The clear benefit of a successful coronectomy is the avoidance of IANI. The disadvantages of this technique include deep periodontal pockets on the distal of the second molars (similar to those after extractions in comparable circumstances), root migration with the possible need of a second procedure, dry sockets, local postoperative infections, postoperative pain and inadvertent root removal, or root walk-out during surgery which may increase the risk of IANI (also known as a failed coronectomy) [6, 7, 17, 21, 22].

Deep pockets and other periodontal damages have been previously reported on the distal of the second molar teeth

TABLE 1: Published prospective trials.

Reference	Author	Article	Published in journal	Year published	*n* subjects	*n* teeth	Study design
[6]	Pogrel et al.	"Coronectomy: a technique to protect the inferior alveolar nerve"	J Oral Maxillofac Surg	2004	41	50	Prospective cohort
[7]	Renton et al.	"A randomised controlled clinical trial to compare the incidence of injury to the inferior alveolar nerve as a result of coronectomy and removal of mandibular third molars"	Br J Oral Maxillofac Surg	2005	128	94	Randomized controlled trial
[8]	Pogrel	"An update on coronectomy"	J Oral Maxillofac Surg	2009	Not available	450	Prospective cohort
[9]	Leung and Cheung	"Safety of coronectomy versus excision of wisdom teeth: a randomized controlled trial"	Oral Surg Oral Med Oral Pathol Oral Radiol Endod	2009	231	171	Randomized controlled trial
[10]	Hatano et al.	"Clinical evaluations of coronectomy (intentional partial odontectomy) for mandibular third molars using dental computed tomography: a case-control study"	J Oral Maxillofac Surg	2009	220	102	Case control study
[11]	Dolanmaz et al.	"A preferable technique for protecting the inferior alveolar nerve: coronectomy"	J Oral Maxillofac Surg	2009	43	47	Prospective cohort
[12]	Cilasun et al.	"Coronectomy in patients with high risk of inferior alveolar nerve injury diagnosed by computed tomography"	J Oral Maxillofac Surg	2011	120	175	Prospective cohort
[13]	Leung and Cheung	"Coronectomy of the lower third molar is safe within the first 3 years"	J Oral Maxillofac Surg	2012	98	135	Prospective cohort

after third molar removal [23–26]. The measurements used in these studies were attachment levels, pocket depth and/or alveolar bone height. Shallower pocket depths postoperatively have been obtained through the debridement of the distal root of the second molar [27, 28]. Grafting following extraction has also minimized the development of second molar periodontal defects in the high-risk group (age ≥ 26 years., preexisting attachment loss ≥ 3 mm, and mesioangular or horizontal impaction) [29, 30] and in the younger patients group (ages 21–26 years) [31]. However, coronectomy in conjunction with grafting and distal root surface of the second molar debridement and demineralization has not been previously reported.

This paper provides a description of a case of a Modified and Grafted Coronectomy (MGC), developed by the authors. The goals of the technique are to decrease the incidence of intraoperative root walkout, to minimize the potential and/or preexisting periodontal pockets distal to the second molar similar to the "Preservation of periodontal health of adjacent teeth" Specific Therapeutic Goal of ParCare 2012 [20], and to decrease the risk of delayed root migration with the possible need for a second surgical procedure, all while preserving the excellent IANI-prevention record of a standard coronectomy. The reduction in pocket depth may also prevent or minimize the need for future periodontal interventions. The following case has met the goals described herein.

2. Clinical Report

A 37-year-old female, a smoker for the past 15 years but otherwise in good general health, was repeatedly referred for extractions of her MTM due to severe localized periodontal disease at the distal of the mandibular second molar (MSM) teeth. She stated that over the last four years she had consulted five oral surgeons who each suggested third molar extraction. The patient was also advised that she would have a higher than normal chance of bilateral permanent paresthesia. She reported that her periodontist warned her about the deteriorating periodontal health of both of her lower second molar teeth. She also reported occasional pressure and intermittent pain associated with the lower right third molar.

At her consultation appointment, the patient presented with a panoramic radiograph and multiple dental treatment plans, all of which included extraction of the MTMs. A new panoramic radiograph was taken (Figure 1) which confirmed bilateral complete bony, horizontally impacted MTMs, Pell and Gregory's [32] class 2C on the lower right and 3C on the lower left with the roots in intimate radiographic proximity to the IAN bundle. The periodontal ligament space appeared sclerotic. The distal of the right MSM was tender to palpation and slightly swollen, which the patient stated had been bothersome for the last few weeks. Immediately prior to the surgical procedure, the periodontal probing depths were

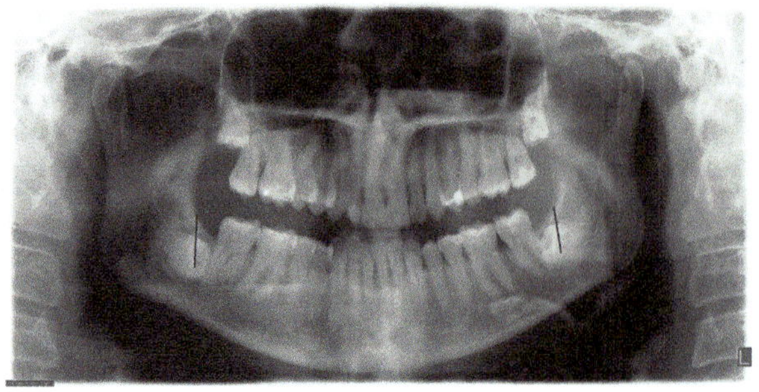

FIGURE 1: Preoperative panoramic radiograph. The direction of the initial cuts is marked.

measured at 13 mm on the distal of right MSM and 8 mm on the distal of left MSM.

The patient was given the options and risks of observation, extractions with grafting, and Modified Grafted Coronectomy. The patient chose to have bilateral MGC performed. The treatment plan was reviewed and her consent was obtained.

Due to the presence of infection, she was placed on oral Clindamycin 150 mg, 40 tablets, QID, and 0.12% chlorhexidine mouth rinse twice a day beginning two days prior to the procedure. The surgery was performed with i.v. sedation and local anesthesia. A lower right full thickness distally released envelope flap was reflected. No lingual retraction was used. A bony window was created for access. An initial vertical cut with a #703 cross cut fissure carbide FG bur, 2.1 mm diameter was made above the CEJ and oriented at a 20° angle to the distal root of the second molar, to facilitate coronal fragment removal. The cut was completed at 3/4 of the tooth diameter to avoid cutting into the lingual wall and/or IAN and to avert possible lingual nerve injury or IANI. The crown was broken off, without excessive apical pressure. After the removal of the first fragment, rest seats were created in the root portion at each of the subsequent steps. These were used to apply gentle apical pressure on the distal section with the sharp end of a Molt 9A periosteal elevator while grinding, cutting, and fracturing off the coronal fragments. This action stabilized the root portion, dampened the vibration, and helped to prevent inadvertent movement and therefore pressure of the remaining root against the IAN. Next, a #10 round carbide HP bur, 2.7 mm diameter was used to grind away the distoocclusal section of the remaining stump above the IAN, well below the bone crest level (Figure 2(a)). Due to insufficient clearance between the third molar stump and the second molar root, an additional cut was performed on the mesial portion of the remaining tooth, at 3/4 of the diameter and it was fractured off with a Schmeckebier #81 straight elevator (Figure 2(b)). A sufficient clearance to the second molar was confirmed with a radiograph (Figure 2(c)). The distal root of the second molar was detoxified and prepared for the bone graft by ultrasonic scaling and by a treatment with a 25% solution of citric acid for five minutes. A resorbable hydroxyapatite (HA) graft was placed into the bleeding site and no membrane was used. The flap was advanced for full coverage of the graft and primary closure and then sutured with 4-0 Vicryl sutures. The

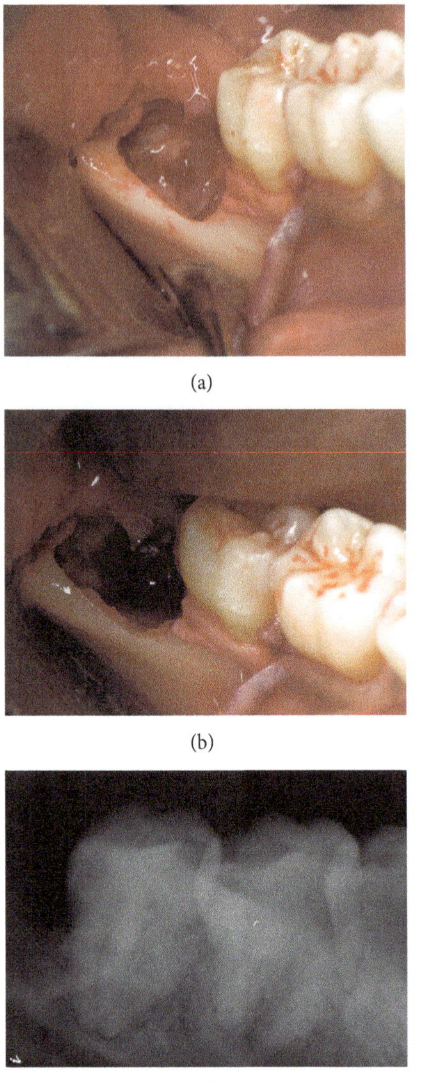

(a)

(b)

(c)

FIGURE 2: Lower right MTM: (a) after amputation of the crown, rotary instruments were used to reduce the distoocclusal section of the remaining stump; (b) after an additional cut and sectioning of the mesial portion of the tooth; (c) sufficient clearance to the second molar confirmed.

surgery on left MTM was carried out in a similar fashion. This side was somewhat more difficult due to less available space mesiodistally and significant resorption of the distal root of left second molar. (Figures 3(b) and 3(c)). Serial progress periapical radiographs were taken.

The patient was seen for a follow-up visit at six days postoperatively. The surgical sites appeared to be healing within normal limits. The absence of paresthesia in the IAN and lingual nerve distribution was assessed by the patient's subjective report of normal sensation with sharp, blunt, and light touch. A follow-up panoramic radiograph was obtained (Figure 4).

Instructions were given for the patient to return for reassessment and radiographs every six months for the first

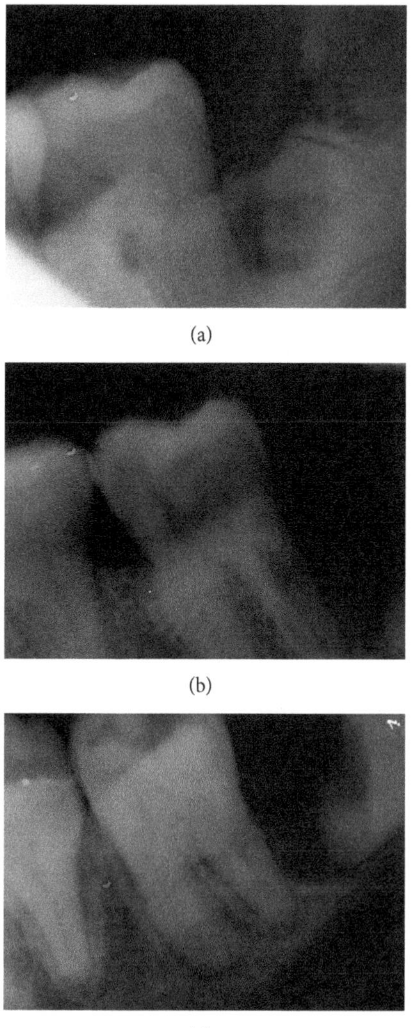

(a)

(b)

(c)

FIGURE 3: Lower left MTM: (a) after amputation of the crown; (b) after reducing the distoocclusal section of the remaining stump; (c) after an additional cut and removal of the mesial portion of the tooth, to create sufficient clearance to the second molar.

two years, and once more after the third year. The patient was advised, if there are no problems found during the first three years, to return only if she experiences any unusual symptoms.

The patient and the referring dentist were advised to exercise special care with the grafted sites for the first six to nine months following treatment by not traumatizing them needlessly and to allow the graft to mature. This included no periodontal pocket charting, scaling on the distal of the second molars, and/or manipulating with any hard objects by the patient. According to the manufacturer, the grafted area becomes radiopaque in comparison to the surrounding bone indicating that the resorbable HA graft has matured.

3. Results

At the two-year follow-up the patient stated the areas felt fine with no sensitivity around the second molars. Periodontal

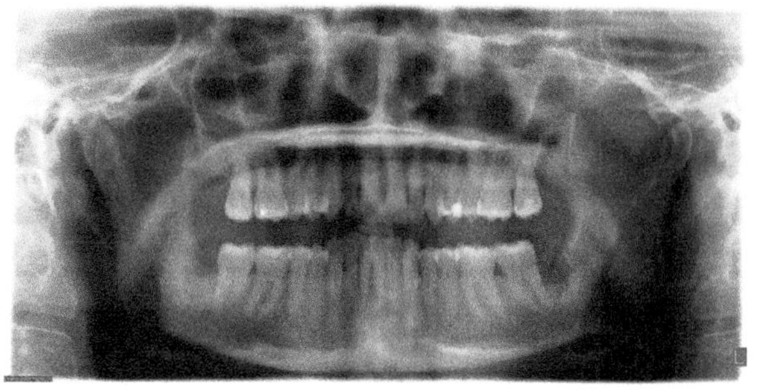

FIGURE 4: Six days postoperatively. Please note that the bone graft is radiolucent at this stage.

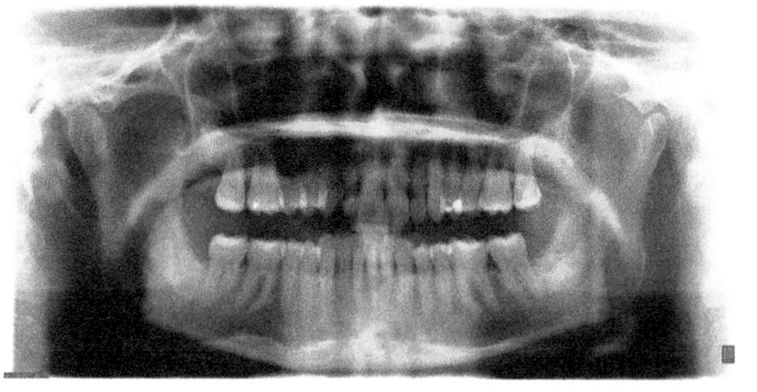

FIGURE 5: A 23-month follow-up with excellent healing.

examination revealed decreased periodontal pocket depths, down to three and four mm. Panoramic radiograph was obtained (Figure 5), displaying good bone fill with excellent periodontal improvement overall. No residual root migration was evident.

4. Discussion

Regular coronectomy is the best studied alternative to the extraction of teeth, which are at a high risk for IANI, as determined by radiographic signs [6, 7, 10, 17, 33–37]. It has now been accepted in USA as a standard and is no longer a controversial treatment option at Third Molar Multidisciplinary Conference in Washington, DC, on October 19, 2010, and AAOMS ParCare 2012 [20, 38]. There are several technique variations to perform a standard coronectomy procedure [6, 7, 9, 10, 14, 16, 17]. While nerve damage is avoided in a successful standard coronectomy, other complications can arise.

IANI was the most serious complication which occurred during some failed coronectomies, where the remaining root was inadvertently mobilized during surgery. This mandated the surgeons to proceed with the extraction of the entire root in 4–38% of the cases [7–9, 17], also resulting in temporary IANI, with an incidence of 8.3–11.1% [7, 8].

Other known complications are deep periodontal pockets on the distal of the second molar, delayed postoperative root migration with the possible need of a second procedure, postoperative pain, dry socket, and infection [7–9, 21, 22].

These drawbacks could be a possible motivation for the recent emergence of additional IANI-risk reducing procedures: staged removal (the removal of a portion of the crown, creating space for the root to erupt away from the IAN, with subsequent removal of the remainder of the root) [39], pericoronal ostectomy (the removal of the overlying bone to allow for the tooth to erupt away from the IAN) [21], and orthodontic extractions (active orthodontic movement of the tooth away from the IAN) [40, 41]. Pericoronal ostectomy and orthodontic extraction allow for bone formation on the distal of the second molar which occurs due to the occlusal extrusion as the MTM moves away from the IAN [21, 41]. While it is obvious that preservation of periodontal health, regenerating bone and preventing or reducing the further need of periodontal surgery at the distal of the lower second molar, is an important advantage for the patients [20], a standard coronectomy procedure lacks this benefit.

With only one recorded case of permanent IANI in its history [17], there is an abundance of evidence that coronectomy has had great success in avoiding IANI. While performing the standard coronectomy since 1995, we have experienced both its IANI avoidance benefits as well as all its negative side effects. In an effort to overcome these, we attempted various modifications to the different steps of the original technique.

Ultimately, the technique used in the case reported above appears to have the most encouraging outcome. In it we introduced a series of amendments to the standard coronectomy procedure and called it a Modified and Grafted Coronectomy.

As with the standard coronectomy, MGC involves the removal of the crown and part of the root/s of an impacted MTM in cases with a high risk of IANI. This modified procedure introduces steps to prevent the complication of inadvertent intraoperative root loosening. It accomplishes this by stabilizing the radicular fragment during cutting as well as when separating the coronal section off, thus overall decreasing the risk of nerve injury. Yet as another modification, to reduce or prevent periodontal pockets on the distal of the second molar, the technique calls for the creation of periodontal "scaffolding," which is achieved through grafting, thus the name Modified and Grafted Coronectomy.

Scaling and debridement [27, 28] as well as root surface demineralization [42–44] with either citric acid or tetracycline of the distal of the second molar were the necessary elements for the reattachment success in all our cases. Of the graft materials we used, only resorbable HA (with or without use of resorbable collagen membrane) or cortical allograft with the membrane gave us satisfactory results.

In our experience with grafting, it is important to create a larger vertical space to allow for bone regeneration. According to Hatano "even if appropriate trimming 2 to 3 mm below the alveolar crest is done, bone coverage on the resected surface is sometimes delayed because of significant root migration" [10]. Combining grafting with the creation of a larger space resulted in a bulkier graft, which worked well in this case. The resulting periodontal healing is very encouraging (Figure 5), as well as the absence of root migration which in turn averts the possible necessity of a second surgical procedure to remove the root fragment. The findings in this paper appear to be promising without the side effects of the standard coronectomy procedure.

MGC appears to be an alternate technique that could be considered for nearly all coronectomy cases of vertical, mesioangular, or horizontal impactions and especially in the cases which have preexisting periodontal lesions or are expected to have large postsurgical defects. A possible additional benefit is the potential prevention for the need of further pocket reduction surgery on the distal of the lower second molar, minimizing the need of subsequent treatments and visits.

Possible considerations of the technique are the additional costs of the graft and the time required to perform the procedure. Further modifications and enhancements could include the use of different graft materials and/or the use of a membrane. Additional research with a large cohort of patients and randomized prospective studies are needed to verify the outcome.

While more research is absolutely necessary, this new technique and/or just some of its steps appears to offer a viable alternative for a coronectomy practitioner, helpful in obtaining superior results in addition to the existing IANI-risk reduction procedures.

Acknowledgments

The authors would like to thank Earl G. Freymiller, D.M.D., M.D., for the editorial guidance; Shankar Iyer, D.D.S., M.D.S., for structural guidance; the late John A. Yagiela, D.D.S, Ph.D., for help with research; Julia Cherney R.D.H., M.S., for editorial assistance.

References

[1] G. W. Bell, "Use of dental panoramic tomographs to predict the relation between mandibular third molar teeth and the inferior alveolar nerve. Radiological and surgical findings, and clinical outcome," *British Journal of Oral and Maxillofacial Surgery*, vol. 42, no. 1, pp. 21–27, 2004.

[2] R. J. Middlehurst, G. R. Barker, and J. P. Rood, "Postoperative morbidity with mandibular third molar surgery: a comparison of two techniques," *Journal of Oral and Maxillofacial Surgery*, vol. 46, no. 6, pp. 474–475, 1988.

[3] V. Lopes, R. Mumenya, C. Feinmann, and M. Harris, "Third molar surgery: an audit of the indications for surgery, post-operative complaints and patient satisfaction," *British Journal of Oral and Maxillofacial Surgery*, vol. 33, no. 1, pp. 33–35, 1995.

[4] Y. Y. Leung, P. P. L. Fung, and L. K. Cheung, "Treatment modalities of neurosensory deficit after lower third molar surgery: a systematic review," *Journal of Oral and Maxillofacial Surgery*, vol. 70, no. 4, pp. 768–778, 2012.

[5] A. Alantar, M. H. Roisin-Chausson, Y. Commissionat et al., "Retention of third molar roots to prevent damage to the inferior alveolar nerve," *Oral Surgery, Oral Medicine, Oral Pathology, Oral Radiology and*, vol. 80, no. 2, p. 126, 1995.

[6] M. A. Pogrel, J. S. Lee, and D. F. Muff, "Coronectomy: a technique to protect the inferior alveolar nerve," *Journal of Oral and Maxillofacial Surgery*, vol. 62, no. 12, pp. 1447–1452, 2004.

[7] T. Renton, M. Hankins, C. Sproate, and M. McGurk, "A randomised controlled clinical trial to compare the incidence of injury to the inferior alveolar nerve as a result of coronectomy and removal of mandibular third molars," *British Journal of Oral and Maxillofacial Surgery*, vol. 43, no. 1, pp. 7–12, 2005.

[8] M. A. Pogrel, "An update on coronectomy," *Journal of Oral and Maxillofacial Surgery*, vol. 67, no. 8, pp. 1782–1783, 2009.

[9] Y. Y. Leung and L. K. Cheung, "Safety of coronectomy versus excision of wisdom teeth: a randomized controlled trial," *Oral Surgery, Oral Medicine, Oral Pathology, Oral Radiology and Endodontology*, vol. 108, no. 6, pp. 821–827, 2009.

[10] Y. Hatano, K. Kurita, Y. Kuroiwa, H. Yuasa, and E. Ariji, "clinical evaluations of coronectomy (intentional partial odontectomy) for mandibular third molars using dental computed tomography: a case-control study," *Journal of Oral and Maxillofacial Surgery*, vol. 67, no. 9, pp. 1806–1814, 2009.

[11] D. Dolanmaz, G. Yildirim, K. Isik, K. Kucuk, and A. Ozturk, "A preferable technique for protecting the inferior alveolar nerve: coronectomy," *Journal of Oral and Maxillofacial Surgery*, vol. 67, no. 6, pp. 1234–1238, 2009.

[12] U. Cilasun, T. Yildirim, E. Guzeldemir, and Z. O. Pektas, "Coronectomy in patients with high risk of inferior alveolar nerve injury diagnosed by computed tomography," *Journal of Oral and Maxillofacial Surgery*, vol. 69, no. 6, pp. 1557–1561, 2011.

[13] Y. Y. Leung and L. K. Cheung, "Coronectomy of the lower third molar is safe within the first 3 years," *JJournal of Oral and Maxillofacial Surgery*, vol. 70, no. 7, pp. 1515–1522, 2012.

[14] J. Ecuyer and J. Debien, "Surgical deductions," *Actualites Odonto-Stomatologiques*, vol. 38, no. 148, pp. 695–702, 1984.

[15] K. Knutsson, L. Lysell, and M. Rohlin, "Postoperative status after partial removal of the mandibular third molar," *Swedish Dental Journal*, vol. 13, no. 1-2, pp. 15–22, 1989.

[16] G. L. Freedman, "Intentional partial odontectomy: review of cases," *Journal of Oral and Maxillofacial Surgery*, vol. 55, no. 5, pp. 524–526, 1997.

[17] B. C. O'Riordan, "Coronectomy (intentional partial odontectomy of lower third molars)," *Oral Surgery, Oral Medicine, Oral Pathology, Oral Radiology and Endodontology*, vol. 98, no. 3, pp. 274–280, 2004.

[18] L. A. Assael, "Coronectomy: a time to ponder or a time to act?" *Journal of Oral and Maxillofacial Surgery*, vol. 62, no. 12, pp. 1445-1446, 2004.

[19] A. Garcia-Garcia, "Is coronectomy really preferable to extraction? [7]," *British Journal of Oral and Maxillofacial Surgery*, vol. 44, no. 1, p. 75, 2006.

[20] S. E. Lieblich, M. A. Kleiman, and J. Zak MJ, "Parameters of care: clinical practice. Guidelines for oral and maxillofacial surgery. (AAOMS ParCare 2012)," *Journal of Oral and Maxillofacial Surgery*, vol. 70, e50, 2012.

[21] L. Tolstunov, B. Javid, L. Keyes, and A. Nattestad, "Pericoronal ostectomy: an alternative surgical technique for management of mandibular third molars in close proximity to the inferior alveolar nerve," *Journal of Oral and Maxillofacial Surgery*, vol. 69, no. 7, pp. 1858–1866, 2011.

[22] G. A. Bonetti, "In reply," *Journal of Oral and Maxillofacial Surgery*, vol. 66, no. 6, p. 1317, 2008.

[23] T. A. Quee, D. Gosselin, E. P. Millar, and J. W. Stamm, "Surgical removal of the fully impacted mandibular third molar. The influence of flap design and alveolar bone height on the periodontal status of the second molar," *Journal of Periodontology*, vol. 56, no. 10, pp. 625–630, 1985.

[24] C. F. Kugelberg, U. Ahlström, S. Ericson, A. Hugoson, and H. Thilander, "The influence of anatomical, pathophysiological and other factors on periodontal healing after impacted lower third molar surgery. A multiple regression analysis," *Journal of Clinical Periodontology*, vol. 18, no. 1, pp. 37–43, 1991.

[25] K. Y. Peng, Y. C. Tseng, E. C. Shen, S. C. Chiu, E. Fu, and Y. W. Huang, "Mandibular second molar periodontal status after third molar extraction," *Journal of Periodontology*, vol. 72, no. 12, pp. 1647–1651, 2001.

[26] W. K. Kwok, J. K. S. Liu, E. C. M. Lo, E. F. Corbet, and W. K. Leung, "Residual periodontal defects distal to the mandibular second molar 6-36 months after impacted third molar extraction: a retrospective cross-sectional study of young adults," *Journal of Clinical Periodontology*, vol. 29, no. 11, pp. 1004–1011, 2002.

[27] W. K. Leung, E. F. Corbet, W. K. Kwok, E. C. M. Lo, and J. K. S. Liu, "A regimen of systematic periodontal care after removal of impacted mandibular third molars manages periodontal pockets associated with the mandibular second molars," *Journal of Clinical Periodontology*, vol. 32, no. 7, pp. 725–731, 2005.

[28] O. Pons-Vicente, E. Valmaseda-Castellón, L. Berini-Aytés, and C. Gay-Escoda, "Effect on pocket depth and attachment level of manual versus ultrasonic scaling of lower second molars following lower third molar extraction: a randomized controlled trial," *Oral Surgery, Oral Medicine, Oral Pathology, Oral Radiology and Endodontology*, vol. 107, no. 3, pp. e11–e19, 2009.

[29] T. B. Dodson, "Management of mandibular third molar extraction sites to prevent periodontal defects," *Journal of Oral and Maxillofacial Surgery*, vol. 62, no. 10, pp. 1213–1224, 2004.

[30] T. B. Dodson, "Third molar socket grafting: is there an indication?" *Journal of Oral and Maxillofacial Surgery*, vol. 64, p. 7, 2006.

[31] G. Sammartino, M. Tia, G. Marenzi, A. Espedito Di Lauro, E. D'Agostino, and P. P. Claudio, "Use of autologous Platelet-Rich Plasma (PRP) in periodontal defect treatment after extraction of impacted mandibular third molars," *Journal of Oral and Maxillofacial Surgery*, vol. 63, no. 6, pp. 766–770, 2005.

[32] G. J. Pell and B. T. Gregory, "Impacted mandibular third molars. Classification and modified techniques for removal," *Dental Digest*, vol. 39, p. 330, 1933.

[33] G. Howe and H. G. Poyton, "Prevention of damage to the inferior dental nerve during the extraction of mandibular third molars," *British Dental Journal*, vol. 109, pp. 355–363, 1960.

[34] J. P. Rood and B. A. A. Nooraldeen Shehab, "The radiological prediction of inferior alveolar nerve injury during third molar surgery," *British Journal of Oral and Maxillofacial Surgery*, vol. 28, no. 1, pp. 20–25, 1990.

[35] B. F. Blaeser, M. A. August, R. B. Donoff, L. B. Kaban, and T. B. Dodson, "Panoramic radiographic risk factors for inferior alveolar nerve injury after third molar extraction," *Journal of Oral and Maxillofacial Surgery*, vol. 61, no. 4, pp. 417–421, 2003.

[36] M. Sedaghatfar, M. A. August, and T. B. Dodson, "Panoramic radiographic findings as predictors of inferior alveolar nerve exposure following third molar extraction," *Journal of Oral and Maxillofacial Surgery*, vol. 63, no. 1, pp. 3–7, 2005.

[37] Y. Y. Leung and L. K. Cheung, "Correlation of radiographic signs, inferior dental nerve exposure, and deficit in third molar surgery," *Journal of Oral and Maxillofacial Surgery*, vol. 69, no. 7, pp. 1873–1879, 2011.

[38] T. B. Dodson, I. D. Cheifetz, W. J. Nelson, and L. K. Rafetto, "Summary of the proceeding of the third molar multidisciplinary conference," *Journal of Oral and Maxillofacial Surgery*, vol. 70, no. 9, supplement 1, pp. S66–S69, 2012.

[39] L. Landi, P. F. Manicone, S. Piccinelli, A. Raia, and R. Raia, "A novel surgical approach to impacted mandibular third molars to reduce the risk of paresthesia: a case series," *Journal of Oral and Maxillofacial Surgery*, vol. 68, no. 5, pp. 969–974, 2010.

[40] A. Hirsch, S. Shteiman, B. D. Boyan, and Z. Schwartz, "Use of orthodontic treatment as an aid to third molar extraction: a method for prevention of mandibular nerve injury and improved periodontal status," *Journal of Periodontology*, vol. 74, no. 6, pp. 887–892, 2003.

[41] G. A. Bonetti, M. Bendandi, L. Laino, V. Checchi, and L. Checchi, "Orthodontic extraction: riskless extraction of impacted lower third molars close to the mandibular canal," *Journal of Oral and Maxillofacial Surgery*, vol. 65, no. 12, pp. 2580–2586, 2007.

[42] A. M. Polson and M. P. Proye, "Effect of root surface alterations on periodontal healing. II. Citric acid treatment of the denuded root," *Journal of Clinical Periodontology*, vol. 9, no. 6, pp. 441–454, 1982.

[43] B. Shetty, A. Dinesh, and H. Seshan, "Comparitive effects of tetracyclines and citric acid on dentin root surface of periodontally involved human teeth: a scanning electron microscope study," *Journal of Indian Society of Periodontology*, vol. 12, no. 1, pp. 8–15, 2008.

[44] A. Polson, K. Gutierrez, B. Frantz et al., "Dentin attachment after treatment with either citric acid or tetracycline," *Journal of Dental Research*, vol. 86, p. 2966, 2007.

Synovial Sarcoma of the Buccal Mucosa: A Rare Case Report

Kumar T. S. Mahesh,[1] Indira Annamalai Ponnuswamy,[2] Maria Priscilla David,[2] Peeyush Shivhare,[1] Mahalakshmi Ikkanur Puttaranganayak,[3] and Pooja Sinha[3]

[1] *Department of Oral Medicine and Radiology, Rajarajeswari Dental College and Hospital, Ramohalli Cross, Kumbalagodu, Mysore Road, Bangalore 560060, Karnataka, India*
[2] *Department of Oral Medicine and Radiology, M. R. Ambedkar Dental College and Hospital, 1/36 Cline Road, Cooke Town, Bangalore 560005, Karnataka, India*
[3] *Department of Oral Medicine and Radiology, Sri Rajiv Gandhi College of Dental Science and Hospital, Chola Nagar, R. T. Nagar, Bangalore 560032, Karnataka, India*

Correspondence should be addressed to Kumar T. S. Mahesh; mahesh_talkad@yahoo.co.in

Academic Editors: C. S. Farah and A. L. S. Guimaraes

Synovial sarcoma (SS) is a rare malignant neoplasm that arises most commonly in joint capsules and articular tendons, but its relationship to the synovium is not always obvious. Synovial sarcoma is a malignant soft tissue tumor representing 5.6% to 10% of all soft tissue sarcomas. They are termed SS because of their histologic resemblance to the synovium, but they rarely involve a synovial structure and are thought to arise from pluripotential mesenchymal cells. The tumor usually occurs in close association with tendon sheaths, bursae, and joint capsules, primarily in the para-articular regions of the extremities, with approximately 9% occurring in the head and neck region. Synovial sarcoma has been reported rarely in the oral cavity. We report a very rare case of Synovial sarcoma of the buccal mucosa in a 24-year-old male patient.

1. Introduction

Synovial sarcoma (SS) is a rare malignant neoplasm that arises most commonly in joint capsules and articular tendons, but its relationship to the synovium is not always obvious. Synovial sarcoma is a malignant soft tissue tumor representing 5.6% to 10% of all soft tissue sarcomas [1]. They are termed SS because of their histologic resemblance to the synovium, but they rarely involve a synovial structure and are thought to arise from pluripotential mesenchymal cells [2, 3].

The tumor usually occurs in close association with tendon sheaths, bursae, and joint capsules, primarily in the para-articular regions of the extremities, with approximately 9% occurring in the head and neck region. Most studies have found that the median age of SS is in the third decade and approximately 66% of the patients are male. The most common sites involved in the head and neck include the hypopharynx, postpharyngeal region, and the parapharyngeal space [4].

The origin of synovial sarcoma remains unknown, but the neoplasm is thought to arise from primitive undifferentiated pluripotential mesenchymal cells unrelated to synovial tissue [5]. Synovial sarcoma has been reported rarely in the oral cavity [6]. We report a case of synovial sarcoma of the buccal mucosa in a 24-year-old male patient.

2. Case Report

A 24-year-old male patient reported to the Department of Oral Medicine and Radiology, with a chief complaint of a swelling on the left side of the face since 2 years. Initially swelling was smaller in size which gradually increased to the present size, associated with difficulty in mouth opening and swallowing. There was a history of weight loss over the last few months. On general physical examination, the patient was moderately built and poorly nourished. All the vital signs were within the normal limits.

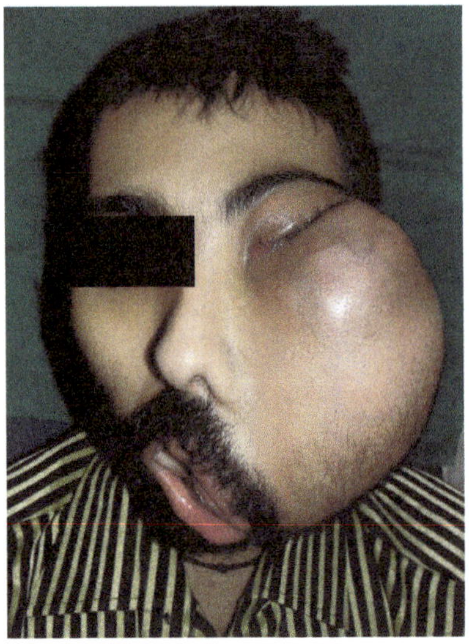

Figure 1: Frontal view.

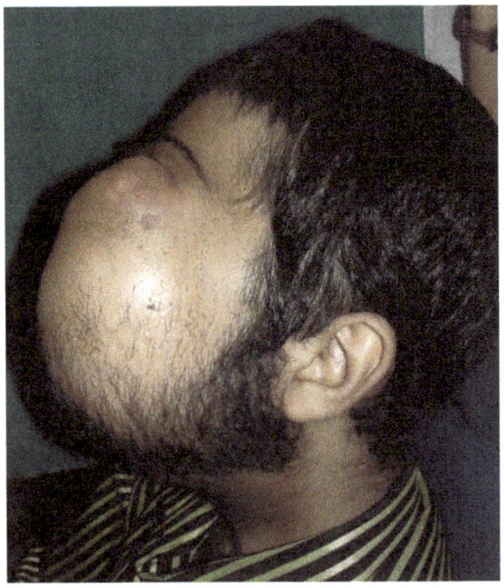

Figure 2: Lateral view.

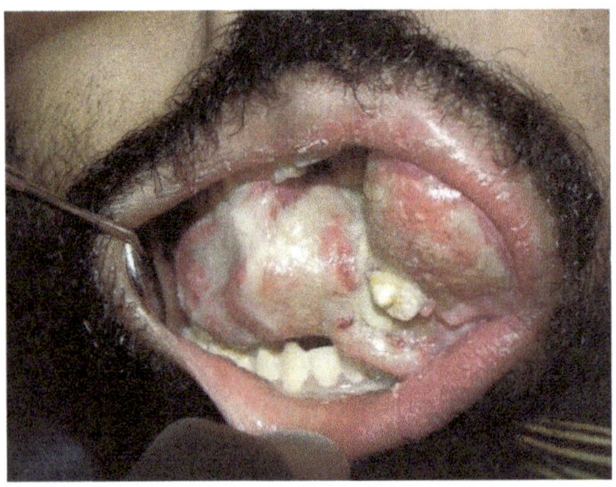

Figure 3: Intraoral view depicting the growth.

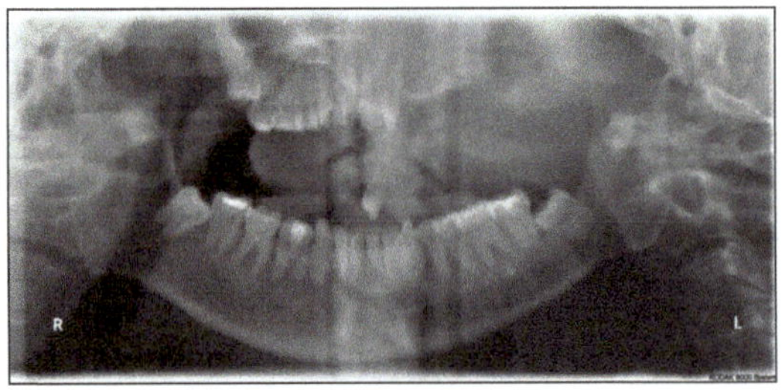

Figure 4: OPG showed erosion of the left maxilla and downward displacement of 24.

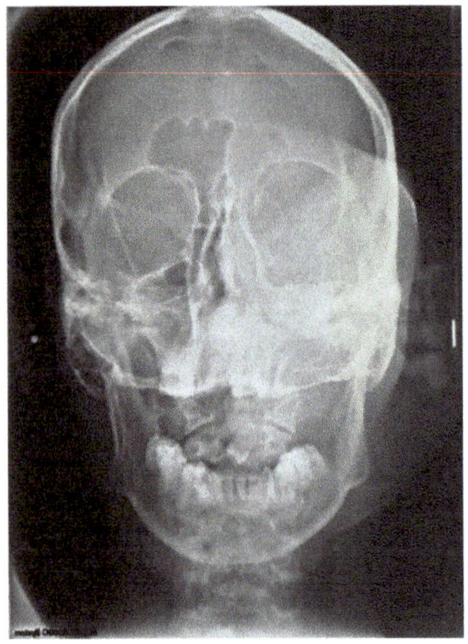

Figure 5: PA view showed erosion of the left maxilla and downward displacement of 24.

Extra oral examination revealed facial asymmetry with a diffuse swelling on left side measuring 22 × 17 cms in dimension. Swelling was extending from lower eyelid superiorly to 2 cm below the lower border of the mandible inferiorly. Medially it extends from the philtrum and lateral wall of the nose to 2 cm anterior to tragus of the ear. Skin over the swelling was stretched, shiny, and erythematous. The nasolabial fold was obliterated and the patient was not able to close his mouth. Swelling was firm to hard in consistency and nontender on palpation (Figures 1 and 2).

Intraoral examination revealed a proliferative growth measuring approximately 12 × 10 cm extending from left buccal mucosa involving upper alveolus, extending downwards crossing the midline, and extending towards the opposite side. Surface of the growth was lobulated, covered with necrotic slough, with pus discharge, and erythematous areas. The growth was firm in consistency and tender on palpation (Figure 3).

Investigations included complete hemogram, panoramic radiograph, skull views, CT scan, and biopsy. The hemogram showed a normal blood count with an elevated total leucocyte count and elevated ESR. Orthopantomograph and posteroanterior views showed erosion of the left maxilla and downward displacement of 24 (Figures 4 and 5). CT scan revealed

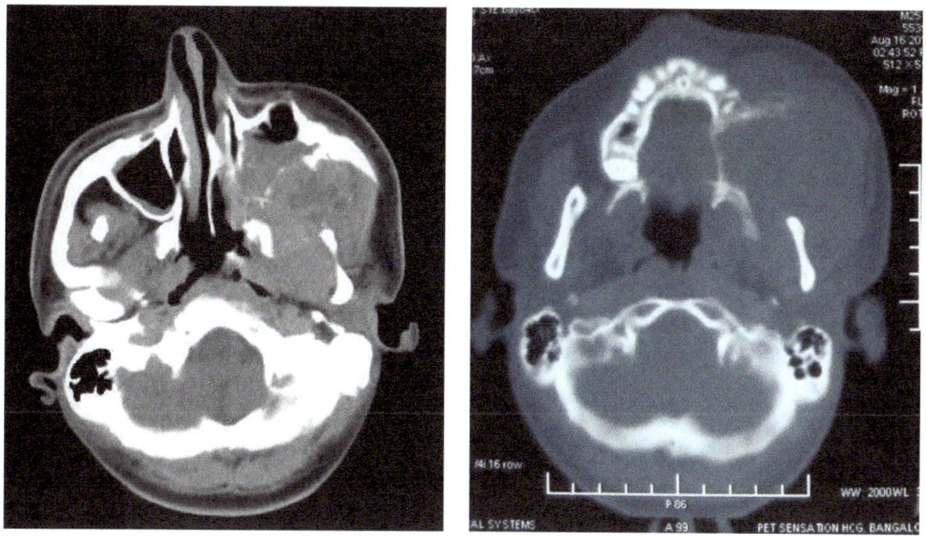

(a) (b)

FIGURE 6: CT showing the extent of the lesion.

a large mass epicentered over the left masticator space with destruction of the posterolateral wall of the maxillary sinus. The mass extended into the sinus cavity anteriorly, the infratemporal fossa laterally, pterygoid muscles posteriorly, and inferiorly the mass caused destruction of alveolar process of maxilla. There was destruction of superior aspect of the anterior wall of the left maxillary sinus adjacent to zygomatic arch, which also extended into orbital floor and anterolateral aspect, posteromedially extended to involve left sphenoid sinus and posterior ethmoid sinuses (Figure 6).

CT of chest revealed emphysematous changes in the lungs and irregular areas of consolidation/atelectasis in the medial aspects of both lower lobes and the inferior lingual. The mediastinal lymph nodes and bilateral axillary lymph nodes were noted and which are not significant by size criteria. Biopsy of the lesion was done under local anesthesia and on histopathological examination revealed sheets of neoplastic cells having round hyperchromatic nuclei with scanty discernible cytoplasm with some cells with clear cytoplasm suggestive of the diagnosis as poorly differentiated small round cell tumor (Figure 7).

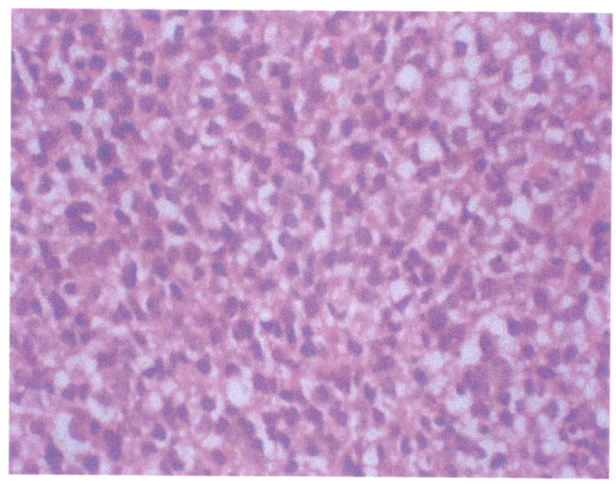

FIGURE 7: Histopathological picture showing sheets of neoplastic cells having round hyper chromatic nuclei with scanty discernible cytoplasm. Some cells have clear cytoplasm.

Immunohistochemistry revealed the neoplastic cells expressing Vimentin, Mic-2, Bcl-2 and are negative for Myf-4, S-100, CK-7, CK-20, SMA, Desmin HMB-45, supporting diagnosis of poorly differentiated small cell variant synovial sarcoma (Figure 8).

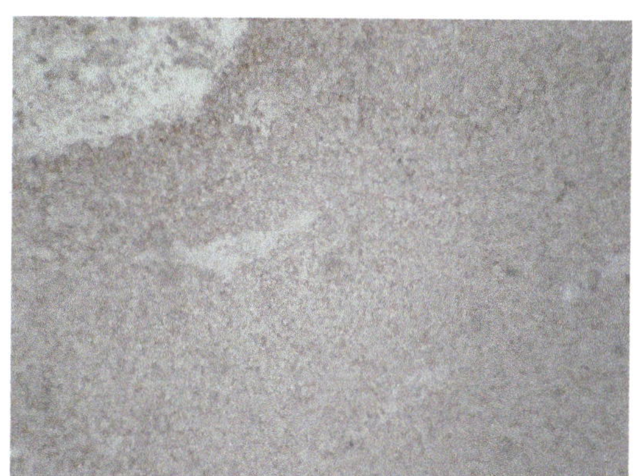

FIGURE 8: IHC revealed, tumor cells express Mic-2 with crisp cytoplasmic positivity.

The patient was referred to the oncologist for surgery, radiotherapy and chemotherapy. But the patient discontinued the treatment and the patient expired within a year.

3. Discussion

Synovial sarcoma is a well-defined clinical and morphological entity that was originally described by Simon in 1865 and was so named in 1934 by Sabrazes et al. [7]. Synovial sarcomas are a tumor of mesenchymal origin that occur predominantly in the juxta-articular regions of the lower limb; however, the cell of origin in general and of this tumor in particular is uncertain. Mainly young adults and adolescents are affected with a male-female ratio of 1.2 : 1 [8, 9]. The patient typically presents with a slow-growing palpable mass, which may grow over weeks or months, thus simulating a benign lesion [10]. More peripheral superficial lesions may be smaller, owing to earlier clinical detection. Deeper lesions might go undetected and become quite large. Lesions ranging from 2 cm to >14 cm are seen [11].

Patient with a head and neck sarcoma might present with dysphagia, hoarseness, or headache, depending on the plane of spread and site of origin of the tumor. In a large study of 672 cases, males and females were affected equally [12]. The growth was staged as stage IVB low grade using RMH Staging System [13] as follows:

Stage IA, low grade, <5 cm;

Stage IB, low grade, ≥5 to <10 cm, intermediate grade, <5 cm;

Stage IIA, low grade, ≥10 to <15 cm, intermediate grade, ≥5 to <10 cm, high grade, <5 cm;

Stage IIB, low grade, ≥15 cm, intermediate grade, ≥10 to <15 cm, high grade, ≥ 5 to <10 cm;

Stage IIIA, intermediate grade, ≥15 cm, high grade, ≥10 to <15 cm;

Stage IIIB, high grade, ≥15 cm;

Stage IVA, any grade, any size, node metastases;

Stage IVB, any grade, any size, distant metastases.

It sometimes appears in locations unrelated to synovium, and thus its origin remains unknown. There are four subtypes of Synovial sarcoma: biphasic tumors, monophasic tumors, monophasic epithelial tumors, and poorly differentiated (round cell) tumors [14, 15].

Variants of synovial sarcomas (SS) are subclassified into three groups: (i) monophasic epithelial type; (ii) monophasic spindle cell type; and (iii) biphasic type with distinct epithelial and spindle cell components. Regardless of the subtype, the conventional clues and immunohistochemical evidence of the epithelial element are characteristic of synovial sarcoma, and have led to the consensus that this tumor should be regarded as a carcinosarcoma of soft tissue origin [16]. In addition to the three subtypes, Enzinger and Weiss have described a "poorly differentiated" type of SS which shows more aggressive behavior [17].

In the present case, histopathological picture showed sheets of neoplastic cells having round hyperchromatic nuclei with scanty discernible cytoplasm. Some cells had clear cytoplasm. Immunohistochemistry revealed that tumor cells express Vimentin, Bcl-2, and Mic-2 with crisp cytoplasmic positivity suggesting the diagnosis as poorly differentiated small cell variant synovial sarcoma. Bcl-2 protein is regularly expressed in synovial sarcomas, and CD99, the product of the MIC2 gene, is seen in 67% of all cases [1].

Wide surgical resection is the primary treatment option for SS. Because complete excision of intraoral tumors is not always possible, a multimodal therapeutic approach consisting of extensive radical local excision, postoperative radiation therapy, and chemotherapy is often recommended. The metastatic potential (29.2%) and recurrence rate (20.8%) of the oral tumors appeared to be lower than those of synovial sarcoma originating at other sites [4]. Multiple recurrences were not rare. Synovial sarcoma most commonly metastasized to the lung, followed by the lymph nodes and the bone marrow [1].

Tumor recurrence typically manifested in the first 2 years after initial therapy. Prognosis is generally poor (5-year survival rate, 55%) [18]. Prognosis is adversely affected by a tumor size of more than 5 cm, tumor site, age over 60 years, high grade malignancy, and the presence of metastatic disease [9].

In the present case, the prognosis was poor; patient expired within a year after diagnosis. Synovial sarcoma is rare in the oral cavity, a feature that may increase the potential for misdiagnosis. These tumors should be considered in histopathologic differential diagnosis of both malignant primary and metastatic spindle cell tumors of the oral cavity.

The rarity of the present case is very rare malignant soft tissue tumor representing 5.6% to 10% of all soft tissue sarcomas, with approximately 9% occurring in the head and neck region, its aggressive nature, and its tendency to metastasize to other sites. This emphasizes on the early diagnosis and management of synovial sarcoma.

References

[1] S. Meer, H. Coleman, and M. Altini, "Oral synovial sarcoma: a report of 2 cases and a review of the literature," *Oral Surgery, Oral Medicine, Oral Pathology, Oral Radiology, and Endodontics*, vol. 96, no. 3, pp. 306–315, 2003.

[2] E. M. Sturgis and B. O. Potter, "Sarcomas of the head and neck region," *Current Opinion in Oncology*, vol. 15, no. 3, pp. 239–252, 2003.

[3] R. Carrillo, J. L. Rodriguez-Peralto, and J. G. Batsakis, "Synovial sarcomas of the head and neck," *Annals of Otology, Rhinology and Laryngology*, vol. 101, no. 4, pp. 367–370, 1992.

[4] C. Koga, H. Harada, J. Kusukawa, and T. Kameyama, "Synovial sarcoma arising in the mandibular bone," *Oral Oncology Extra*, vol. 41, no. 3, pp. 45–48, 2005.

[5] W. Grayson, S. J. Nayler, and G. P. Jena, "Synovial sarcoma of the parotid gland. A case report with clinicopathological analysis and review of the literature," *South African Journal of Surgery*, vol. 36, no. 1, pp. 32–35, 1998.

[6] J. J. Mitcherling, E. M. Collins, C. E. Tomich, R. P. Bianco, and W. K. Cooper, "Synovial sarcoma of the neck: report of a case," *Journal of Oral Surgery*, vol. 34, no. 1, pp. 64–69, 1976.

[7] J. Sabrazes, E. Loubat, R. de Grially, and J. Magendie, "Synovial sarcoma," *Gazette Hebdomadaire de Science Médicale de Bordeaux*, vol. 55, pp. 754–762, 1934.

[8] C. A. Perez, "Unusual nonepithelial tumors of head and neck," *Principles and Practice of Radiation Oncology*, vol. 43, pp. 1125–1134, 1998.

[9] P. J. Ameerally, S. K. Sira, A. W. Barrett, and P. Hollows, "Synovial sarcoma of the hard palate," *British Journal of Oral and Maxillofacial Surgery*, vol. 42, no. 3, pp. 261–263, 2004.

[10] M. J. Kransdorf, "Malignant soft-tissue tumors in a large referral population: distribution of diagnoses by age, sex, and location," *American Journal of Roentgenology*, vol. 164, no. 1, pp. 129–134, 1995.

[11] U. Tateishi, T. Hasegawa, Y. Beppu, M. Satake, and N. Moriyama, "Synovial sarcoma of the soft tissues: prognostic significance of imaging features," *Journal of Computer Assisted Tomography*, vol. 28, no. 1, pp. 140–148, 2004.

[12] T. Ishida, T. Iijima, S. Moriyama, C. Nakamura, T. Kitagawa, and R. Machinami, "Intra-articular calcifying synovial sarcoma mimicking synovial chondromatosis," *Skeletal Radiology*, vol. 25, no. 8, pp. 766–769, 1996.

[13] R. C. Ramanthan, R. A'Hern, C. Fisher et al., "Modified staging system for extremity soft tissue sarcomas," *Annals of Surgical Oncology*, vol. 6, no. 1, pp. 57–69, 1999.

[14] C. A. Ewing, M. F. Zakowski, and O. Lin, "Monophasic synovial sarcoma: a cytologic spectrum," *Diagnostic Cytopathology*, vol. 30, no. 1, pp. 19–23, 2004.

[15] R. Rong, E. E. Doxtader, J. Tull, G. de la Roza, and S. Zhang, "Metastatic poorly differentiated monophasic synovial sarcoma to lung with unknown primary: a molecular genetic analysis," *International Journal of Clinical and Experimental Pathology*, vol. 3, no. 2, pp. 217–221, 2010.

[16] J. M. Lopes, B. Bjerkehagen, R. Holm, O. Bruland, M. Sobrinho-Simoes, and J. M. Nesland, "Immunohistochemical profile of synovial sarcoma with emphasis on the epithelial-type differentiation. A study of 49 primary tumours, recurrences and metastases," *Pathology Research and Practice*, vol. 190, no. 2, pp. 168–177, 1994.

[17] S. W. Weiss and J. Goldblum, "Malignant soft tissue tumors of uncertain type," in *Enzinger and Weiss's Soft Tissue Tumors*, S. W. Weiss and J. R. Goldblum, Eds., pp. 1483–1571, CV Mosby, St. Louis, Mo, USA, 2001.

[18] P. H. Wright, F. H. Sim, E. H. Soule, and W. F. Taylor, "Synovial sarcoma," *Journal of Bone and Joint Surgery A*, vol. 64, no. 1, pp. 112–122, 1982.

32

Cemento-Ossifying Fibroma in a Patient with End-Stage Renal Disease

Divya Gopinath,[1] V. T. Beena,[2] G. Sugirtharaj,[2] K. Vidhyadharan,[2] K. Salmanul Faris,[2] and Sajai J. Kumar[2]

[1] *Department of Oral Pathology & Microbiology, Government of Dental College, Calicut, Kerala 673008, India*
[2] *Department of Oral & Maxillofacial Pathology, Government of Dental College, Trivandrum Kerala 695011, India*

Correspondence should be addressed to Divya Gopinath; drdivyakmenon@gmail.com

Academic Editors: R. Crespi, M. Feichtinger, T. Hata, E. F. Wright, and U. Zilberman

The presence of chronic renal disease (CRD) is a predisposing factor for the occurrence of soft and hard tissue lesions in the oral cavity. The cemento-ossifying fibroma (COF) is an uncommon benign fibroosseous lesion composed of fibrocellular component and calcified materials like cementum and woven bone. A 37-year-old female patient undergoing chronic haemodialysis reported to our institution with a complaint of slow growing, nontender swelling of mandible of 6-month duration. Computed tomography disclosed an ill-defined lesion showing thinning and expansion of buccal as well as lingual cortical plate with flecks of radiopacity in centre. Incision biopsy revealed histological characteristics consistent with cemento-ossifying fibroma. The lesion was excised under local anesthesia. The histopathological examination revealed irregularly shaped bone and cementum-like hard tissue calcifications contained within hypercellular fibrous tissue stroma, leading to a confirmation of the diagnosis of cemento-ossifying fibroma. This paper aims to provide light to the fact that the soft and hard tissues of the oral region may become susceptible to the development of pathological growths in case of some particular systemic conditions.

1. Introduction

Chronic renal disease (CRD) can be defined as the progressive and irreversible decline in kidney functions and up to 90% of patients having renal insufficiency may present with oral signs and symptoms in soft and hard tissues either as a result of the disease itself or the treatment protocol [1]. Halitosis, altered taste and sensation, bone demineralization, loss of lamina dura, deep periodontal pockets, changes in saliva and poor oral hygiene are often associated with this condition, based on individual predisposition and the severity of the disease [1]. The knowledge of bone-related oral lesions in CRD patients is limited.

Cemento-ossifying fibroma (COF) is a distinct form of benign fibroosseous lesions of the mandible and maxilla containing fibrous tissue and varying amounts of calcified tissue resembling bone, cementum, or both [2]. The pathologic nature of COF is not yet clearly understood. It is included under neoplastic group of fibro osseous lesions thought to arise from periodontal ligament [2]. The aim of this report is therefore to present a case of COF who was also suffering from CRD and describe clinical characteristics of these conditions.

2. Case Report

A 37-year-old patient reported to outpatient department of our institution with a complaint of swelling of the lower jaw of six-month duration. There was neither a history of trauma or teeth extraction related to the swelling nor any similar swelling in other parts of the body. Patient's history revealed that she had been suffering from chronic renal Disease for the past six years. She had also been undergoing hemodialysis once a week for the past two years. On further questioning, Patient revealed that she was suffering from pain in all joints. patient was having hypertension secondary to the declining kidney function, for which she was under constant medication. The patient was manual labourer in farms for the past 20 years. Because of her declining physical condition she had stopped her work for the past four years.

Extra oral findings were nonremarkable. Intraoral examination revealed a nontender bony hard swelling of size 1.5 × 2 cm on the right mandibular body extending from central incisor to the first premolar with buccal cortical plate expansion. The overlying mucosa appeared to be normal. Pulp vitality of the teeth adjacent to the lesion proved positive. Orthopantomogram revealed an ill-defined radiolucency with radio-opaque specks located in the mandibular body. Root resorption was noted for the right canine and first premolar. Axial imaging showed the lesion to cause thinning and expansion of buccal as well as lingual cortical plate (Figure 1). Likewise, the core region of the lesion showed flecks of radiopacity. 3D reformatted computed tomography illustrated size and location of the well-defined tumor (Figures 2 and 3). A sample of the lesion was obtained for histopathological study, which revealed the presence of a fibrocellular stroma containing cementum-like hard tissue calcifications and other areas presenting recently formed osteoid with peripheral osteoblasts and signs of progressive calcification (Figure 4). There were no atypia or mitotic figures. The diagnosis was suggestive of cemento-ossifying fibroma. After medical clearance, surgical excision was carried out under local anaesthesia. The lesion was present as tiny irregular granulated fibrous tissue and pieces of bone-like immaturely calcified material. Teeth associated with the lesion were extracted, and curettage was performed to remove all fragments which were firmly attached to the underlying bone structure. The patient was clinically and radiographically symptom-free at the 18-month followup. Patient was advised orthopedic consultation for any other bony lesions, but the reports were inconclusive. But her renal condition was worse than before, and she was undergoing dialysis twice a week.

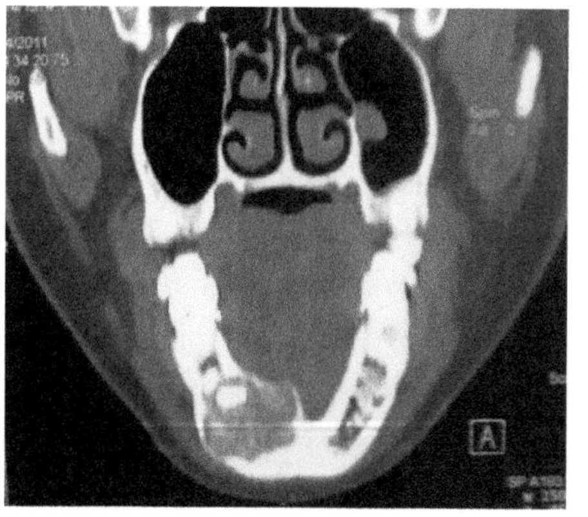

Figure 1: Axial CT image showing the lesion causing thinning and expansion of buccal as well as lingual cortical plate.

3. Discussion

The concept of "fibroosseous lesions" of bone evolved over the last several decades to include two major entities: fibrous dysplasia and ossifying fibroma as well as the other less common. It is a slow-growing lesion most often seen in women between the third and fourth decades of life. Both jawbones can be affected, although 62% to 89% of the lesions arise in the mandible, involving premolar and molar regions in 77% of cases. While one-half of all cases are asymptomatic, the growth of the tumor over time may lead to facial asymmetry, with the appearance of a mass causing discomfort or mandibular expansion and the possible displacement of dental roots.

Cemento-ossifying fibroma is a thought to have its origin from arises from the periodontal membrane [3]. The periodontal membrane is the layer of fibrous connective tissue surrounding the roots of teeth. It contains multipotent cells capable of forming cementum, lamellar bone, and fibrous tissue [4, 5]. However, lesions with similar histopathological features have been reported in other craniofacial structures and in long bones which do not contain cementum [6]. In addition, bone and cementum are both originated from mesenchymal stem cells. Accordingly, the classification of the World Health Organization suggested the term ossifying fibroma and considered it as a nonodontogenic neoplasm [7]. But cementum forming cells have been demonstrated to be phenotypically distinct from bone forming osteoblasts, and immunohistochemical staining differences have been reported with cementocytes being positive for fibromodulin and lumican whilst the bone forming cells are negative [8, 9]. Cementum lacks the lamellar architecture of mature bone and has been described as resembling a primitive, fetal type woven bone [10].

Cemento-ossifying fibroma is a slow growing lesion composed of cellular fibroblastic tissue containing basophilic masses of cementum-like tissue. In addition, a varying amount of bony trabeculae is interspersed within the lesion, giving it its characteristic appearance [11]. Reed used the presence or absence of woven and lamellar bone in histopathological section to differentiate the cement-ossifying fibroma from the other osseous lesions [12]. Fibrous dysplasia contains no lamellar bone but rather has a woven bone. On the other hand, cemento-ossifying fibroma and the ossifying fibroma contain woven bone that is often rimmed by osteoblasts that have laid down layers of lamellar bone [13]. Additionally, cemento-ossifying fibroma may have areas of cementum, appearing as psammoma bodies embedded in a benign fibrous stroma [13].

Radiological findings suggests that the lesion is usually well circumscribed and demarcated from surrounding bone, in contrast to true fibrous dysplasia. The central cementifying fibroma and the central ossifying fibroma, have a centrifugal growth pattern rather than a linear one. Therefore, lesions grow by expansion equally in all direction and present as round tumor masses.

The association of ossifying fibromas with renal diseases can be observed in hyperparathyroidism-jaw tumor syndrome, in which the patients suffer from familial parathyroid adenomas, ossifying fibroma of the jaws, renal cysts, and Wilms tumors [2, 14]. The HRPT2 gene has been found to be mutated in this syndrome, and it inactivates the

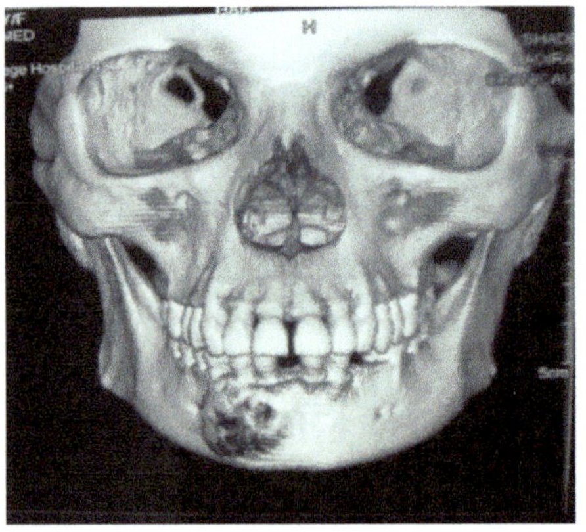

FIGURE 2: 3D reformatted CT illustrating size and location of the well-defined tumor.

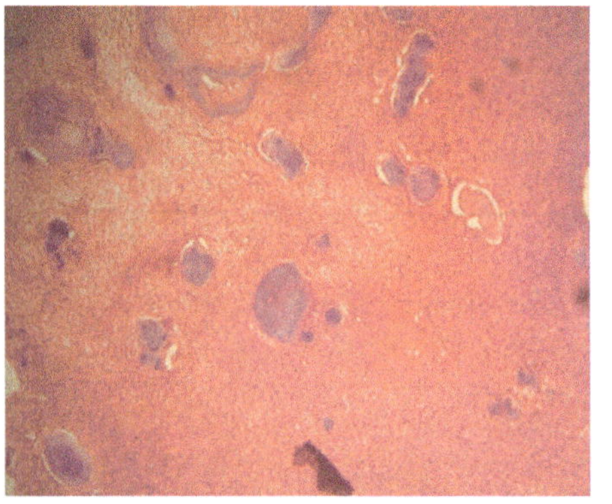

FIGURE 4: Fibro-cellular stroma containing cementum-like hard tissue calcifications (H&E stained section 10x)

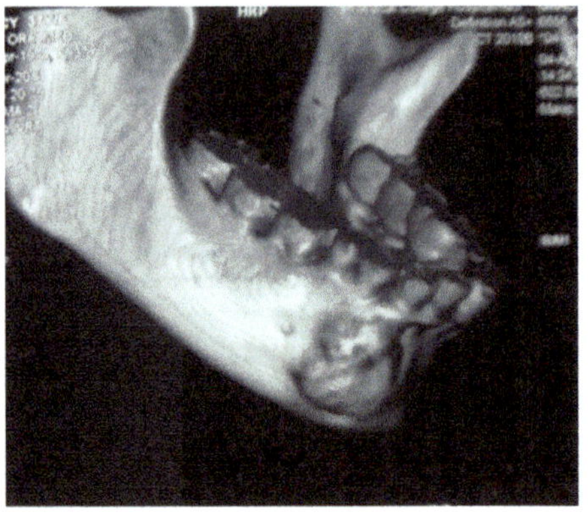

FIGURE 3: 3D reformatted CT illustrating size and location of the well-defined tumor.

parafibromin protein which has antiproliferative properties [14]. More recent studies have found perturbations in this gene among nonsyndrome associated ossifying fibromas of the jaws [15]. But only one case report describes an association of cementoossifying fibroma with end-stage renal disease [14]. The findings were similar to ours with normal PTH levels and no sign of parathyroid adenoma. Renal osteodystrophy, the term used to describe the skeletal complications of end-stage renal disease, is a multifactorial disorder of bone remodelling. Oral manifestations of the CRD due to renal osteodystrophy are late sign of renal disease and are usually due to alterations in calcium and phosphorum metabolism, abnormal metabolism of vitamin D, and the compensatory hyperactivity of parathyroid glands (secondary hyperparathyroidism). It is characterized by the following signs: bone demineralization, decreased trabeculation, decreased thickness of cortical bone, ground-glass appearance of bone, metastatic soft-tissue calcifications, radiolucent fibrocystic lesions, radiolucent giant cell lesions, lytic areas of bone, jaw fracture (spontaneous or after dental procedures), abnormal bone healing after extraction, and, sometimes, dental mobility as a consequence of the loss of substance in the bone [16]. But in the earlier stages of CRD, little is known about changes in bone metabolism and the effect of disturbed mineral metabolism on bone histology [17]. In the incipient stages of CRD, normal or mildly elevated PTH concentrations have until recently seldom resulted in therapy and thus may have mitigated the demand for bone biopsy; however, it has become evident that disturbances in bone metabolism present very early in CRD [17]. Humoral factors that are involved in the maintenance of normal bone homeostasis are usually perturbed as soon as the GFR (glomerular filtration rate) drops below 60 to 70 mL/min [18]. Serum FGF-23 (fibroblast growth factor) levels increase as soon as the GFR decreases below 60 mL/min, even before the development of hyperphosphatemia and hyperparathyroidism [19]. Moreover, additional studies have shown that the maximal tubular reabsorption of phosphate negatively correlates with serum concentrations of FGF-23 in stage 3 CRD, whereas in advanced CRD, this correlation is mitigated [19, 20]. Nevertheless, the increased FGF-23 further aggravates calcitriol deficiency by directly inhibiting the renal 1α-hydroxylase activity [20]. Both FGF-23 and calcitriol are important regulators of bone homeostasis [21]. Calcitriol and its receptor, the vitamin D receptor (VDR), are critical for normal bone metabolism, because appropriate activation of the VDR is necessary for normal osteoblastic bone formation and osteoclastic bone resorption, as well as for the coupling of osteoblastic and osteoclastic activity [21]. Studies have shown that FGF-23 overexpression is associated with severe skeletal phenotype characterized by disturbed mineralization process and growth plate architecture; however, they could not differentiate between local skeletal action and systemic effects of FGF-23 [22]. In addition, recently published data suggests that FGF-23 is a negative regulator of PTH mRNA expression and secretion in vitro as well [23]. Thus, a possible association of high FGF-23 with low PTH and calcitriol concentrations coupled with down regulation of the VDR may adversely affect bone metabolism, resulting in impaired bone turnover in the early CRD stages [17]. This speculation requires further validation. But whether there is a possible relation between FGF associated bone changes in CRD and the COF remains to be elucidated.

Due to the good delimitation of the COF, surgical removal and curettage is the treatment of choice. In the case of very large lesions with important tissue ablation, the challenge is to replace the affected tissue. The prognosis is usually good, since recurrences are not frequent.

4. Conclusion

Like any other systemic disease, CRD can also present with oral manifestations. Bony alterations in CRD are usually related to renal osteodystrophy. Further studies are needed to elucidate the pathogenesis of ossifying fibroma in patients with CRD.

References

[1] S. A. Summers, W. M. Tilakaratne, F. Fortune, and N. Ashman, "Renal disease and the mouth," *American Journal of Medicine*, vol. 120, no. 7, pp. 568–573, 2007.

[2] R. Eversole, L. Su, and S. ElMofty, "Benign fibro-osseous lesions of the craniofacial complex. A review," *Head and Neck Pathology*, vol. 2, no. 3, pp. 177–202, 2008.

[3] G. R. Huebner, C. V. Brenneise, and J. Ballenger, "Central ossifying fibroma of the anterior maxilla: report of case," *The Journal of the American Dental Association*, vol. 116, no. 4, pp. 507–510, 1988.

[4] B. Bertrand, P. Eloy, J. P. Cornelis, S. Gosseye, J. Clotuche, and C. Gilliard, "Juvenile aggressive cemento-ossifying fibroma: case report and review of the literature," *Laryngoscope*, vol. 103, no. 12, pp. 1385–1390, 1993.

[5] J. E. Hamner, P. M. Lightbody, A. S. Ketcham, and H. Swerdlow, "Cemento-ossifying fibroma of the maxilla," *Oral Surgery, Oral Medicine, Oral Pathology*, vol. 26, no. 4, pp. 579–587, 1968.

[6] L. R. Eversole, A. S. Leider, and K. Nelson, "Ossifying fibroma: a clinicopathologic study of sixty-four cases," *Oral Surgery Oral Medicine and Oral Pathology*, vol. 60, no. 5, pp. 505–511, 1985.

[7] L. Barnes, J. Eveson, P. Reichardt, and D. Sidransky, *World Health Organization Classification of Tumours. Pathology and Genetics Head and Neck Tumours*, IARC Press, Lyon, France, 2005.

[8] W. J. Grzesik, H. Cheng, J. S. Oh et al., "Cementum-forming cells are phenotypically distinct from bone-forming cells," *Journal of Bone and Mineral Research*, vol. 15, no. 1, pp. 52–59, 2000.

[9] D. D. Bosshardt, "Are cementoblasts a subpopulation of osteoblasts or a unique phenotype?" *Journal of Dental Research*, vol. 84, no. 5, pp. 390–406, 2005.

[10] G. Hall, "Fibro-osseous lesions of the head and neck," *Diagnostic Histopathology*, vol. 18, no. 4, pp. 149–158, 2012.

[11] A. J. Kuta, C. M. Worley, and G. E. Kaugars, "Central cementoossifying fibroma of the maxillary sinus: a review of six cases," *American Journal of Neuroradiology*, vol. 16, no. 6, pp. 1282–1286, 1995.

[12] R. J. Reed, "Fibrous dysplasia of bone. A review of 25 cases," *Archives of Pathology*, vol. 75, pp. 480–495, 1963.

[13] T. M. Voytek, J. Y. Ro, J. Edeiken, and A. G. Ayala, "Fibrous dysplasia and cemento-ossifying fibroma: a histologic spectrum," *American Journal of Surgical Pathology*, vol. 19, no. 7, pp. 775–781, 1995.

[14] Y. Sirin, N. Kahraman, and V. Olgac, "Maxillary cemento-ossifying fibroma in a male patient with end-stage chronic renal disease," *International Journal of Clinical Dental Science*, vol. 2, no. 3, pp. 33–37, 2011.

[15] F. J. Pimenta, L. F. Gontijo Silveira, G. C. Tavares et al., "HRPT2 gene alterations in ossifying fibroma of the jaws," *Oral Oncology*, vol. 42, no. 7, pp. 735–739, 2006.

[16] S. S. de Rossi and M. Glick, "Dental considerations for the patient with renal disease receiving hemodialysis," *Journal of the American Dental Association*, vol. 127, no. 2, pp. 211–219, 1996.

[17] A. Gal-Moscovici and S. M. Sprague, "Role of bone biopsy in stages 3 to 4 chronic kidney disease," *Clinical Journal of the American Society of Nephrology*, vol. 3, supplement 3, pp. S170–S174, 2008.

[18] N. A. T. Hamdy, J. A. Kanis, M. N. C. Beneton et al., "Effect of alfacalcidol on natural course of renal bone disease in mild to moderate renal failure," *British Medical Journal*, vol. 310, no. 6976, pp. 358–363, 1995.

[19] T. Shigematsu, J. J. Kazama, T. Yamashita et al., "Possible involvement of circulating fibroblast growth factor 23 in the development of secondary hyperparathyroidism associated with renal insufficiency," *American Journal of Kidney Diseases*, vol. 44, no. 2, pp. 250–256, 2004.

[20] O. Gutierrez, T. Isakova, E. Rhee et al., "Fibroblast growth factor-23 mitigates hyperphosphatemia but accentuates calcitriol deficiency in chronic kidney disease," *Journal of the American Society of Nephrology*, vol. 16, no. 7, pp. 2205–2215, 2005.

[21] D. K. Panda, D. Miao, I. Bolivar et al., "Inactivation of the 25-hydroxyvitamin D 1alpha-hydroxylase and vitamin D receptor demonstrates independent and interdependent effects of calcium and vitamin D on skeletal and mineral homeostasis," *Journal of Biological Chemistry*, vol. 279, no. 16, pp. 16754–16766, 2004.

[22] T. Larsson, R. Marsell, E. Schipani et al., "Transgenic mice expressing fibroblast growth factor 23 under the control of the α1(I) collagen promoter exhibit growth retardation, osteomalacia, and disturbed phosphate homeostasis," *Endocrinology*, vol. 145, no. 7, pp. 3087–3094, 2004.

[23] T. Krajisnik, P. Björklund, R. Marsell et al., "Fibroblast growth factor-23 regulates parathyroid hormone and 1α-hydroxylase expression in cultured bovine parathyroid cells," *Journal of Endocrinology*, vol. 195, no. 1, pp. 125–131, 2007.

33

Unicystic Mural Ameloblastoma: An Unusual Case Report

V. Nagalaxmi, Mithare Sangmesh, Kotya Naik Maloth, Srikanth Kodangal, Vani Chappidi, and Stuti Goyal

Sri Sai College of Dental Surgery, H. No. 5-5-47/1, Mustafa Nagar, Khammam 507 001, Vikarabad, Andhra Pradesh, India

Correspondence should be addressed to Kotya Naik Maloth; dr.kotyanaik.maloth@gmail.com

Academic Editors: J. J. Segura-Egea and N. Shah

Ameloblastoma is a benign odontogenic neoplasm which frequently affects the mandible. The term ameloblastoma includes several clinicoradiological and histological types. Apart from the most commonly encountered clinicopathologic models, there are few variants, whose biological profile is unknown or not elicited. Among these types, unicystic ameloblastoma is the least encountered variant of the ameloblastoma. Unicystic ameloblastoma refers to those cystic lesions that show clinical, radiographic, or gross features of a jaw cyst but on histologic examination show a typical ameloblastomatous epithelium lining the cyst cavity, with or without luminal and/or mural tumor proliferation. Unicystic ameloblastoma is a less encountered variant of the ameloblastoma and is believed to be less aggressive. As this tumor shows considerable similarities with dentigerous cysts, both clinically and radiographically, the biologic behaviour of this tumor group was reviewed. Moreover, recurrence of unicystic ameloblastoma may be long delayed, and a long-term postoperative followup is essential for proper management of these patients. Here we are presenting a case of unicystic ameloblastoma in an 18-year-old female patient.

1. Introduction

Many benign lesions cause mandibular swellings, and these can be divided into odontogenic and nonodontogenic origin. The most common tumor of odontogenic origin is ameloblastoma which develops from epithelial cellular elements and dental tissues in their various phases of development. More than 80% of all ameloblastomas are solid or multicystic variants, with unicystic ameloblastoma being an important clinicopathologic form of ameloblastoma and occupying the remaining 20% of the cases along with peripheral ameloblastoma [1]. Unicystic ameloblastoma, a variant of ameloblastoma, was first described by Ackermann et al. in 1988 [2]. Unicystic ameloblastoma (UCA) is the most common term used to designate its different pathological entities. Sometimes these can present as a multilocular radiolucency which makes the use of the term "cystic ameloblastoma" more appropriate. However, some authors still believe that the notion that cystic ameloblastomas can have a "true" clinically multicystic pattern is arguable and contend with the use of the term "unicystic ameloblastoma" [3, 4].

The unicystic ameloblastoma is a less encountered variant of the ameloblastoma, referring to those cystic lesions that show clinical and radiographic characteristics of an odontogenic cyst but in histologic examination show a typical ameloblastomatous epithelium lining part of the cyst cavity, with or without luminal and/or mural tumor proliferation [5]. This paper illustrates a case of unicystic (mural) ameloblastoma of the mandible in an 18-year-old female.

2. Case Report

An 18-year-old female patient reported to our outpatient department with a chief complaint of swelling in the lower left front teeth region, for 3 months. Patient was apparently well 3 months back and noticed a swelling and displacement of teeth in the left lower front tooth region and reports of having pain in the same region, for 3 months. Pain was of dull aching type, which was intermitted, and it aggravates on putting mastication and relieves on rest. Pain was not associated with fever and no medication was taken. On extraoral examination a diffuse swelling was seen on the lower third of the face extending onto the left side with mild obliteration of mentolabial sulcus which is measuring about app 4 × 3 cm in size. Overlying skin was normal; no visible pulsations and no discharge were seen. On palpation, the swelling was firm in

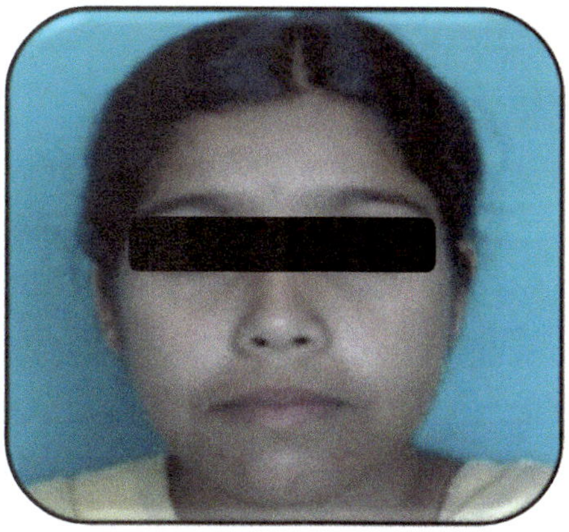

FIGURE 1: Preoperative extraoral photograph.

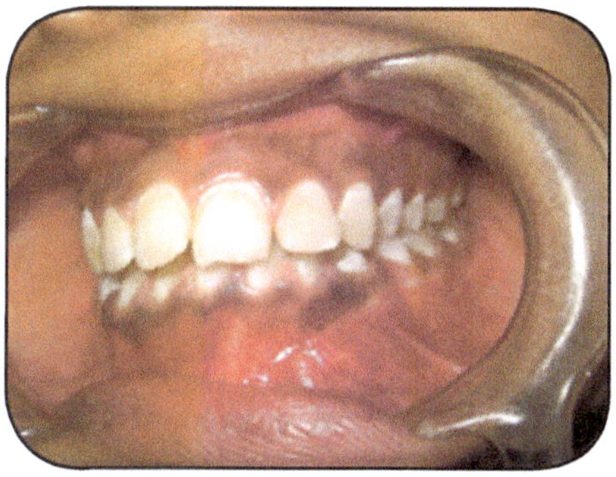

FIGURE 2: Preoperative intraoral photograph.

consistency and tender; no local rise of temperature was felt. It was nonpulsatile and noncompressible, and no discharge was present. A single left submandibular lymph node of size measuring about 0.5 × 0.5 cms in size was palpable, which was firm in consistency, mobile, and nontender (Figure 1). On intraoral examination, a single diffuse swelling was seen in the mandibular left buccal vestibule irt 31, 32, 33, and 34 regions measuring approximately 4 × 2 cms. It extends anterioposteriorly—from the mandibular labial frenum to 35 and superior-inferiorly from the attached gingival to the labial vestibule. Expansion of the lingual cortical plate was seen irt to 31, 32, and 33 (33 is missing). Neither discharge nor pulsations were seen. On palpation, crepitus was felt on the lingual cortical plate. Tenderness was elicited on palpation irt 33, 34, and 35. The swelling was firm in consistency, and surface was smooth. It was nonfluctuant and nonreducible and no discharge was noticed, non were pulsations felt (Figure 2). On needle aspiration, brown yellow fluid was aspirated. Based on the patient's history and clinical finding, the diagnosis was given as dentigerous cyst.

3. Differential Diagnosis

In differential diagnosis, ameloblastoma, calcifying epithelial odontogenic tumor (CEOT), odontogenic keratocyst (OKC), central giant cell granuloma (CGCG), odontogenic myxoma were considered but features like old age, site, multilocularity

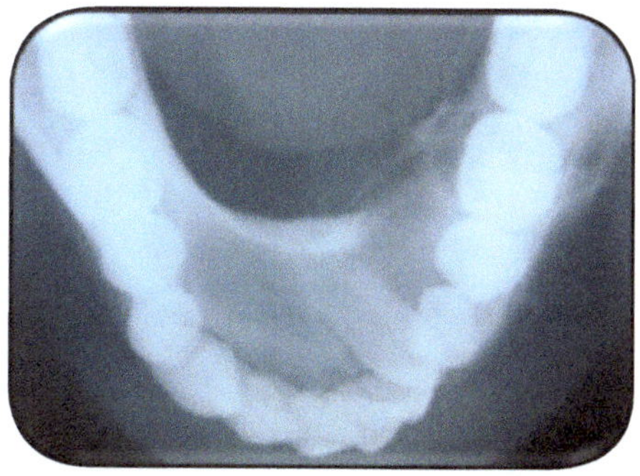

FIGURE 3: Occlusal radiograph.

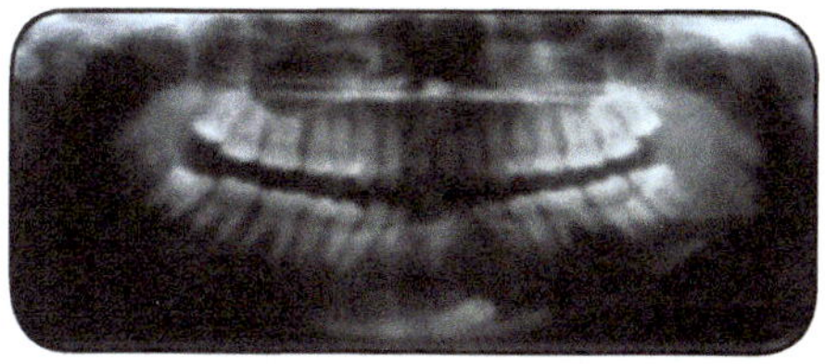

FIGURE 4: OPG radiograph.

of ameloblastoma, and impacted lower canine made us deviate from ameloblastoma. In CEOT focal areas of calcifications are seen, but in our case we see unilocular radiolucency without any radio opaque flecks. Linear expansion of OKC through medullary spaces without any buccolingual expansion ruled out OKC. Lesions like CGCG and odontogenic myxoma were also ruled out based on their clinical and radiological features [6–8].

4. Investigations

Routine investigations like complete blood picture were done, which were normal. On FNAC, a brown yellow fluid was aspirated. Radiographs were taken. Mandibular occlusal view reveals impacted 33 and expansion of lingual cortical plates irt 32, 33, 34, 35, and 36 and mild expansion of buccal cortical plate (Figure 3). OPG reveals a well-defined multilocular radiolucency with internal bony septae formation and impacted 33. Displacements of teeth irt 35, 34, 32, 31, 41, 42, and 43 were seen, with root resorption of 36 (Figure 4). A lateral cephalogram reveals a clear multilocular radiolucency with septae formation (Figure 5). A CT scan reveals expansion and perforation of the cortical plates and the extent of lesion (Figure 6). Incisional biopsy was done and submitted for histopathological examination. The biopsy tissue shows multiple cystic lesions and collagenous wall of varying thickness. The cyst is lined by odontogenic squamous epithelium of varying thickness with nuclear palisading along the margins and loose stellate reticulum. They contain moderate to abundant pale acidophilic vacuolated cytoplasm and round to oval vesicular nucleus. There are thin plates of lamellar bone with focal osteoid deposition and patchy areas of hemorrhage. There are focal epithelial invaginations associated with desmoplastic fibrosis (Figure 7). Based upon

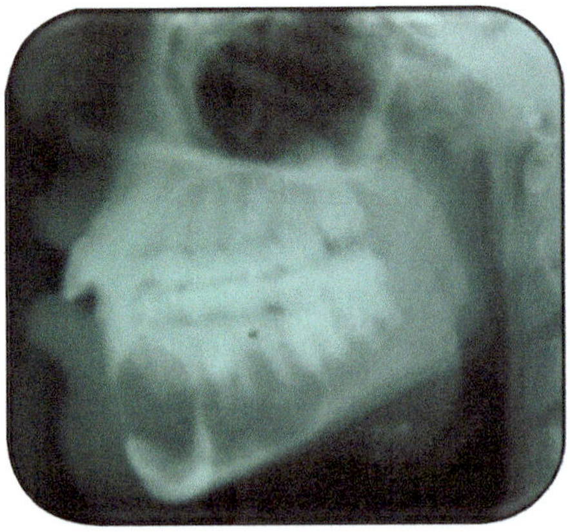

Figure 5: Lateral cephalogram radiograph.

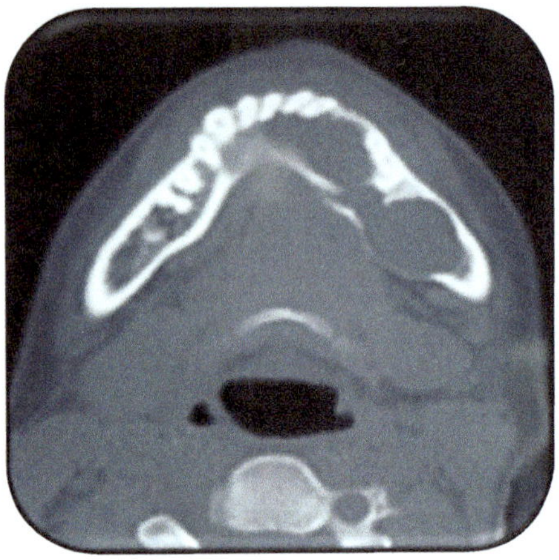

Figure 6: CT scan (axial view).

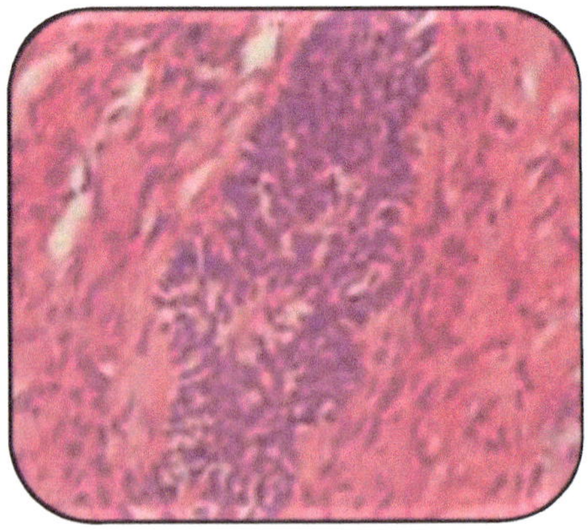

Figure 7: Histopathology.

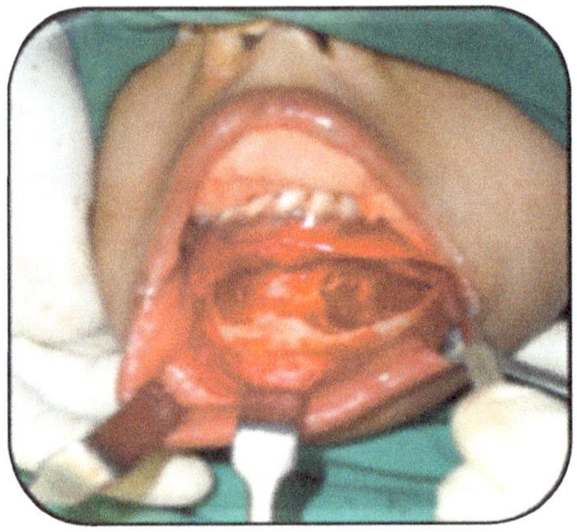

Figure 8: Intraoperative enucleation.

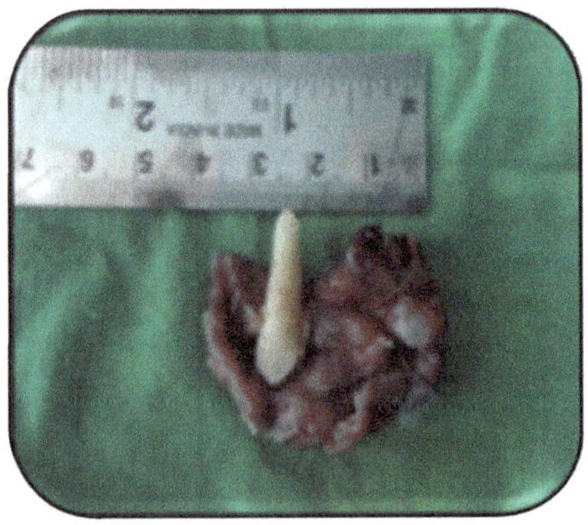

Figure 9: Intraoperative enucleation.

the radiological and histopathological report, the case was diagnosed as mural ameloblastoma.

5. Treatment

The lesion was treated conservatively with careful *enucleation* (Figures 8 and 9).

6. Discussion

Ameloblastoma is a benign, locally aggressive odontogenic neoplasm with variable clinical expression and accounts for 1% of all cysts/tumors of jaws and 18% of all odontogenic neoplasms. It is typically slow growing, locally aggressive and rarely metastasizes but has a high rate of recurrence (55–90%) if not removed adequately.

As per the WHO system of 2003, ameloblastoma is classified based on differences in biologic behavior, treatment plan and recurrence rate as follows:

(1) classic solid/multicystic ameloblastoma,

(2) unicystic ameloblastoma,

(3) peripheral ameloblastoma,

(4) desmoplastic ameloblastoma, including the so-called hybrid lesions [3].

Unicystic ameloblastoma (UCA) is a rare type of ameloblastoma, accounting for about 6% of ameloblastomas. It usually occurs in a younger age group of 16–20 years, with about 50% of the cases occurring in the second decade of life as in our case [9, 10]. The gender distribution shows a slight male predilection with a male to female ratio of 1.6 : 1.

However, when the tumor is not associated with an unerupted tooth, the gender ratio is reversed to a male to female ratio of 1:1.8 [11]. More than 90% are located in the mandible in the posterior region, followed by the parasymphysis region, the anterior maxilla, and the posterior maxilla [9]. UCA is usually asymptomatic, although a large tumor may cause painless swelling of the jaws with facial asymmetry [9]. Mucosal ulceration is rare but may be caused by continued growth of the tumor [12]. The clinical and radiographic findings in most cases of unicystic ameloblastoma suggest that the lesion is an odontogenic cyst, particularly dentigerous cyst. However, few are not associated with impacted teeth which are called nondentigerous variant [12]. The mean age of nonimpacted tooth-related cystic ameloblastoma was 5 years in comparison to 16.5 years for the impacted tooth-related variant [2]. Most of the UCAs are associated with an impacted tooth, the mandibular third molar being involved most often. But in our case it was associated with impacted mandibular canine, and it is a dentigerous variant. These findings correlate with those reported by Philipsen et al. and Ackermann et al.

The radiographic appearance of UCAs has been divided into 2 main patterns: unilocular and multilocular, and these have clear preponderance for the unilocular pattern. This preponderance is predominantly marked for the dentigerous variant, where the unilocular to multilocular ratio is 4.3:1, and for the nondentigerous type, this ratio is 1.1:1 [4, 13]. The involved teeth show varying degrees of root resorption [3].

Eversole et al. and Paikkatt et al. identified predominant radiographical patterns for UCA: unilocular, scalloped macromultilocular, pericoronal, interradicular, or periapical expansile radiolucencies [4, 14]. Our case study had a peculiar radiographic presentation of multilocular radiolucency crossing the midline of the mandible. The early ameloblastic changes within the cyst wall were first described by Vickers and Gorlin in 1970, and their histologic criteria for the diagnosis of unicystic ameloblastoma includes a cyst lined by ameloblastic epithelium with a tall columnar basal layer, subnuclear vacuoles, reverse polarity of hyperchromatic nucleus, and a thin layer of oedematous, degenerating stellate reticulum-like cells on the surface [15]. The mural extension into the cystic wall is the frequently seen feature, and the term mural UCA is used when the thickened lining (either plexiform or follicular) penetrates the adjacent capsular tissue [1, 9].

In a clinicopathologic study of 57 cases of unicystic ameloblastoma, Ackermann classified this entity into the following three histologic groups [2, 16]:

Group I—luminal UA (tumor confined to the luminal surface of the cyst);

Group II—intraluminal/plexiform UA (nodular proliferation into the lumen without infiltration of tumor cells into the connective tissue wall);

Group III—mural UA (invasive islands of ameloblastomatous epithelium in the connective tissue wall not involving the entire epithelium). According to this classification, our case study belongs to Group III.

Histologic subgrouping by Philipsen and Reichart has also been described:

Subgroup 1—luminal UA;

Subgroup 1.2—luminal and intraluminal;

Subgroup 1.2.3—luminal, intraluminal and intramural;

Subgroup 1.3—luminal and intramural.

A definitive diagnosis of unicystic ameloblastoma can only be done by histological examination of the entire lesion and cannot be predicted preoperatively on clinical or radiographic grounds. As preoperative incisional biopsy is not representative of the entire lesion, it may result in an incorrect classification. The epithelial lining of a UCA is not always uniformly characteristic and is often lined partly by a nonspecific thin epithelium that mimics the dentigerous cyst lining. Thus, true nature of the lesion becomes evident only after enucleation when the entire specimen is available for microscopy [12]. The pathogenesis of cystic ameloblastomas remains obscure. Whether UCA originates *de novo* as a neoplasm or whether it is a result of neoplastic transformation of nonneoplastic cyst epithelium has long been debated. Some investigators believe that UCA arises from preexisting odontogenic cysts, in particular a dentigerous cyst, while others maintain that it arises *de novo*. Ackermann et al. (1988) and Robinson and Martinez (1977) argued that as the epithelium of odontogenic cysts and ameloblastomas have a common ancestry, a transition from a nonneoplastic to a neoplastic one could be possible, even though it occurs infrequently [2, 17].

Leider et al. (1985) proposed three pathogenic mechanisms for the evolution of UA [18].

(1) The reduced enamel epithelium which is associated with a developing tooth undergoes ameloblastic transformation with subsequent cystic development.

(2) Ameloblastomas arise in dentigerous cysts or in others in which the neoplastic ameloblastic epithelium is preceded temporarily by a nonneoplastic stratified squamous epithelial lining.

(3) A solid ameloblastoma undergoes cystic degeneration of the ameloblastic islands, with subsequent fusion of multiple microcysts and develops into unicystic lesions.

Several attempts have been made in the past to distinguish the lining of the UCAs from that of odontogenic cysts. However, immunohistochemical markers like lectins (*Ulex europaeus* agglutinin I and *Bandeiraea simplicifolia* agglutinin I) and proliferating cells (proliferating cell nuclear antigen (PCNA) and Ki-67) may assist in their differential diagnosis [19]. However, Eversole et al. contend that currently unaided histologic assessment for UCA remains the gold standard for diagnosis, because of a variable response of UCA to tissue markers. Histologically, the minimum criteria for diagnosing a lesion as UCA are the demonstration of a single cystic sac lined by odontogenic (ameloblastomatous) epithelium often seen only in focal areas [20]. Treatment planning depends on the histological type of UA. The UA which is diagnosed as

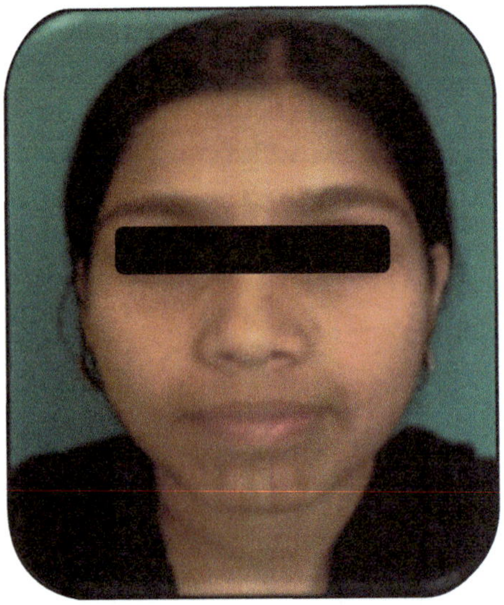

FIGURE 10: Postoperative photograph.

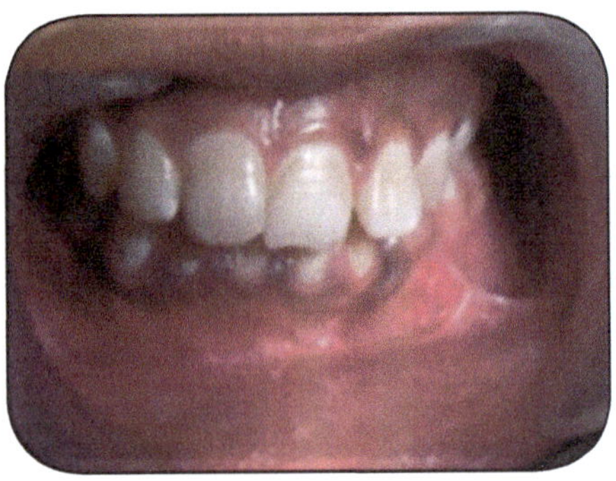

FIGURE 11: Postoperative photograph.

subgroups 1 and 1.2 may be treated conservatively (careful enucleation), whereas Subgroups 1.2.3 and 1.3 should be treated aggressively [11]. The histological typing of the current case was 1.2 and hence, the lesion was treated conservatively with careful enucleation. The recurrence rate for UAs after conservative surgical treatment (curettage or enucleation) is generally reported to be 10–20% [11] and on average, less than 25% [10]. This is considerably less than 50–90% recurrence rates which are noted after the curettage of conventional solid or multicystic ameloblastomas [11, 21]. Lau and Samman reported recurrence rates of 3.6% for resection, 30.5% for enucleation alone, 16% for enucleation followed by Carnoy's solution application, and 18% by marsupialisation followed by enucleation (where the lesion is reduced in size) [22].

Whatever surgical approach the surgeon decides to take, long-term followup is mandatory as recurrence of unicystic ameloblastoma may be long delayed. The case was followed for 9 months; there was no recurrence noted till now (Figures 10 and 11).

7. Conclusion

The diagnosis of unicystic ameloblastoma was based on clinical, radiological, histopathologic, and CT features. It is a tumor with a strong propensity of recurrence, especially when the ameloblastic focus penetrates the adjacent tissue from the wall of the cyst. Radiographically, most of ameloblastomas show multilocularity, whereas unicystic ameloblastomas show a single large unilocular radiolucency. Very rarely, we come across a case with presentation of both multilocular and unicystic type in the same person crossing midline. Unicystic variant of ameloblastoma with aggressive histologic behaviour also might be successfully treated with marsupialisation with subsequent enucleation, and this approach can be considered as an alternative to resection.

References

[1] H. P. Philipsen and P. A. Reichart, "Unicystic ameloblastoma. A review of 193 cases from the literature," *Oral Oncology*, vol. 34, no. 5, pp. 317–325, 1998.

[2] G. L. Ackermann, M. Altini, and M. Shear, "The unicystic ameloblastoma: a clinicopathological study of 57 cases," *Journal of Oral Pathology*, vol. 17, no. 9-10, pp. 541–546, 1988.

[3] P. A. Reichart and H. P. Philipsen, *Odontogenic Tumors and Allied Lesions*, Quintessence, Hanover, Germany, 2004.

[4] L. R. Eversole, A. S. Leider, and D. Strub, "Radiographic characteristics of cystogenic ameloblastoma," *Oral Surgery Oral Medicine and Oral Pathology*, vol. 57, no. 5, pp. 572–577, 1984.

[5] T. J. Li, Y. T. Wu, S. F. Yu, and G. Y. Yu, "Unicystic ameloblastoma: a clinicopathologic study of 33 Chinese patients," *American Journal of Surgical Pathology*, vol. 24, no. 10, pp. 1385–1392, 2000.

[6] S. C. White and M. J. Pharoah, *Oral Radiology: Principles and Interpretation*, Mosby, St. Louis, Mo, USA, 5th edition, 2004.

[7] R. P. Langlais, O. E. Langland, and C. J. Nortje, *Multilocular Radiolucencies, Chapter-3, Diagnostic Imaging of Jaws*, Williams & Wilkins, 1995.

[8] R. Rajendran and B. Sivapathasundharam, *Shafer's Textbook of Oral Pathology*, Elsevier, New Delhi, India, 5th edition, 2006.

[9] K. R. K. Kumar, G. B. George, S. Padiyath, and S. Rupak, "Mural unicystic ameloblastoma crossing the midline: a rare case report," *International Journal of Odontostomatology*, vol. 6, no. 1, pp. 97–103, 2012.

[10] D. G. Gardner and R. L. Corio, "Plexiform unicystic ameloblastoma. A variant of ameloblastoma with a low-recurrence rate after enucleation," *Cancer*, vol. 53, no. 8, pp. 1730–1735, 1984.

[11] B. W. Neville, D. D. Damm, C. M. Allen, and J. E. Bouquot, "Odontogenic cysts and tumors," in *Oral and Maxillofacial Pathology*, pp. 610–618, W. B. Saunders, St. Louis, Mo, USA, 2nd edition, 2002.

[12] R. E. Roos, E. J. Raubenheimer, and W. F. van Heerden, "Clinico-pathological study of 30 unicystic ameloblastomas," *The Journal of the Dental Association of South Africa*, vol. 49, no. 11, pp. 559–562, 1994.

[13] A. Peter, P. A. Reichart, and H. P. Philipsen, "Unicystic ameloblastoma," in *Odontogenic Tumors and Allied Lesions*, pp. 77–86, Quintessence, London, UK, 2004, editorial and consensus conference held in Lyon, France (WHO,IARD) in July 2003 in conjunction with preparation of new WHO Blue Book, Pathology and genetics of tumors of head and neck.

[14] V. J. Paikkatt, S. Sreedharan, and V. P. Kannan, "Unicystic ameloblastoma of the maxilla: a case report," *Journal of Indian Society of Pedodontics and Preventive Dentistry*, vol. 25, no. 2, pp. 106–110, 2007.

[15] E. Braunshtein, M. Vered, S. Taicher, and A. Buchner, "Clear cell odontogenic carcinoma and clear cell ameloblastoma: a single clinicopathologic entity? A new case and comparative analysis of the literature," *Journal of Oral and Maxillofacial Surgery*, vol. 61, no. 9, pp. 1004–1010, 2003.

[16] H. P. Philipsen and P. A. Reichart, *Classification of Odontogenic Tumors and Allied Lesions*, Odontogenic tumors and allied lesions Quintessence, 2004.

[17] L. Robinson and M. G. Martinez, "Unicystic ameloblastoma: a prognostically distinct entity," *Cancer*, vol. 40, no. 5, pp. 2278–2285, 1977.

[18] A. S. Leider, L. R. Eversole, and M. E. Barkin, "Cystic ameloblastoma. A clinicopathologic analysis," *Oral Surgery Oral Medicine and Oral Pathology*, vol. 60, no. 6, pp. 624–630, 1985.

[19] T. J. Li, R. M. Browne, and J. B. Matthews, "Expression of proliferating cell nuclear antigen (PCNA) and Ki-67 in unicystic ameloblastoma," *Histopathology*, vol. 26, no. 3, pp. 219–228, 1995.

[20] H. Konouchi, J. I. Asaumi, Y. Yanagi et al., "Usefulness of contrast enhanced-MRI in the diagnosis of unicystic ameloblastoma," *Oral Oncology*, vol. 42, no. 5, pp. 481–486, 2006.

[21] P. Ameerally, M. McGurk, and O. Shaheen, "Atypical ameloblastoma: report of 3 cases and a review of the literature," *British Journal of Oral and Maxillofacial Surgery*, vol. 34, no. 3, pp. 235–239, 1996.

[22] S. L. Lau and N. Samman, "Recurrence related to treatment modalities of unicystic ameloblastoma: a systematic review," *International Journal of Oral and Maxillofacial Surgery*, vol. 35, no. 8, pp. 681–690, 2006.

A Case of Sublingual Ranula That Responded Successfully to Localized Injection Treatment with OK-432 after Healing from Drug Induced Hypersensitivity Syndrome

Kunio Yoshizawa,[1] Akinori Moroi,[1] Shuichi Kawashiri,[2] and Koichiro Ueki[1]

[1] *Department of Oral and Maxillofacial Surgery, Division of Medicine, Interdisciplinary Graduate School of Medical and Engineering, University of Yamanashi, 1110 Shimokato, Chuo, Yamanashi 409-3898, Japan*
[2] *Department of Oral and Maxillofacial Surgery, Kanazawa University Graduate School of Medical Science, 13-1 Takaramachi, Kanazawa, Ishikawa 920-8641, Japan*

Correspondence should be addressed to Kunio Yoshizawa; yoshizawak@yamanashi.ac.jp

Academic Editor: Eugenio Maiorano

A ranula is a mucus retention cyst or pseudocyst caused by leakage of mucus from the sublingual gland and generally occurs in the oral floor. In addition, drug induced hypersensitivity syndrome (DIHS) is a rare but well-recognized serious adverse effect characterized by fever, skin rashes, generalized lymphadenopathy, hepatitis, and hepatosplenomegaly and oral stomatitis. This paper presents the first case of successfully treated sublingual ranula with localized injection of OK-432 after healing from drug induced hypersensitivity syndrome, which has previously been unreported in the literature. We present the case of a 38-year-old Japanese woman with sublingual ranula that responded successfully to localized injection treatment with OK-432 after healing from drug induced hypersensitivity syndrome. She was affected with cutaneous myositis and interstitial lung disease when she was 26 years old. At the age 34 years, she received additional oral treatment of diaminodiphenyl-sulfone due to deterioration of the cutaneous myositis, which resulted in drug induced hypersensitivity syndrome (DIHS) with severe oral stomatitis. Local injection of OK-432 to the ranula may be a very safe and useful treatment method even if the patient has a history of drug allergy and has connective tissue disease such as cutaneous myositis.

1. Introduction

Drug induced hypersensitivity syndrome (DIHS) is a rare but well-recognized serious adverse effect characterized by fever, skin rashes, generalized lymphadenopathy, hepatitis, and hepatosplenomegaly and oral stomatitis [1, 2]. A ranula is a mucus retention cyst or pseudocyst caused by leakage of mucus from the sublingual gland and generally occurs in the oral floor. OK-432 (Picibanil®, Chugai Pharmaceutical Co., Tokyo, Japan), which is a lyophilized streptococcal preparation made from the low virulence Su strain of A-group *Streptococcus pyogenes* incubated with penicillin, is useful to treat ranula [3].

First, complete enucleation of the ranula by surgery is a challenge because its wall is so thin that it is liable to rupture during the procedure, rendering the surgery inadequate [4, 5]. Secondly, the risk of causing damage to the surrounding lingual nerve and Wharton's duct may increase because operative field is too narrow and adjoining to the tissue [6]. Considering the high rate of recurrence and potential complications of surgical management of a sublingual ranula, local injection of OK-432 is reasonable. Benefits of this therapy as compared with other procedures are summarized as follows. (1) With regard to cost performance, no hospitalization is required. (2) The treatment is painless and the time required for the procedure is brief, which means it can be well tolerated by children and nervous patients. (3) No local anesthesia is required during the procedure. (4) Nerve injury and cosmetic problems are avoided. (5) Secondary infection and hemorrhage are rare. (6) Recurrences are less frequent.

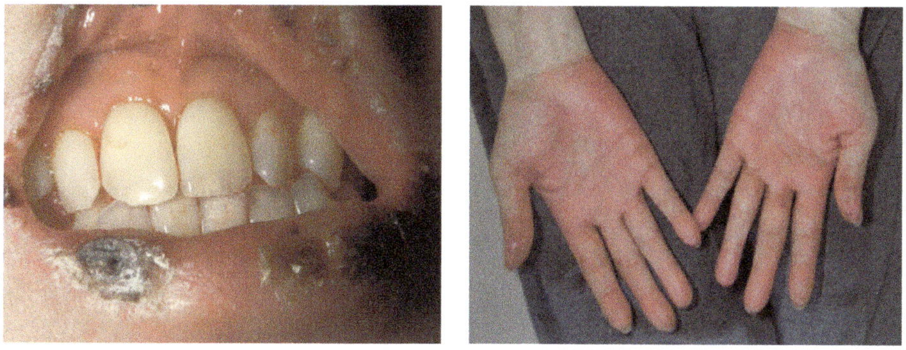

(a) (b)

FIGURE 1: DIHS shows a systemic mucocutaneous disease. (a) Severe erosion with haphalgesia in the entire mouth. (b) Palmar lesion with reddening.

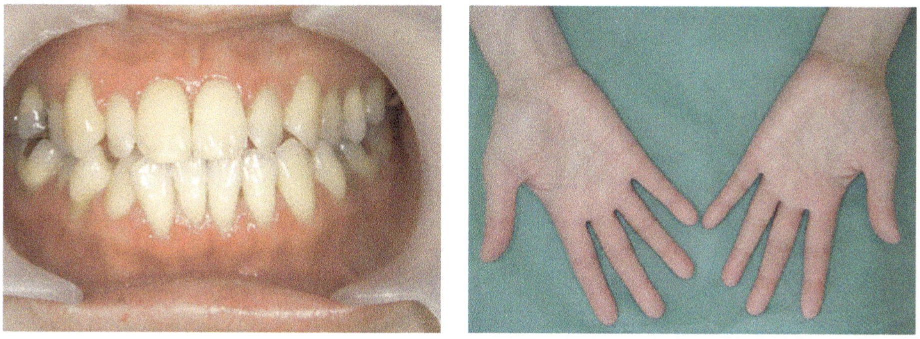

(a) (b)

FIGURE 2: Healed state of the mouth and hand after treatment for DIHS.

(7) The response does not appear to extend beyond the cystic cavity, avoiding any difficulty or increased morbidity of subsequent surgeries [3, 7]. Many authors that have reported on the use of OK-432 injection to treat ranula have indicated it to be a very effective treatment for both intraoral and plunging ranulas. Fukase et al. [8] reported disappearance of the ranula after injection therapy in 97% of cases.

This paper presents the first case of successfully treated sublingual ranula with localized injection of OK-432 after healing from drug induced hypersensitivity syndrome, which has previously been unreported in the literature.

2. Case Report

We present the case of a 38-year-old Japanese woman with sublingual ranula that responded successfully to localized injection treatment with OK-432 (Picibanil, Chugai Pharmaceutical Co., Tokyo, Japan) after healing from drug induced hypersensitivity syndrome. She was affected with cutaneous myositis and interstitial lung disease when she was 26 years old. Therefore, she was treated with oral prednisolone 60 mg, and in 2008, at the age 34 years, she received additional oral treatment of diaminodiphenyl-sulfone (dapsone) (Lectisol®, Mitsubishi Tanabe Pharma Co., Osaka, Japan) due to deterioration of the cutaneous myositis. She received oral treatment of dapsone for a few days, which resulted in drug induced hypersensitivity syndrome (DIHS) with severe oral stomatitis. She presented with these symptoms on her first visit for oral and maxillofacial surgery (Figure 1). By replacing the offending drug with Lectisol and starting her on steroid pulse therapy, the DIHS and oral stomatitis were resolved (Figure 2).

However, in 2012 December at 38 years of age, she developed oral ranula and visited our department with sublingual swelling and pain as chief complaints. Swelling size was 50 m × 30 mm. T2 weighted magnetic resonance imaging (MRI) showed a high-intensity area in the right sublingual regions (Figure 3). The aspirated content from the cystic lesion was yellowish and mucinous. The findings confirmed the diagnosis of right sublingual ranula. The patient experienced reexpansion a few weeks after treatment by aspiration. After receiving a detailed explanation of available treatments including ranula excision, marsupialization, combined ranula and sublingual gland excision, and OK-432 intracystic injection, the patient selected the OK-432 treatment. We familiarized ourselves with the procedure for locally injecting OK-432 solution (0.7 KE/0.3 mL) using a 27-gauge (G) needle, which was inserted inside the cyst in February 2013, according to the method previously reported by Fukase et al. [9]. However, we could not confirm the effect of treatment in the absence of an inflammatory reaction for nine consecutive days. Thus, we additionally performed the following procedure

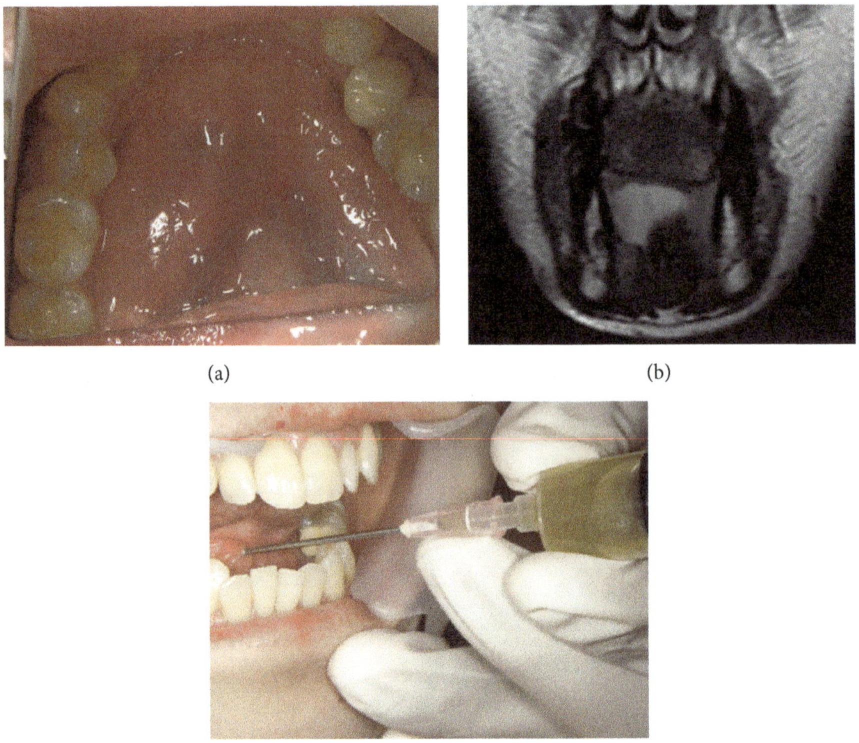

(a) (b) (c)

FIGURE 3: Appearance of the ranula at the first medical examination shows swelling of the anterior floor of the mouth (using mirror) (a). T2-weighted magnetic resonance images before treatment, showing the high-intensity areas in the right sublingual regions (b). The aspirated content from the cystic lesion was yellowish and mucinous (c).

which consisted of a series of punctures and injections. The cystic tumor was punctured using an 18 G needle, and the maximum possible amount of mucus (10 mL) was aspirated. OK-432 solution (0.2 Klinische Einheit [KE] per millimeter; 0.02 mg/mL, total 1 KE/5 mL) was then injected using the same needle, which was fixed inside the cyst, in order to avoid rapture or fluid spillage until the end of the procedure as reported previously by Ogita et al. [10] (Figure 4). On the day when the second injection was administered, the patient had mild inflammation and tenderness around the area of injection for 2 weeks and slight fever of 37.5–38°C for a few days. The ranula disappeared completely without severe complications such as interstitial lung disease and severe allergen reactions at 2 weeks after the second injection. No recurrence was observed during the 30-month postinjection period until presently (Figure 5).

3. Discussion

OK-432 exerts a sclerosing effect by immediately evoking inflammation into cystic space. When OK-432 is administered locally, inflammatory cells, such as neutrophils and monocytes, infiltrate the cyst and various cytokines, including IL-6, IL-8, IFN-γ, and TNF-α, are secreted [11]. Although fluid drainage and fibrotic adhesion induced by inflammation with OK-432 may be considered effective against abnormal exfiltration of saliva, the mechanism whereby OK-432 produces a better effect on ranula is not clearly understood.

In the present case, though we were concerned about the onset of severe complications due to her current and anamnestic history such as cutaneous myositis, interstitial lung disease, and DIHS, there was none. Dapsone is a drug of choice in the treatment of leprosy and other dermatoses including cutaneous myositis [1]. Dapsone hypersensitivity syndrome is a rare but well-recognized serious adverse effect characterized by fever, skin rashes, generalized lymphadenopathy, hepatitis, and hepatosplenomegaly and oral stomatitis [1, 12]. It may be caused by metabolites of dapsone forming haptens with the formation of anti-dapsone antibodies [13]. Thus, one may suggest that local injection of OK-432 was a secure and appropriate option as no adverse events such as drug allergy, which can be expected in cases of autoimmune skin disease and DIHS, occurred. Also, the findings in this case were similar to those of previous reports on OK-432 where serious adverse events and complications were avoided [8, 10, 14]. Moreover, we have reported this case report as the first case of successfully treated sublingual ranula with localized injection of OK-432 after healing from drug induced hypersensitivity syndrome. However, rigorous management after the injection procedure is important from the point view of Poldervaart et al. who reported that such treatment should always take place in

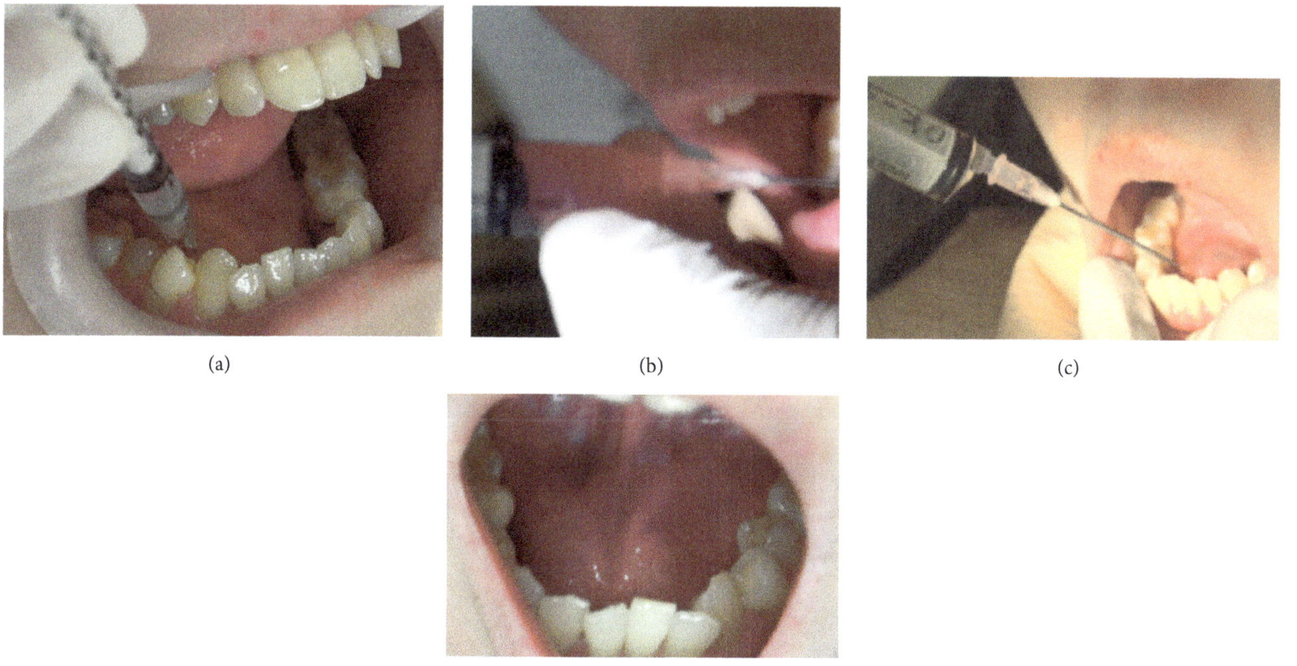

(a) (b) (c) (d)

Figure 4: Procedure of first local injection of OK-432 solution (0.7 KE/0.3 mL) using a 27-G needle (a). The cyst showed no inflammation after the first procedure. Nine consecutive days later, we punctured the cyst using an 18 G needle, and the maximum possible amount of mucus (10 mL) was aspirated immediately (b). OK-432 solution (0.2 Klinische Einheit [KE] per millimeter; total 1 KE/5 mL) was then injected using the same needle (c). There was mild spontaneous pain and swelling with redness around the injected region over the center-line of the mouse at eight days after the second injection of OK432 (1 KE/5 mL) (d).

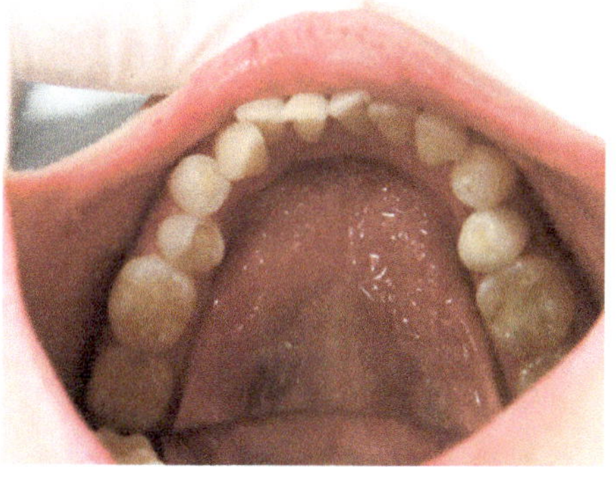

Figure 5: Ranula in the healed state following two treatments of local injection of OK-432.

treatment facilities specialized in the procedure for treating lymphatic malformations with OK-432 [14].

Leakage of the injected OK-432 could be a reason for the poor response to the first injection. Such leakage occurs due to increased swelling of the cyst as the inner pressure of the cyst may be too high. Another reason is that the amount of OK-432 (0.7 KE) was too low to evoke an adequate inflammatory reaction. Therefore, to avoid raising the internal pressure in the second treatment, the quantity of diluted OK-432 (5 mL) was adjusted to the half and allowed to be absorbed in the cystic cavity. This procedure was previously reported by Ohta et al. [11]. The intralesional fluid was highly viscous, so it was necessary to use a relative larger needle (18 G) to aspirate the fluid even though a smaller 27 G needle was preferred to avoid leakage of OK-432 from the cystic lesion. Our role is to seek a safe and effective method for administering OK-432 into an intraoral ranula.

4. Conclusions

We successfully treated sublingual ranula with localized injection of OK-432 after healing from drug induced hypersensitivity syndrome. Local injection of OK-432 to the ranula may be a very safe and useful treatment method without serious systemic adverse effect even if the patient has a history of drug allergy such as DIHS and has connective tissue disease such as cutaneous myositis.

Consent

Written informed consent was obtained from the patient for publication of this case report and any accompanying images.

Competing Interests

The authors declare that they have no competing interests.

References

[1] S. Agrawal and A. Agarwalla, "Dapsone hypersensitivity syndrome: a clinico-epidemiological review," *Journal of Dermatology*, vol. 32, no. 11, pp. 883–889, 2005.

[2] S. J. Sultan, F. Sameem, and M. Ashraf, "Drug reaction with eosinophilia and systemic symptoms: manifestations, treatment, and outcome in 17 patients," *International Journal of Dermatology*, vol. 54, no. 5, pp. 537–542, 2015.

[3] N. Ohta, S. Fukase, Y. Suzuki, A. Ishida, and M. Aoyagi, "Treatments of various otolaryngological cystic diseases by OK-432: its indications and limitations," *Laryngoscope*, vol. 120, no. 11, pp. 2193–2196, 2010.

[4] M. H. Rho, D. W. Kim, J. S. Kwon et al., "OK-432 sclerotherapy of plunging ranula in 21 patients: it can be a substitute for surgery," *American Journal of Neuroradiology*, vol. 27, no. 5, pp. 1090–1095, 2006.

[5] J.-L. Roh, "Primary treatment of ranula with intracystic injection of OK-432," *Laryngoscope*, vol. 116, no. 2, pp. 169–172, 2006.

[6] S. Garofalo, V. Briganti, S. Cavallaro et al., "Nickel gluconate-mercurius heel-potentised swine organ preparations: a new therapeutical approach for the primary treatment of pediatric ranula and intraoral mucocele," *International Journal of Pediatric Otorhinolaryngology*, vol. 71, no. 2, pp. 247–255, 2007.

[7] M. Kinoshita, W. Kida, and H. Nakahara, "Plunging ranula intruding into the parapharyngeal space treated with OK-432," *American Journal of Otolaryngology-Head and Neck Medicine and Surgery*, vol. 33, no. 3, pp. 345–348, 2012.

[8] S. Fukase, N. Ohta, K. Inamura, and M. Aoyagi, "Treatment of ranula with intracystic injection of the streptococcal preparation OK-432," *Annals of Otology, Rhinology and Laryngology*, vol. 112, no. 3, pp. 214–220, 2003.

[9] S. Fukase, N. Ohta, K. Inamura, S. Gon, and M. Aoyagi, "Indications and Limitations of OK-432 intracystic injection therapy for head and neck cystic diseases," *Japan Society of Immunology & Allergology in Otolaryngology*, vol. 19, no. 4, pp. 19–23, 2001.

[10] S. Ogita, T. Tsuto, K. Tokiwa, and T. Takahashi, "Intracystic injection of OK-432: a new sclerosing therapy for cystic hygroma in children," *British Journal of Surgery*, vol. 74, no. 8, pp. 690–691, 1987.

[11] N. Ohta, S. Fukase, T. Watanabe, T. Ito, and M. Aoyagi, "Effects and mechanism of OK-432 therapy in various neck cystic lesions," *Acta Oto-Laryngologica*, vol. 130, no. 11, pp. 1287–1292, 2010.

[12] K. Yoshizawa, K. Ueki, S. Takatsuka, K. Nakagawa, and E. Yamamoto, "A case of drug-induced hypersensitivity syndrome (DIHS) accompanied by severe stomatitis caused by diaminodiphenyl sulphone (DDS)," *Japanese Journal of Oral Diagnosis/Oral Medicine*, vol. 24, no. 1, pp. 30–35, 2011.

[13] J. P. Uetrecht, "Idiosyncratic drug reactions: possible role of reactive metabolites generated by leukocytes," *Pharmaceutical Research*, vol. 6, no. 4, pp. 265–273, 1989.

[14] M. T. Poldervaart, C. C. Breugem, L. Speleman, and S. Pasmans, "Treatment of lymphatic malformations with ok-432 (picibanil): review of the literature," *Journal of Craniofacial Surgery*, vol. 20, no. 4, pp. 1159–1162, 2009.

Nonsyndromic Familial Oligodontia with Multiple Dens Invaginatus: A Case Report of an Unusual Case

D. P. Vinuth,[1] Poonam Agarwal,[2] Gunjan Dube,[3] S. Abhilash,[4] and Pallavi Dube[5]

[1] *Department of Oral Pathology and Microbiology, Hitkarini Dental College and Hospital, Jabalpur 482005, India*
[2] *Department of Oral Medicine Diagnosis and Radiology, Hitkarini Dental College and Hospital, Jabalpur 482005, India*
[3] *Department of Oral and Maxillofacial Surgery, Hitkarini Dental College and Hospital, Jabalpur 482005, India*
[4] *Department of Conservative Dentistry, Hitkarini Dental College and Hospital, Jabalpur, Madhya Pradesh 482005, India*
[5] *Dube Surgical & Dental Hospital, Jabalpur, Madhya Pradesh 482005, India*

Correspondence should be addressed to Poonam Agarwal; dr.poonam.agarwal@gmail.com

Academic Editors: C. S. Farah, M. M. Kassab, and K. Nakamori

Oligodontia is a rare dental anomaly with a prevalence of 0.3% in permanent teeth and much less frequency in the primary dentition. Familial oligodontia represents an absence of varying numbers of primary and/or secondary teeth as an isolated trait. It is a complex and multifactorial condition. Many explanations—evolutionary, genetic, and environmental—have been proposed as the etiology. Simultaneous with oligodontia are often the different positional changes of the existing teeth, their morphology, size, and growth disturbances of the maxillofacial skeleton. Early recognition is vital to provide adequate treatment and prevent squeal. Multidisciplinary referral or consultation is thus important in treatment planning to improve function and esthetics. The present paper reports a rare case of familial oligodontia associated with multiple dense invaginatus and microdontia.

1. Introduction

Tooth agenesis is the most common craniofacial malformations. Its prevalence in permanent dentition reaches 20%, and its expressivity ranges from only one tooth, usually a third molar, to the whole dentition [1]. The term "severe hypodontia" (or oligodontia) is defined as agenesis of six or more permanent teeth, excluding the third molar (Schalk van der Weide, 1992) [2]. It is found in about one in 15 hypodontia patients [3]. Oligodontia can be isolated (oligodontia/I), as the only phenotypic alteration in a person, or associated to other alterations as part of a syndrome (oligodontia/S). Isolated, nonsyndromic agenesis can be sporadic or familial, and it may be inherited in Mendelian dominant or recessive autosomal mode or X-linked. Penetrance has been traditionally considered as incomplete but high. The expressivity of the various forms is quite variable, with a wide range of missing teeth [4].

Several factors have been proposed for the etiology of oligodontia [5]. It is basically caused by the complex interactions between genetic, epigenetic, and environmental factors during the long process of dental development [6]. The prevalence of hypodontia has been shown to be higher within the extended family circle than in the general population, which supports a hereditary tendency [4]. Familial oligodontia represents an absence of varying numbers of primary and/or secondary teeth as an isolated trait. A large number of candidate genes have been provided from studies in the mouse, but only a few of them have been identified in human family pedigrees affected by hypodontia. This suggests that in many cases, familial human hypodontia may represent a more complex and multifactorial condition [7]. Oligodontia has serious implications for the patient in terms of masticatory function, malocclusion, speech impairment, and psychological impact. As such, severe hypodontia can have a dramatic effect on a patient's (oral health-related) quality of life [2].

The present report describes an unusual case of nonsyndromic familial oligodontia coexistent with multiple dens invaginatus seen clinically and radiographically. Of interest to the author was the consistent presence of multiple dens invaginatus in the siblings of a family associated with oligodontia. To the authors' best of knowledge, no such case has been reported, and this rarity prompted to report the case.

2. Case Report

A 21-year-old male patient was referred to our outpatient department with a chief complaint of several missing teeth. Dental history revealed no evidence of extensive extractions; however, past dental records were not available for verification. The patient's medical history revealed that he was born of a full-term pregnancy and was delivered by forceps. The patient's mother gave no history of exposure to radiation and did not take any medications during pregnancy. Patient was born to nonconsanguineous parents. No history of orofacial trauma or unusual childhood diseases was reported. Drug history was not significant. The family history was positive for missing teeth in the father and two (24 years old male & 16 years old female) of the five siblings.

Physical examination revealed a moderately built and nourished young man with height and weight within the normal range for his age and sex. In view of the oligodontia of permanent teeth, a detailed examination was done to rule out syndromes associated with oligodontia. His hearing and vision appeared to be normal. The hair of the scalp, eyebrows, and eyelashes was normal in distribution, density, and texture. Skin and nails were of normal appearance. Sweating, lacrimal, and salivary secretions were within normal limits. Both history and general examination findings were essentially similar in the affected siblings. The clinical examination of the other available members of the family revealed that the mother and the other two siblings had a full complement of teeth with no associated dental anomalies, while the father was completely edentulous (history of presence of only few permanent teeth since the beginning). None of them had clinical ectodermal abnormalities.

Sibling 1: 21 Years/Male

Clinical Findings. Extraoral examination revealed a bilaterally symmetrical face with a straight profile. There was reduction of the lower facial height and protuberance of lips caused by the loss of vertical dimension as a result of oligodontia. Intraorally, soft tissues appeared normal in color and texture. Oral hygiene and gingival status were good and no caries was found. Alveolar bone height was reduced where the teeth were missing. The bone was otherwise healthy and robust looking. Examination of teeth revealed presence of only nine erupted permanent teeth—17, 16, 13, 11, 21, 26, 27, 36, and 46. The remaining permanent teeth were missing clinically (i.e., 19 teeth were congenitally missing excluding the third molars). Of the primary dentition, the retained 54 tooth was present. Abnormal crown morphology was appreciated with 17. The maxillary central incisors were shovel shaped with deep lingual pits. Mild attrition was present with mandibular molars (Figures 1(a), 1(b), and 1(c)).

Radiographic Findings. Suspecting the congenital absence of permanent teeth, panoramic radiograph was taken which confirmed congenital absence of all permanent teeth that clinically were not present (Figure 1(d)). Intraoral periapical radiograph was taken in relation to 11 and 21 which revealed the presence of Oehlers type II dens in dente (dens invaginatus) with the central incisors (Figure 1(e)).

Sibling 2: 16 Years/Female

Clinical Findings. Clinical examination showed facial symmetry with a convex profile. Intraoral examination revealed a faulty prosthesis (fixed with acrylic resin to the adjacent teeth) in the mandibular anterior tooth region. There was moderate localized gingivitis associated with the prosthesis. Hard tissue examination was carried out following the removal of the faulty prosthesis. The bony structure of the upper and lower jaw appeared normal. The following permanent teeth were present and erupted: 17, 16, 12, 11, 21, 22, 24, 25, 26, 27, 36, 37, 32, 42, 44, and 46 (i.e., 12 congenitally missing teeth excluding the third molars). Several retained deciduous teeth were present—55, 53, 73, 74, 75, and 83. The maxillary central and lateral incisors were shovel shaped with deep lingual pits. Mild generalized attrition was present. Mesial rotation was noted with 32 and 42. Generalized microdontia with spacing in the permanent dentition was appreciable (Figures 2(a), 2(b), and 2(c)).

Radiographic Findings. Panoramic radiograph disclosed congenital absence of all permanent teeth that were missing on clinical examination with generalized spacing (Figure 2(d)). On periapical radiography, Oehlers type I dens in dente was seen in relation to all maxillary incisors (Figure 2(e)).

Sibling 3: 24 Years/Male

Clinical Findings. Extraoral examination revealed bilaterally symmetrical face. Patient had a concave profile. There was reduction of the lower facial height and protuberant lips caused by the loss of vertical dimension as a result of oligodontia. Intraoral examination revealed an overdenture with the mandibular arch. Dental history disclosed presence of multiple retained primary teeth in the lower arch which were extracted due to mobility. However, past dental records were not available for verification. Examination of the maxillary arch revealed the presence of following permanent teeth: 17, 16, 15, 14, 11, 21, 24, 25, 26, and 27. Microdontia was present with the premolars. Shovel-shaped crown morphology was appreciable with 21, with associated deep lingual pit (Figures 3(a) and 3(b)).

Radiographic Findings. Panoramic radiography confirmed the congenital absence of following permanent teeth: 13, 12, 22, and 23 (Figure 3(c)). Oehlers Type I dens in dente was detected with 21 on periapical radiograph (Figure 3(d)).

Our clinical & radiographic examinations and interviews of the kindred revealed that all affected members were missing more than 6 teeth and had not the other systemic abnormality. They were diagnosed for nonsyndromic oligodontia.

3. Discussion

Characteristic dental findings of oligodontia are a reduced number of teeth, smaller teeth, malformation of the teeth, and the delayed eruption [8]. In the present cases, along with

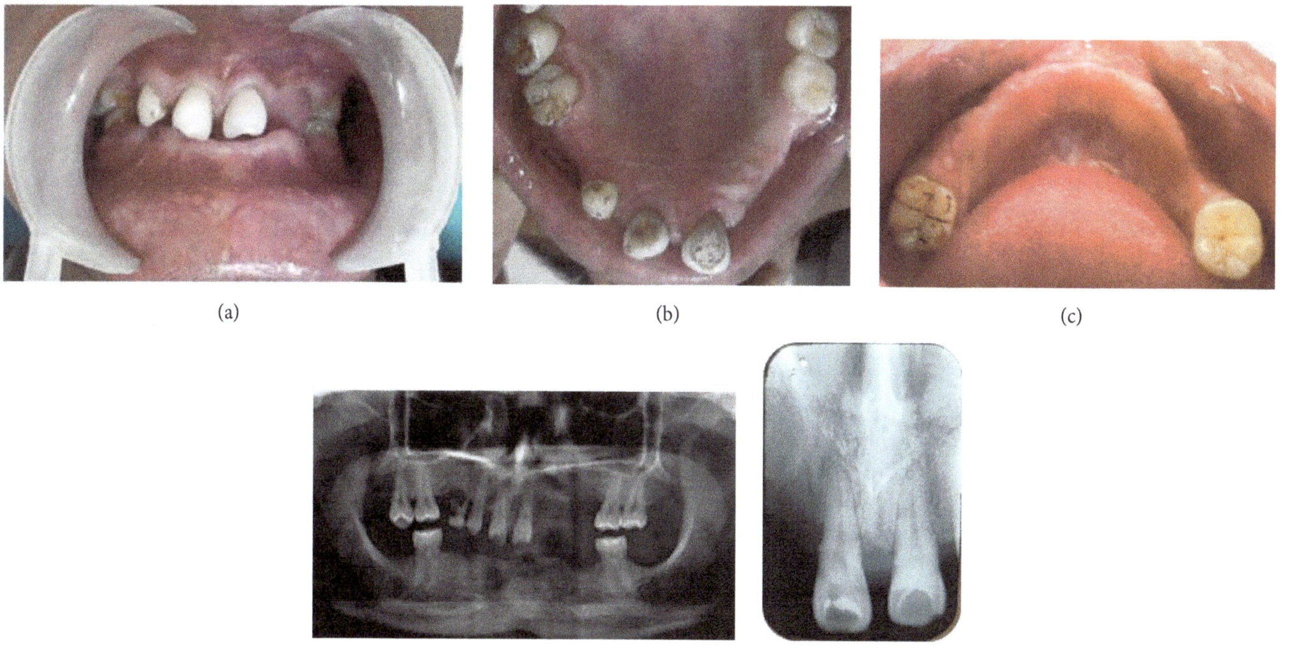

(a) (b) (c) (d) (e)

FIGURE 1: (a) Intraoral photograph of Sibling 1. (b) Intraoral photograph of maxillary arch of Sibling 1. (c) Intraoral photograph of mandibular arch of Sibling 1. (d) OPG of Sibling 1. (e) IOPA of Sibling 1 showing dens invaginatus in both the central incisors.

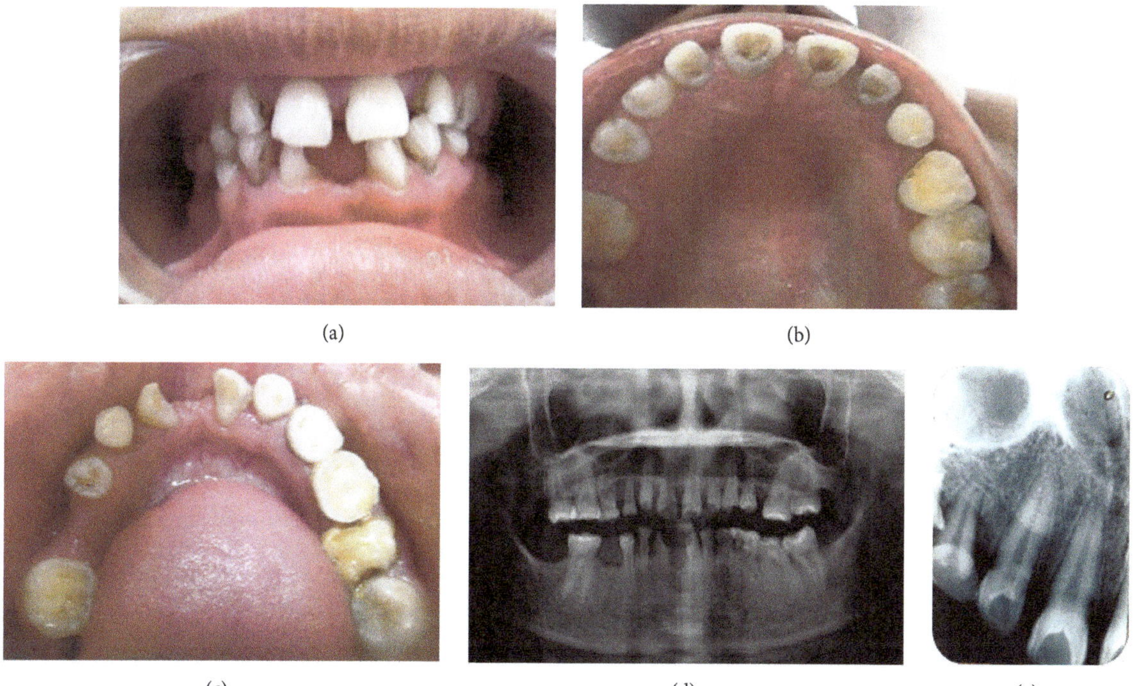

(a) (b) (c) (d) (e)

FIGURE 2: (a) Intraoral photograph of Sibling 2. (b) Intraoral photograph of maxillary arch of Sibling 2. (c) Intraoral photograph of mandibular arch of Sibling 2. (d) OPG of Sibling 2. (e) IOPA of Sibling 2 showing shovel-shaped incisors with dens invaginatus.

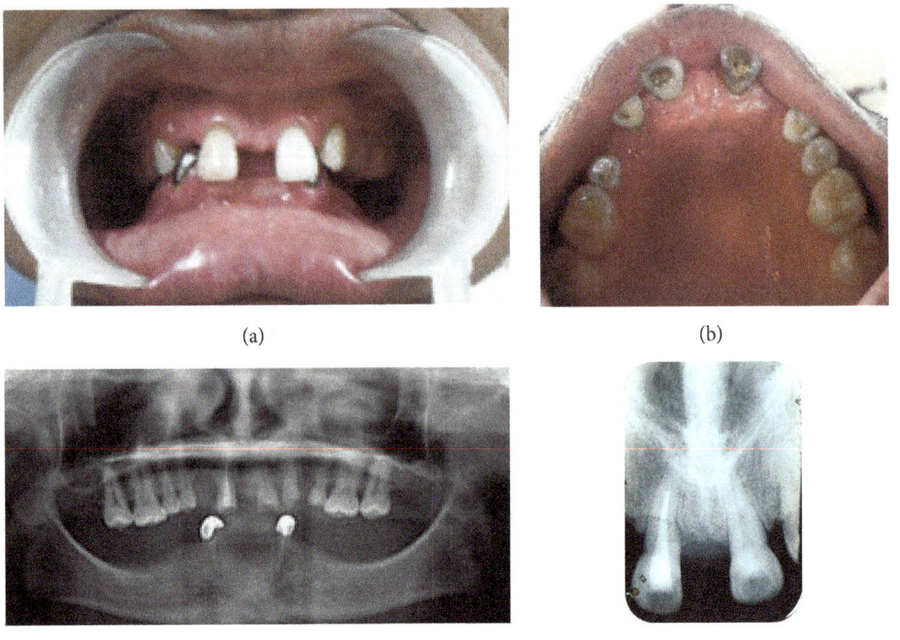

FIGURE 3: (a) Intraoral photograph of Sibling 3. (b) Intraoral photograph of maxillary arch of Sibling 3. (c) OPG of Sibling 3. (d) IOPA of Sibling 3 showing incisor with dens invaginatus.

oligodontia, the patients exhibited malformation of teeth in the form of dens invaginatus and microdontia. However, no evidence of delayed eruption was noted.

When looking at the association of the number and type of missing teeth amongst siblings, no consistency in pattern was seen. Studies of families suggest that genetic factors may play an important role in oligodontia. Recently investigators favor the hypothesis of a polygenically determined, quasicontinuous type of inheritance. However, environmental factors cannot be ignored. Some of the genes already identified are MSX1, PAX9, and AXIN. There is evidence to suggest that PAX9 and MSX1 interact during tooth development [7]. Interaction of such genes along with epigenetic and environmental factors may together be important in determining the expression of this trait. Hence the etiology can be described as being multifactorial and may account for the different teeth missing in the affected individuals of the same family with the same mutation [9].

In the present cases, more teeth were missing in the mandible than the maxilla with more or less bilateral symmetry. There was no consistent pattern of agenesis in various tooth groups except for the third molars. Studies have shown that the most common pattern in the lower arch involved agenesis of all mandibular premolars. Other common patterns in the lower arch were agenesis of the incisors, canine, both premolars, and the second molar. In the maxilla, the most common patterns involved were agenesis of the maxillary lateral incisor and both premolars, whereas in the mandible it was agenesis of all mandibular premolars [2].

A recent study showed that tooth agenesis may be a symmetrical phenomenon [10]. The relatively high-degree of left versus the right-side symmetry of the patterns may indicate a possible common genetic cause. The relatively low-symmetry of upper versus lower arch tooth agenesis may suggest that different mechanisms are responsible for tooth agenesis in the upper and lower arches.

With regard to the association of the location of hypodontia among the siblings, the similarity amongst offspring may indicate that hypodontia affecting different tooth types is caused by different genetic factors. However, the differences of offspring expressing hypodontia in different locations to each other suggest that the combinations of genes and the epigenetic and environmental factors are important in determining expression of hypodontia.

A reduction in tooth dimensions which is as appreciable in siblings in the present case has been documented by previous studies in cases of hypodontia as well as oligodontia. Continuous traits such as height and tooth size typically have a multifactorial mode of inheritance. Brook and Bailit suggested that hypodontia is an example of a "quasicontinuous" trait with a threshold mechanism. The accepted explanation of discontinuous multifactorial variation rests on the assumption that there is an underlying scale of continuous variation, this being, in the case of hypodontia, tooth size. The distribution curve of relatives appears to be to the left of that of the general population. The position of an individual on the scale depends upon a combination of numerous genetic and environmental factors. Proportionally more family members of index patients exceed the threshold for tooth agenesis. The model also suggests that first-degree relatives of index patients will have reduced mean tooth dimensions compared to the general population, even if they do not have hypodontia [11–13].

Dens invaginatus of different grades is appreciated in the central and/or lateral incisors of the siblings which were bilaterally present. Dens invaginatus is most frequently seen in maxillary lateral incisors, but other teeth involvement have also been reported [14]. Some evidence suggests that the problem may be symmetrical [15].

The absence of certain molecules can result in abnormally shaped teeth as well as defects in the developing tooth germ. For this reason the proposal that genetic factors may be the cause of that dens invaginatus has some credibility. The support comes from the study conducted by Grahnen et al. on 3020 Swedish children that reported 2.7% of patients with dens invaginatus, and 43% of their parents and 32% of siblings also had evidence of the condition. Additional support for a genetic influence is drawn from the fact that the invaginations appear to have a limited variation and can occur in a number of teeth in the same individual or in siblings [15]. This partly explains the consistent findings of multiple dens invaginatus in combination with oligodontia in the present cases.

Causative genes, MSX1 and PAX9, can be proposed by the observation that mutations of these genes cause familial and sporadic forms of selective tooth agenesis. PAX9 defect was shown to be responsible for "molar oligodontia". In contrast, the developmental absence of maxillary and mandibular second bicuspids and maxillary first bicuspids, whilst most mandibular first bicuspids are retained, appears to be the pattern of tooth agenesis that best indicates the presence of an MSX1 mutation [16].

The changes are that the increasing number of missing permanent teeth cause is limited to the dental and soft tissue parameters. As the number of missing teeth increased, there was a trend for a decrease in the mandibular plane angle, an increase in the facial axis, and a reduction in the lower anterior facial height. This has not been reported in studies with lower prevalence of hypodontia. The typical dentofacial structure seen in persons with severe hypodontia is due to dental and functional compensation rather than to an altered growth pattern [17].

The unesthetic appearance, missing teeth, and overclosure in patients with oligodontia may cause depression and psychosocial problems. Therefore, the main treatment goal is to improve appearance, mastication, and speech. Treatment in such cases is typically multidisciplinary. A wide and expanding range of prosthetic, orthodontic, restorative and surgical therapies are currently employed. The prosthetic treatment of oligodontia varies and includes removable partial dentures, fixed partial dentures, attachment dentures, and overdentures. The choice is dependent on the condition of the remaining teeth [5]. From the orthodontic aspect, the consequences of missing teeth are numerous and depend on the number and type of teeth that are missing. Surgical therapy for such patients can include various aspects, such as autotransplantation, insertion of osteointegrated implants, or orthognathic surgery [18]. Commonly a combined orthodontic-restorative-surgical approach is necessary with orthodontic treatment needed to relocate space in preparation for later conventional fixed prostheses or implants [19].

Although dens invaginatus is common, it may be easily overlooked because of absence of any significant clinical signs of the anomaly. This is unfortunate as the presence of an invagination is considered to increase the risk of caries, pulpal pathosis, and periodontal inflammation. Treatment ranges from conservative restorative procedures (if diagnosed early) to nonsurgical root canal therapy, surgery, or extraction. Root canal treatment of such teeth is often complicated by the unusual forms and location of invaginated and pulpal spaces that complicate thorough debridement [15].

4. Conclusion

The consequences of missing teeth are numerous and depend on the number and type of teeth that are missing. Most frequently speech and masticatory functional disorders occur and, the aesthetic problems are caused by disturbed growth and development of the orofacial area, which can manifest outside the mouth. In the case of patients with oligodontia, prompt and accurate diagnosis is necessary as well as the careful planning of treatment, with a preconception of the final solution. This can only be achieved by multidisciplinary cooperation, which usually includes the following specialists: orthodontist, endodontist, oral surgeon, and prosthetist.

To conclude, it is suggested that detailed studies of oligodontia cases are required to investigate the prevalence and location of missing teeth, the size and morphology of remaining teeth in the dentition, and also the pattern of tooth size, shape, and number in relatives of affected individuals. Such studies may aid in better understanding of underlying factors that are involved in the pathogenesis. The presentation of the dentition in oligodontia being very heterogenous, formulation of universal treatment strategy could be a challenge as homogenous, comparable subgroups of patients are not available.

References

[1] F. J. Kolenc Fusé, "Tooth agenesis: in search of mutations behind failed dental development," *Medicina Oral, Patologia Oral y Cirugia Bucal*, vol. 9, no. 5, pp. 385–395, 2004.

[2] S. P. K. Tan, A. J. Van Wijk, and B. Prahl-Andersen, "Severe hypodontia: identifying patterns of human tooth agenesis," *European Journal of Orthodontics*, vol. 33, no. 2, pp. 150–154, 2011.

[3] S. O. Adeboye, B. O. I. Cole, R. S. Hobson, and M. J. Wright, "Severe hypodontia in a set of triplets," *British Dental Journal*, vol. 201, no. 2, pp. 93–96, 2006.

[4] M. A. Créton, M. S. Cune, J. W. Verhoeven, and G. J. Meijer, "Patterns of missing teeth in a population of oligodontia patients," *International Journal of Prosthodontics*, vol. 20, no. 4, pp. 409–413, 2007.

[5] S. Shilpa, A. Mohapatra, C. P. Reddy, and N. Sivakumar, "Congenital absence of multiple primary teeth," *Journal of Indian Society of Pedodontics and Preventive Dentistry*, vol. 28, no. 4, pp. 319–321, 2010.

[6] A. H. Brook, "Multilevel complex interactions between genetic, epigenetic and environmental factors in the aetiology of anomalies of dental development," *Archives of Oral Biology*, vol. 54, no. 1, pp. S3–S17, 2009.

[7] M. T. Cobourne, "Familial human hypodontia—is it all in the genes?" *British Dental Journal*, vol. 203, no. 4, pp. 203–208, 2007.

[8] Y. Schalk-van der Weide, F. A. Beemer, J. A. Faber, and F. Bosman, "Symptomatology of patients with oligodontia," *Journal of Oral Rehabilitation*, vol. 21, no. 3, pp. 247–261, 1994.

[9] M. Rasool, J. Schuster, M. Aslam et al., "A novel missense mutation in the EDA gene associated with X-linked recessive isolated hypodontia," *Journal of Human Genetics*, vol. 53, no. 10, pp. 894–898, 2008.

[10] J.-W. Kim, J. P. Simmer, B. P.-J. Lin, and J. C.-C. Hu, "Novel MSX1 frameshift causes autosomal-dominant oligodontia," *Journal of Dental Research*, vol. 85, no. 3, pp. 267–271, 2006.

[11] A. H. Brook, "A unifying aetiological explanation for anomalies of human tooth number and size," *Archives of Oral Biology*, vol. 29, no. 5, pp. 373–378, 1984.

[12] H. F. McKeown, D. L. Robinson, C. Elcock, M. Al-Sharood, and A. H. Brook, "Tooth dimensions in hypodontia patients, their unaffected relatives and a control group measured by a new image analysis system," *European Journal of Orthodontics*, vol. 24, no. 2, pp. 131–141, 2002.

[13] N. Parkin, C. Elcock, R. N. Smith, R. C. Griffin, and A. H. Brook, "The aetiology of hypodontia: the prevalence, severity and location of hypodontia within families," *Archives of Oral Biology*, vol. 54, no. 1, pp. S52–S56, 2009.

[14] H. Ikeda, T. Yoshioka, and H. Suda, "Importance of clinical examination and diagnosis: a case of dens invaginatus," *Oral Surgery, Oral Medicine, Oral Pathology, Oral Radiology and*, vol. 79, no. 1, pp. 88–91, 1995.

[15] A. Alani and K. Bishop, "Dens invaginatus—part 1: classification, prevalence and aetiology," *International Endodontic Journal*, vol. 41, no. 12, pp. 1123–1136, 2008.

[16] K. Xuan, F. Jin, Y.-L. Liu et al., "Identification of a novel missense mutation of MSX1 gene in Chinese family with autosomal-dominant oligodontia," *Archives of Oral Biology*, vol. 53, no. 8, pp. 773–779, 2008.

[17] B. Øgaard and O. Krogstad, "Craniofacial structure and soft tissue profile in patients with severe hypodontia," *American Journal of Orthodontics and Dentofacial Orthopedics*, vol. 108, no. 5, pp. 472–477, 1995.

[18] Z. Muretic, "Marija magdalenic mestrovic, damir zarkovic an interdisciplinary approach to the treatment of oligodontia," *Acta Stomatologica Croatica*, vol. 35, pp. 117–120, 2001.

[19] C. McNamara, T. Foley, and C. M. McNamara, "Multidisplinary management of hypodontia in adolescents: case report," *Journal of the Canadian Dental Association*, vol. 72, no. 8, pp. 740–746, 2006.

Disseminated Intravascular Coagulation after Surgery for Facial Injury

Hisashi Ozaki, Hirohiko Tachibana, Shigeo Ishikawa, Kazuyuki Yusa, Kenichirou Kitabatake, and Mitsuyoshi Iino

Department of Dentistry, Oral and Maxillofacial-Plastic and Reconstructive Surgery, Faculty of Medicine, Yamagata University, 2-2-2 Iida-Nishi, Yamagata 990-9585, Japan

Correspondence should be addressed to Hisashi Ozaki; ozahisa19@yahoo.co.jp

Academic Editor: Mohammad Hosein K. Motamedi

A case of disseminated intravascular coagulation (DIC) presenting after surgery for facial trauma associated with multiple facial bone fractures is described. With regard to the oral and maxillofacial region, DIC has been described in the literature following head trauma, infection, and metastatic disease. Until now, only 5 reports have described DIC after surgery for facial injury. DIC secondary to facial injury is thus rare. The patient in this case was young and had no medical history. Preoperative hemorrhage or postoperative septicemia may thus induce DIC.

1. Introduction

Disseminated intravascular coagulation (DIC) is a dynamic pathologic process in which thrombin forms within the vascular system [1]. DIC is commonly associated with malignant neoplasm, major trauma, head injury, infection, and obstetric complications [2]. With regard to the oral and maxillofacial region, DIC has been described in the literature following head trauma, infection, and metastatic disease [3]. However, a review of literature shows only a small number of reports describing DIC in relation to oral and maxillofacial surgery [4]. In particular, few reports have mentioned DIC after surgery for facial injury. We report herein a rare case of DIC after surgery for facial trauma associated with multiple facial bone fractures.

2. Case Presentation

A 21-year-old man was brought to the emergency department at Yamagata University Hospital after becoming involved in a traffic accident while riding a motorbike. On arrival, he was fully conscious and complained of facial pain. Clinical examination showed facial swelling, persistent intraoral and nasal hemorrhage, and bloody otorrhea from the left ear. He showed gross malocclusion associated with discontinuity and mobilization of the maxillary and mandibular dentitions. He had no significant medical history and had been healthy before the accident. Computed tomography (CT) and plain radiography revealed right pulmonary contusion, fractures of a second rib and the right radius, and airway narrowing. In the maxillofacial region, bilateral condylar and mandibular fractures, LeFort II-type fracture, and blow-out fracture of the orbit were recognized (Figure 1). Airway control was achieved by awake orotracheal intubation. Hemostasis was performed by suture compression for oral hemorrhage and by gauze tamponade for nasal hemorrhage under local anesthesia, although nasal hemostasis proved extremely difficult to achieve. Respiratory management with a ventilator was conducted under intravenous sedation until general condition was stable. After another 2 days, the tracheal tube was removed, because no airway narrowing or obstruction was evident. Six days after the accident, tracheotomy and repositioning and fixation of the fractured facial bones, including the mandible, maxilla, zygoma, and blow-out fracture of the orbit, were performed under general anesthesia (Figure 1). Surgery lasted 7 h 16 min, with 30 mL of intraoperative bleeding. Intraoperatively, the patient received blood transfusion of 2 units of red blood cell concentrate due to low hemoglobin levels (7.3 g/dL). The postoperative course was uneventful. On postoperative day 5, however, fever over 39.0°C and shivering

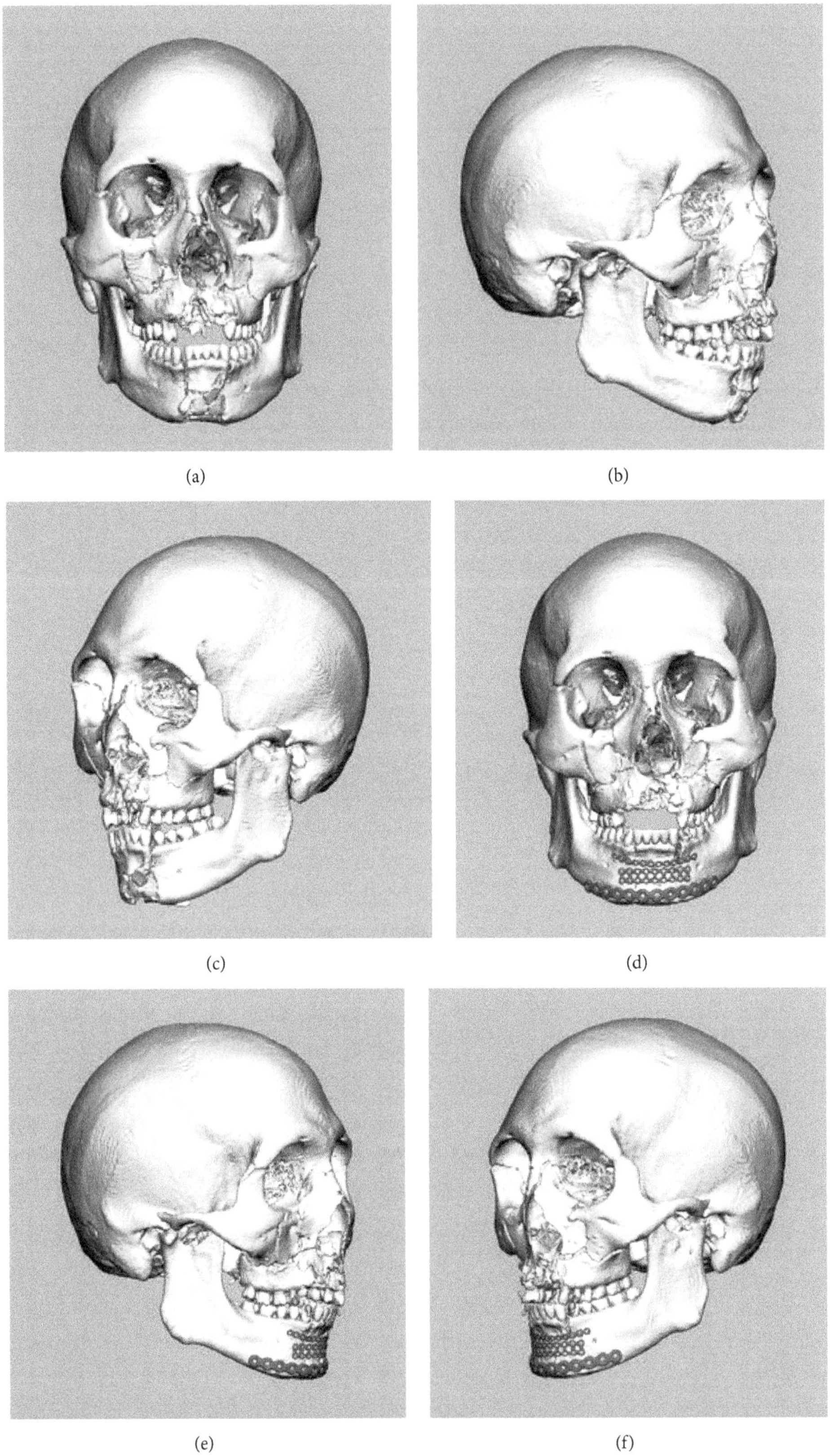

FIGURE 1: Images from preoperative and postoperative 3D-CT. (a)–(c) showed that bilateral condylar and mandibular fractures, LeFort II-type fracture, and blow-out fracture of orbit are apparent. (d)–(f) showed that mandibular fracture was fixed by titanium plates and LeFort II-type fracture and blow-out fracture of the orbit were fixed by absorbable plates. (a) Preoperative frontal view. (b) Preoperative lateral view of the right. (c) Preoperative lateral view of the left. (d) Postoperative frontal view. (e) Postoperative lateral view of the right. (f) Postoperative lateral view of the left.

Table 1: Laboratory data.

Examination	First visit	Preoperative	POD 5	POD 6 (preshock)	POD 13
WBC ($\times 10^3/\mu$L)	17.71	10.09	14.06	10.17	12.16
RBC ($\times 10^6/\mu$L)	4.69	2.33	2.91	2.7	2.55
Hemoglobin (g/dL)	14.7	7.3	9.0	8.2	7.7
Hematocrit (%)	44	22.3	26.4	25	24.1
Platelets ($\times 10^4/\mu$L)	23.8	9.8	13.1	4.6	17.5
CRP (mg/dL)	<0.10	3.82	12.10	23.9	4.09
TBIL (mg/dL)	0.8	0.4	—	2.1	0.6
Crea (mg/dL)	0.94	0.64	0.76	0.97	0.67
BUN (mg/dL)	16	14	20	30	13
Lactate (mmol/L)	4.07	—	—	4.07	—
Glucose (mg/dL)	169	—	—	118	—
PT (s)	—	11	—	21.7	13.7
PT (%)	—	110	—	43	79
PT-INR	—	0.94	—	1.86	1.17
aPTT (s)	—	27.8	—	35	30.4
Fbg (mg/dL)	—	—	—	664	624
FDP (μg/mL)	—	—	—	10.8	5.3
D-dimer (μg/mL)	—	—	—	6.4	5.07

POD: postoperative day.

were noted. Laboratory examination showed increases in the white blood cell count to 14,060/μL and C-reactive protein (CRP) to 12.1 mg/dL and a decrease in platelets to $131 \times 10^3/\mu$L (down from $238 \times 10^3/\mu$L at the time of the accident). CT revealed no abnormalities other than those at the surgical sites. The next day, the patient showed preshock status with a significant decrease in blood pressure, fever over 39.0°C, and transient loss of consciousness. Emergency laboratory tests showed increases in CRP to 23.9 mg/dL, TBIL to 2.1 mg/dL, creatinine to 0.97 mg/dL, lactate to 4.07 mmol/L, prothrombin time to 21.7 s, FDP (fibrin degradation product) to 10.8 μg/mL, and PT-INR (prothrombin time-international normalized ratio) to 1.86, along with a decrease in platelets to $46 \times 10^3/\mu$L (Table 1). The bacteria was not detected in several tests of blood culture. In the evaluation of respiratory system, PaO2 was 68.2 mmHg, PaCO2 was 28.2 mmHg in blood gas analysis, and PaO2/FiO2 was 341. In circulatory dynamics, noradrenaline was administered sustainably by 0.04γ for keeping of blood pressure. In the evaluation of central nervous system, Glasgow Coma Scale was E4V5M6 and a total of 15. Therefore, SOFA (sequential organ failure assessment) score was 9. From the above results, septic shock was diagnosed and the patient was sent to the intensive care unit (ICU). According to the scoring algorithm criteria established by the Japanese Association for Acute Medicine (JAAM) for DIC [21], the patient scored 5. DIC was therefore diagnosed and treatment was initiated. To treat severe infection, cefozopran hydrochloride and freeze-dried polyethylene glycol-treated human normal immunoglobulin were applied by intravenous injection empirically. A total of 38,840 units of thrombomodulin α was administered for the treatment of DIC. After another 7 days, laboratory tests showed a return to nearly normal state, with CRP of 4.09 mg/dL; TBIL of 0.6 mg/dL, Crea of 0.67 mg/dL, WBC of 12,160/μL; platelet count of $175 \times 10^3/\mu$L; prothrombin time of 13.7 s; FDP of 5.3 μg/mL; and PT-INR of 1.17 (Table 1). The patient was then moved to a general ward and the subsequent course was uneventful.

3. Discussion

In the oral and maxillofacial region, several reports have described DIC in patients with oral cancer [17], infection [11], injury [3, 13, 16, 17], orthognathic surgery [12], and tooth extraction [5–10, 14, 15, 18, 19]. To the best of our knowledge, however, the English literature contains only 19 reports of DIC in relation to oral and maxillofacial surgery except for oral cancer (Table 2). This means that DIC associated with oral and maxillofacial surgery is uncommon. Of these 19 cases, the most frequent surgery associated with DIC was tooth extraction, in 10 cases. On the other hand, including our case, only 5 cases involved facial injury related to DIC. Table 2 also shows the diseases underlying DIC, with prostatic adenocarcinoma and aortic aneurysm in 4 cases each, and septicemia in 3 cases. Among the 5 cases of facial injury, each patient showed prostatic adenocarcinoma, abruption, septicemia, or no underlying disease. In the remaining cases, Morimoto et al. [17] did not discuss the causative underlying disease. The present patient had no medical history before the traffic accident and preoperative hemostatic function tests yielded normal results. Two reasons could explain DIC in the present case. One is septicemia associated with severe postoperative systemic inflammatory response syndrome (SIRS). Postoperative stress seemed to not only induce SIRS but also increase its severity. Under severe SIRS, DIC may have developed from hypercoagulability because of

Table 2: DIC relevant to oral and maxillofacial surgery.

Number	Author	Year	Age	Sex	Surgery	Underlying disease	Progress
1	Falace and Kelly [5]	1976	85	M	Extraction of 6 anterior teeth	Occult prostatic adenocarcinoma	Alive
2	Rawson et al. [6, 7]	1976	45	F	Extraction of a third molar and submandibular abscess	Septicemia	Dead
3	Samman [3]	1984	28	F	Forehead, lip, and tongue laceration from traffic accident	Abruption (38-week pregnancy)	Alive
4	McKechnie [8]	1989	59	M	Extraction of maxillary first molar	Occult prostatic adenocarcinoma	Dead
5	Chishiro [9]	1989	86	M	Extraction of maxillary molar	Known abdominal aortic aneurysm	Dead
6	Marshall et al. [10]	1993	24	F	Extraction of 3 third molars	Unknown	Dead
7	Currie and Ho [11]	1993	31	M	Acute dentoalveolar abscess	Septicemia	Dead
8	Christiansen and Soudah [12]	1993	19	M	LeFort I osteotomy	None	Alive
9	McLoughlin et al. [13]	1994	62	M	Lower lip laceration	Occult prostatic adenocarcinoma, multiple bone metastases	Alive
10	Herold and Falworth [14]	1994	73	M	Extraction of upper canine	Occult abdominal aortic aneurysm	Alive
11	Mehra et al. [4]	1997	65	M	Scaling, parotitis	Unknown	Alive
12	Sawaki et al. [15]	1999	62	M	Extraction of maxillary premolar and molar	Occult prostatic adenocarcinoma, multiple bone metastases	Alive
13	Cbo et al. [16]	2001	28	F	Fracture of mandible	None	Alive
14	Morimoto et al. [17]	2001	37	F	Infection after tooth extraction	Unknown	Alive
15	Morimoto et al. [17]	2001	25	M	Multiple injuries of the mandible	None	Alive
16	Ita et al. [18]	2001	22	F	Extraction of mandibular third molar	KTW syndrome	Alive
17	Peters et al. [19]	2005	82	M	Extraction of anterior tooth	Aortic aneurysm	Alive
18	Imai et al. [20]	2010	88	M	Spontaneous hemorrhage	Aortic aneurysm	Alive
19	Ozaki et al.	2016	21	M	Multiple facial injury from traffic accident	Septicemia	Alive

abnormally high activity of a chemical mediator [22]. The other is persistent intraoral and nasal hemorrhage after the accident. Laboratory testing showed prominent decreases in hemoglobin (14.7 g/dL to 7.3 g/dL) and platelets ($23.8 \times 10^4/\mu L$ to $9.8 \times 10^4/\mu L$) between the first visit and the surgery. DIC was possibly triggered in the patient from the large volume of blood loss, consumption of platelets and coagulation factors by acute massive hemorrhage, and a high volume of blood transfusion within a short period [22, 23]. Under such general conditions, the patient had already been in a chronic state of DIC before surgery, and this served to aggravate the symptoms.

The occurrence of DIC is difficult to predict in cases involving young patients with no underlying disease, as in the present case. Over the last 20 years, no fatal cases of DIC have been reported in association with oral and maxillofacial surgery (Table 2). Therefore, in cases with facial injury, symptoms must be detected and progression of DIC prevented by careful perioperative management.

Consent

Informed consent was obtained from the patient for publication of this case report and accompanying images.

Competing Interests

The authors declare that there are competing interests regarding the publication of this paper.

References

[1] J. A. Spero, J. H. Lewis, and U. Hasiba, "Disseminated intravascular coagulation. Findings in 346 patients," *Thrombosis and Haemostasis*, vol. 43, no. 1, pp. 28–33, 1980.

[2] H. Wada, J. Thachil, M. Di Nisio et al., "Guidance for diagnosis and treatment of disseminated intravascular coagulation from harmonization of the recommendations from three guidelines," *Journal of Thrombosis and Haemostasis*, vol. 11, no. 4, pp. 761–767, 2013.

[3] N. Samman, "Disseminated intravascular coagulation and facial injury," *British Journal of Oral and Maxillofacial Surgery*, vol. 22, no. 4, pp. 295–300, 1984.

[4] P. Mehra, A. Caiazzo, and J. Cataudella, "Disseminated intravascular coagulation associated with parotitis: a case report and review," *Journal of Oral and Maxillofacial Surgery*, vol. 55, no. 12, pp. 1478–1482, 1997.

[5] D. A. Falace and D. E. Kelly, "Disseminated intravascular coagulation and fibrinolysis as a cause of postextraction hemorrhage. Report of a case," *Oral Surgery, Oral Medicine, Oral Pathology*, vol. 41, no. 6, pp. 718–725, 1976.

[6] D. W. Rawson, J. B. Harrison, C. C. Alling, and M. K. Hamilton, "Clinicopathological conference. Case 13, part 1," *Journal of Oral Surgery*, vol. 34, no. 1, pp. 62–63, 1976.

[7] D. W. Rawson, J. B. Harrison, C. C. Alling, and M. K. Hamilton, "Clinicopathological conference. Case 13, part 2. Disseminated intravascular coagulation," *Journal of Oral Surgery*, vol. 34, no. 2, pp. 173–177, 1976.

[8] J. McKechnie, "Prostatic carcinoma presenting as a haemorrhagic diathesis after dental extraction," *British Dental Journal*, vol. 166, no. 8, pp. 295–296, 1989.

[9] T. Chishiro, "A case of disseminated intravascular coagulation thought to be caused by tooth extraction in the hypercoagulable condition due to abdominal aortic aneurysm," *Nippon Naika Gakkai Zasshi*, vol. 78, no. 12, pp. 1777–1778, 1989.

[10] D. A. S. Marshall, C. Berry, and A. Brewer, "Fatal disseminated intravascular coagulation complicating dental extraction," *British Journal of Oral and Maxillofacial Surgery*, vol. 31, no. 3, pp. 178–179, 1993.

[11] W. J. R. Currie and V. Ho, "An unexpected death associated with an acute dentoalveolar abscess—report of a case[a/t]," *British Journal of Oral and Maxillofacial Surgery*, vol. 31, no. 5, pp. 296–298, 1993.

[12] R. L. Christiansen and H. P. Soudah, "Disseminated intravascular coagulation following orthognathic surgery," *The International Journal of Adult Orthodontics and Orthognathic Surgery*, vol. 8, no. 3, pp. 217–224, 1993.

[13] P. McLoughlin, S. Chen, and J. G. Phillips, "Disseminated intravascular coagulation presenting as perioral haemorrhage," *British Journal of Oral and Maxillofacial Surgery*, vol. 32, no. 2, pp. 94–95, 1994.

[14] J. Herold and M. A. Falworth, "Disseminated intravascular coagulopathy presenting as a bleeding tooth socket," *British Dental Journal*, vol. 177, no. 1, pp. 21–22, 1994.

[15] Y. Sawaki, M. Yamada, Y. Kasuya, and M. Ueda, "Disseminated intravascular coagulation presenting as hemorrhage after tooth extraction," *Journal of Oral and Maxillofacial Surgery*, vol. 57, no. 3, pp. 341–344, 1999.

[16] Y.-S. Cbo, K.-W. Kim, and S.-N. Yang, "Disseminated intravascular coagulation after a surgery for a mandibular fracture," *Journal of Oral and Maxillofacial Surgery*, vol. 59, no. 1, pp. 98–102, 2001.

[17] Y. Morimoto, M. Ikeuchi, K. Yamamoto, T. Kirita, and M. Sugimura, "Clinical study of disseminated intravascular coagulation in oral and maxillofacial regions—predictors of onset and prognosis," *Oral Diseases*, vol. 7, no. 5, pp. 291–295, 2001.

[18] M. Ita, M. Okafuji, Y. Maruoka, and F. Shinozaki, "An unusual postextraction hemorrhage associated with Klippel-Trenaunay-Weber syndrome," *Journal of Oral and Maxillofacial Surgery*, vol. 59, no. 2, pp. 205–207, 2001.

[19] K. A. Peters, P. T. Triolo Jr., and D. L. Darden, "Disseminated intravascular coagulopathy: manifestations after a routine dental extraction," *Oral Surgery, Oral Medicine, Oral Pathology, Oral Radiology and Endodontology*, vol. 99, no. 4, pp. 419–423, 2005.

[20] T. Imai, M. Michizawa, H. Shimizu, Y. Yura, and Y. Doi, "Spontaneous intraoral hemorrhage as manifestation of thoracoabdominal aortic aneurysm-associated disseminated intravascular coagulation: case report and review," *Journal of Oral and Maxillofacial Surgery*, vol. 68, no. 1, pp. 195–200, 2010.

[21] S. Gando, T. Iba, Y. Eguchi et al., "A multicenter, prospective validation of disseminated intravascular coagulation diagnostic criteria for critically ill patients: comparing current criteria," *Critical Care Medicine*, vol. 34, no. 3, pp. 625–631, 2006.

[22] R. I. Handin, "Disorders of platelet and vessel wall," in *Harrison's Principles of Internal Medicine*, K. J. Issel Bacher and E. Brauwald, Eds., pp. 1798–1804, McGraw-Hill, New York, NY, USA, 13th edition, 1994.

[23] H. Wada, K. Minamikawa, Y. Wakita et al., "Hemostatic study before onset of disseminated intravascular coagulation," *American Journal of Hematology*, vol. 43, no. 3, pp. 190–194, 1993.

Immediate Nonfunctional Loading of Two Single-Maxillary Postextractive Implants: 6-Year Postloading Results of Two Case Reports

Vincenzo Ariano,[1] Manuele Mancini,[1] Andrea Cardi,[2] Roberta Condò,[1] Loredana Cerroni,[1] and Guido Pasquantonio[1]

[1] *Department of Dental Materials, University of Rome "Tor Vergata", Viale Oxford 81, 00133 Rome, Italy*
[2] *Private Practice, Rome, Italy*

Correspondence should be addressed to Manuele Mancini; manuele.mancini@uniroma2.it

Academic Editor: Jamil A. Shibli

Objectives. The aim of the study was to evaluate and compare crestal bone loss of single-maxillary immediate postextractive implants and immediate nonfunctional loading (INFL) during 72 months of follow-up. *Material and Methods.* Two single titanium implants (Certain Prevail, Biomet 3I, USA) were placed in two patients using INFL technique. Implant stability and crestal bone level were measured on periapical radiographs at 1, 3, and 6 months after surgery. *Results.* All osseointegrated implants were clinically successful after 6 years of functional loading. *Conclusion.* Within the limit of the present case report, the paper supports the concept that INFL of single dental implant can be a successful treatment procedure.

1. Introduction

Loss of teeth involves a physiological remodelling of the alveolar bone [1–3] with consequent soft tissues modification. Bone atrophy can be equal to 50% after 5-6 months [4] affecting mainly the horizontal dimension, predominantly on the buccal side, with respect to the vertical dimension [1], continuing slowly but steadily throughout life [5]. Bone reabsorption may lead to a narrower and shorter ridge, thus compromising the functional and aesthetic rehabilitation [6]. Therefore, postextractive hard tissue reabsorption should be avoided. Despite conflicting studies, it could be stated that positioning an implant into a postextractive socket can considerably reduce crestal bone reabsorption [7–9]. Moreover, if the implant is quickly loaded, crestal bone resorption seems to be reduced [10, 11]. Some authors showed that the thickness of the residual bone walls combined with an immediate postextractive implant influences the hard tissue recovery [7–9]. To reduce working time, morbidity, and patient discomfort, many authors stated to immediately insert temporary crowns that can be either loaded or not [12, 13]. The predictability of this technique is guaranteed by the correct treatment plan [14]. This paper shows two case reports of first maxillary premolars replaced by postextractive implants with immediate nonfunctional loading.

2. Material and Methods

Two nonsmoking patients were selected: a 59-year-old man (Case 1) and a 77-year-old woman (Case 2), in good physical and psychological conditions. Both patients had tooth 1.4 fractured without acute inflammatory events. After a clinical and radiographic evaluation (Figures 1 and 2), two postextractive implants with immediate nonfunctional loading were planned, due to the aesthetic position of the teeth. Teeth were planned for extraction because the remaining sound tooth and the request of endodontic retreatment and postendodontic build-up were not giving higher percentage of success than the placement of an INFL implant. Gingival biotype was evaluated before the surgery. Soft tissue in both patients was healthy and sound. A preoperative antibiotic and

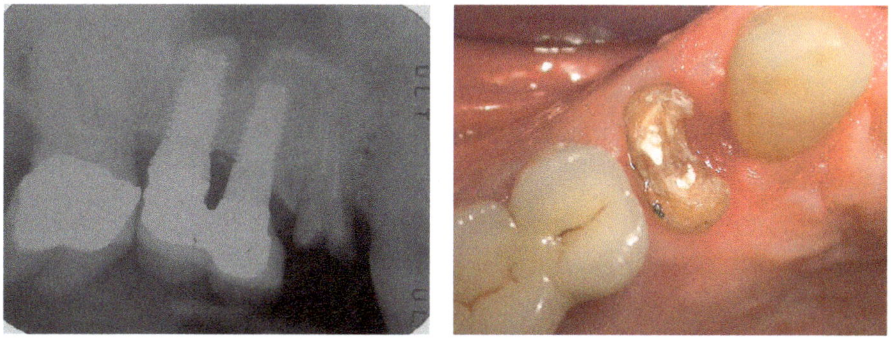

Figure 1: Case 1: clinical and radiographic evaluation before the extraction.

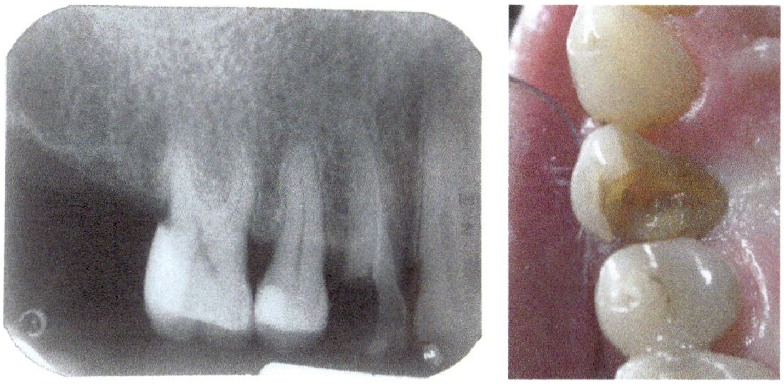

Figure 2: Case 2: clinical and radiographic evaluation before the extraction.

analgesic therapy with amoxicillin 875 mg with clavulanic acid 125 mg (Neoduplamox, Procter & Gamble, USA), 1 tablet every 12 hours for six days starting on the evening before the surgery, and ketoprofen 80 mg (Oki, Dompè Spa, Italy), 2 times a day for 2 days after surgery, was given. Oral disinfection was performed using a 0.2% chlorhexidine mouthwash (Curasept, Curaden Healthcare, Italy) and after surgery a 0.3% chlorhexidine gel (Clexidin Gel Forhans, Uragme, Italy) was added for the 10 days, two times per day. After local anaesthesia with articaine 2% with adrenalin 1 : 100000 (Citocartin, Molteni Dental, Italy) a minimally traumatic flapless extraction of the two elements was performed. After the removal of granulation tissue, an inspection of the alveolar bone to control the presence of any fenestrations was made. Facial bone was intact and it was more than 1 mm thick (Figures 3 and 4). The socket was drilled 3-4 mm over the apical end of the extracted tooth. Moreover the position of fixture was guided by the hollow socket: slightly palatal, 3-4 mm over the apical end of the extracted tooth, and centered between the adjacent teeth. Two fixtures (Certain Prevail, Biomet 3I, USA) previously selected were manually placed to better control their positions (Figures 5 and 6). In Case 1 a 4 × 13 mm fixture and in Case 2 a 4 × 11 mm fixture were used. After connecting the impression transfer (Figure 5), a polyether impression (Impregum Penta, 3M, USA) was taken with a custom tray prepared by the dental laboratory. Subsequently, sites were washed thoroughly with sterile saline and absence of impression material debris was verified. In Case 1, a grafting with hydroxyapatite particles, collagen, and glycosaminoglycans (Biostite, Gaba, Therwil, Switzerland) was placed in the peri-implant space. Healing fixtures were inserted and 4/0 silk sutures (Ethicon, Johnson & Johnson Medical, Rome, Italy) were positioned (Figure 6). After 24 hours the healing fixture was removed; the two resin temporary crowns, built around a PEEK (polyetheretherketone) abutment, were tightened to the fixture without any contact. Screw-retained temporary crowns were chosen to avoid cement that may lead to inflammation (Figures 7 and 8). Patients were instructed to maintain a liquid diet for 3 days and a semisolid diet for about a month avoiding chewing in that side. Both patients reported no pain during the first two weeks and the whole period before the final prosthetic rehabilitation. Sutures were removed after ten days. After four months provisionals were removed. A gold-ceramic crown was luted on a standard titanium abutment in Case 1. In Case 2, a full ceramic crown cemented on a zirconia abutment (Atlantis, Astra Tech Dental System, Mölndal, Sweden) was cemented (Figures 9 and 10). After one year the full crown of Case 2 was replaced by a zirconium ceramic one due to accidental fracture. A sixty-month follow-up was chosen, with clinical evaluation of the soft tissues and radiographic check for any bone resorption in the peri-implant site (Figures 11 and 12). Radiographies were taken with Rinn® (Dentsply-Rinn, York, USA) centering system.

3. Results

A 6-year periapical X-ray follow-up showed a good maintenance of crestal bone in Case 1 and a moderate crestal

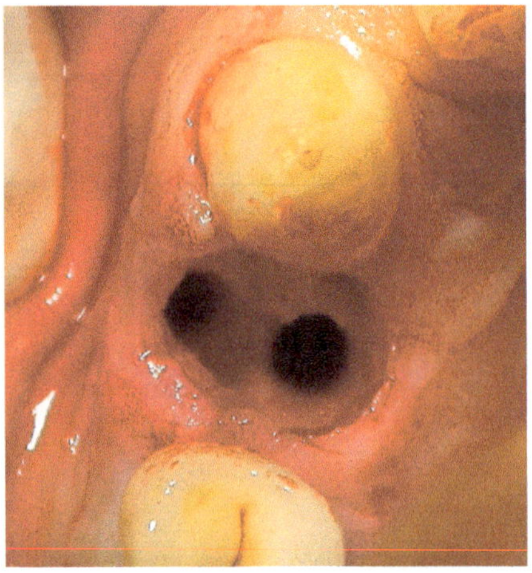

FIGURE 3: Case 1: extraction with the preservation of the buccal bone.

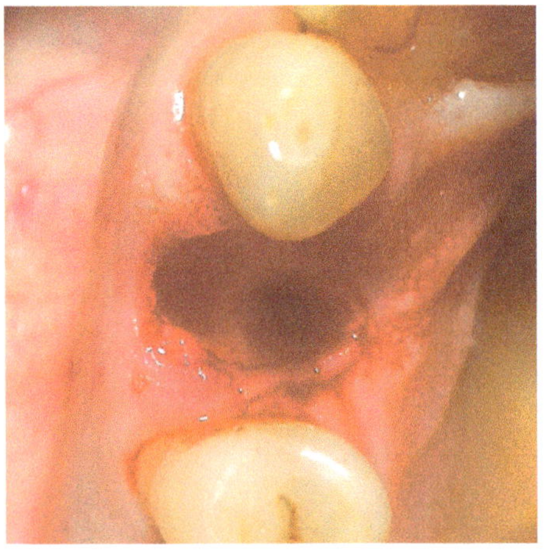

FIGURE 4: Case 2: extraction with the preservation of the buccal bone.

bone resorption (<2 mm) in Case 2. Case 1 shows a good preservation of gingival architecture with a discrete presence of mesial papilla (justified by the presence of tooth 1.3); the distal papilla is underrepresented, for the unfavorable presence of an implant replacing tooth 1.5. In Case 2 mesial and distal papilla is well preserved as good as the gingival margin, showing a slight vertical discharge not affecting aesthetics.

4. Discussion

The loss of a tooth is followed by a major alveolar bone reabsorption compromising any future implant-prosthetic rehabilitation. Therefore, bone volume preservation should always be the main goal, even though bone volume augmentation and short and small-diameter implants are nowadays safe and validated alternatives [15–17]. Long-term predictability [9, 18, 19] of immediate-loaded postextractive implants brings advantages to both patients and dentists: reduced postoperative time to finalization, increased patient comfort, reduced morbidity, and good preservation of gingival architecture [20]. Immediate postextractive implants showed osseointegration rates similar to those of delayed implants, with survival rates varying from 90 to 100% [21, 22] with similar histological healing [23]. Many studies on immediate postextractive implants were carried out, but results on physiological crestal bone resorption are controversial [23–27]. Immediate-loading implants seem to promote conservative bone remodelling; in fact, it was shown that implants stimulate bone formation influencing the early stage of the osteointegration. Moreover, they increase mineralized bone at the bone-implant interface [26, 28]. Conversely, some authors showed that immediate-loading postextractive implants do not prevent physiological bone resorption [29, 30]. Those different results can be explained by many factors such as implant positions, implant diameter [31], surface treatment, thickness of residual alveolar crestal bone [7, 8], and type of surgery [32]. Many authors showed the long-term success of immediate-loaded postextractive implants [9, 18, 19]. The scheduling of this rehabilitation technique should be very precise, from patients' selection to surgery [24]. An accurate radiological examination is of paramount importance selecting the fixture: morphology and position of contiguous teeth roots, distance between them, and the remaining bone are essential to reduce micromovements that should be less than 50 microns [10, 31, 33]. Surgery should be very precise [34]. Performing a flapless technique could be useful to further reduce bone resorption [35], even though some authors showed that this technique does not increase benefits [36]. An atraumatic extraction of the selected tooth, respecting both hard and soft tissues, will be crucial [14, 37, 38]. Looking for fenestrations and fractures of the bone socket is important [10] as well as the evaluation of the gingival biotype, its dimension, and the distance between gingival margin and the residual bone crest level. All these data are important to choose the correct drilling depth before positioning the right fixture to obtain good aesthetics of the soft tissue [39]. To assure sufficient tissue tropism distance from contiguous roots should be at least 1.5 mm [37, 40]. The gap between implant and cortical bone does not necessarily need to be filled with bone grafts when it is shorter than 1.5 mm [23, 25, 41, 42]. However, some authors showed that it is better to fill the gap to maintain a greater volume of buccal tissue [43]. In order to reduce gingival dimensional changes and to obtain a long-term success, profiling emergence of the abutment, temporary, and final crowns should be well-finished and should present a concave contour [44, 45]. Contraindications of immediate-loaded postextractive implants are related to all conditions in which primary stability with torque values higher than 35 N/cm cannot be obtained, like insufficient apical bone or the presence of bone gaps [46, 47] and the absence of intact peri-implant bone walls [32, 38, 48]. Benefits of immediate nonfunctional loaded postextractive implant surgery can be listed as good preservation of gingival architecture, reduction of surgical and prosthetic phases with a significant shortening of time, reduced morbidity, reduced costs, improved patient's comfort, and satisfaction [14].

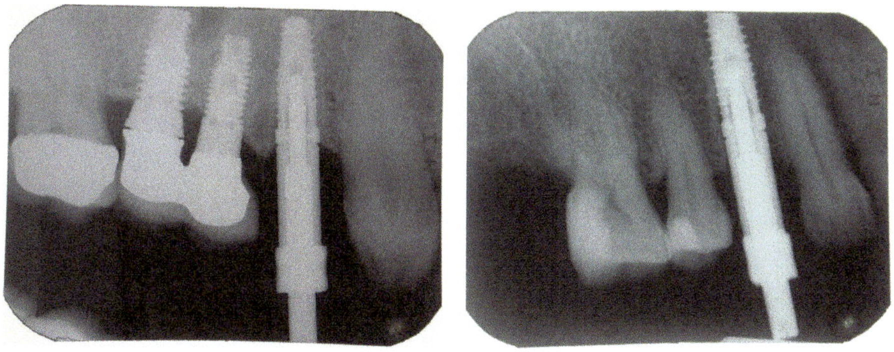

FIGURE 5: Case 1 and Case 2: after implant placement and connection of the impression transfer periapical radiograph.

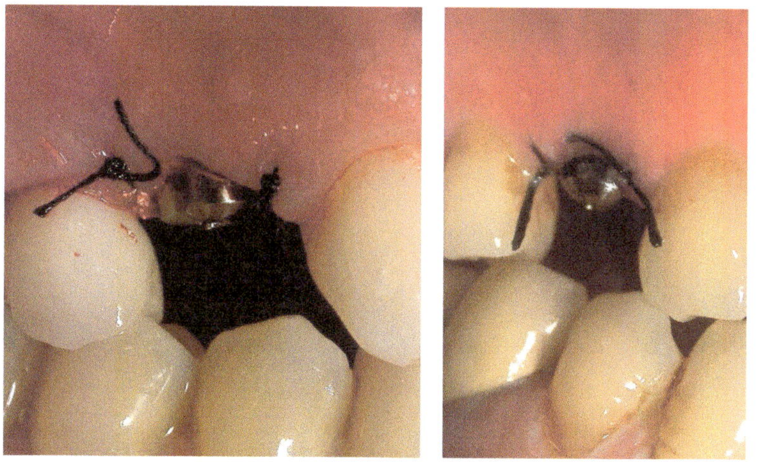

FIGURE 6: Case 1 and Case 2: placement of healing fixtures and sutures.

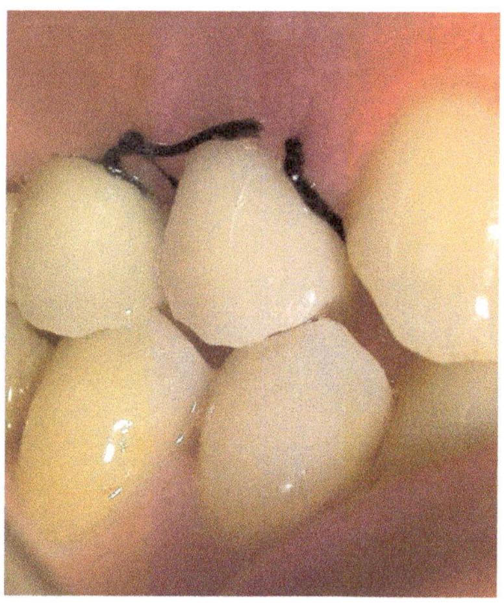

FIGURE 7: Case 1: connection of the provisional restoration.

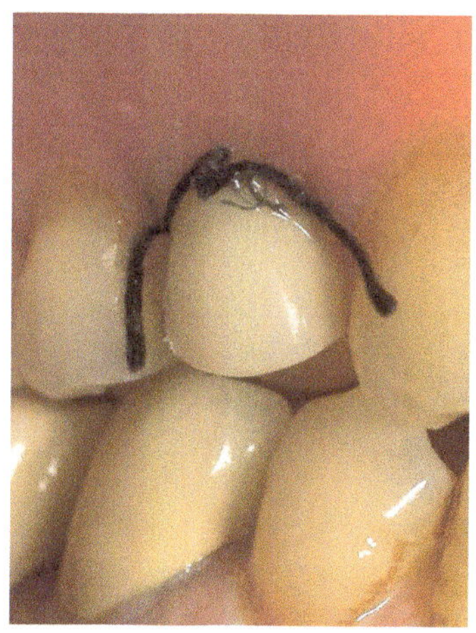

FIGURE 8: Case 2: connection of the provisional restoration.

5. Conclusion

Within the limits of the present study, the two case reports showed good and satisfactory long-term clinical results using immediate nonfunctional loaded postextractive implants as widely reported by many authors.

Disclosure

The authors affirm that they have no financial affiliation (e.g., employment, direct payment, stock holdings, retainers, consultantships, patent licensing arrangements, or honoraria) or involvement with any commercial organization with direct

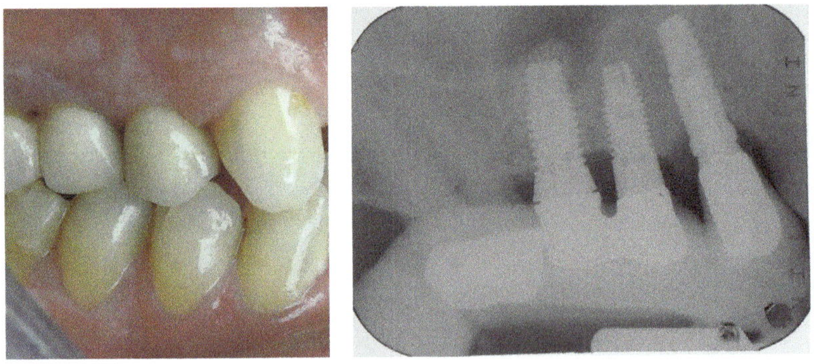

Figure 9: Case 1: definitive prosthetic restoration with periapical radiograph.

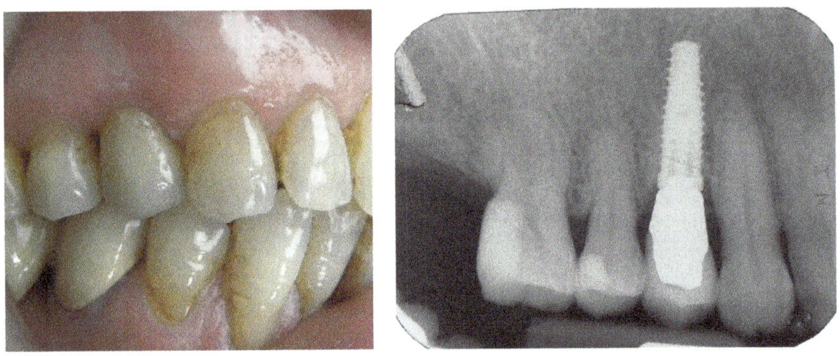

Figure 10: Case 2: definitive prosthetic restoration with periapical radiograph.

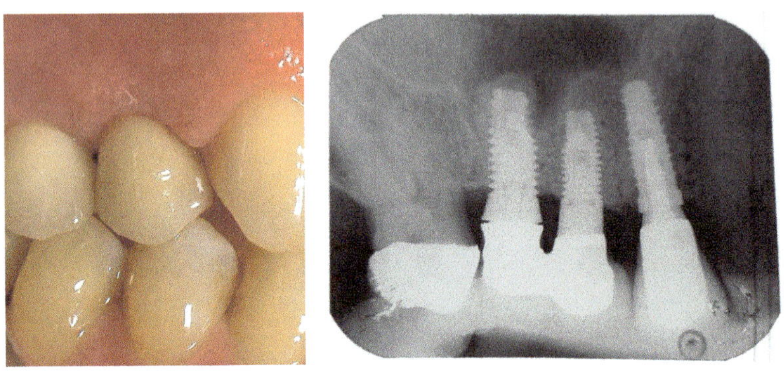

Figure 11: Case 1: 6 years of follow-up and radiographic control.

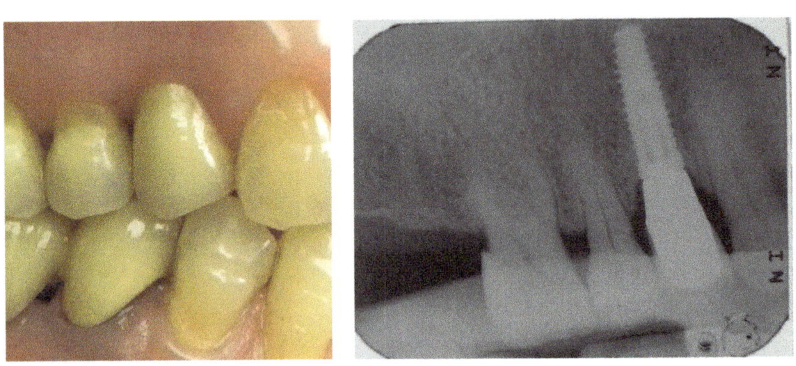

Figure 12: Case 2: 6 years of follow-up and radiographic control.

financial interest in the subject or materials discussed in this paper nor have any such arrangements existing in the past three years.

Competing Interests

The authors declare that they have no competing interests.

References

[1] F. Van der Weijden, F. Dell'Acqua, and D. E. Slot, "Alveolar bone dimensional changes of post-extraction sockets in humans: a systematic review," *Journal of Clinical Periodontology*, vol. 36, no. 12, pp. 1048–1058, 2009.

[2] J. Pietrokovski and M. Massler, "Alveolar ridge resorption following tooth extraction," *The Journal of Prosthetic Dentistry*, vol. 17, no. 1, pp. 21–27, 1967.

[3] M. G. Araújo and J. Lindhe, "Dimensional ridge alterations following tooth extraction. An experimental study in the dog," *Journal of Clinical Periodontology*, vol. 32, no. 2, pp. 212–218, 2005.

[4] L. Schropp, A. Wenzel, L. Kostopoulos, and T. Karring, "Bone healing and soft tissue contour changes following single-tooth extraction: a clinical and radiographic 12-month prospective study," *International Journal of Periodontics and Restorative Dentistry*, vol. 23, no. 4, pp. 313–323, 2003.

[5] L. Jahangiri, H. Devlin, K. Ting, and I. Nishimura, "Current perspectives in residual ridge remodeling and its clinical implications: a review," *The Journal of Prosthetic Dentistry*, vol. 80, no. 2, pp. 224–237, 1998.

[6] O. Hoffmann, B. K. Bartee, C. Beaumont, A. Kasaj, G. Deli, and G.-G. Zafiropoulos, "Alveolar bone preservation in extraction sockets using non-resorbable dPTFE membranes: a retrospective non-randomized study," *Journal of Periodontology*, vol. 79, no. 8, pp. 1355–1369, 2008.

[7] C. Tomasi, M. Sanz, D. Cecchinato et al., "Bone dimensional variations at implants placed in fresh extraction sockets: a multilevel multivariate analysis," *Clinical Oral Implants Research*, vol. 21, no. 1, pp. 30–36, 2010.

[8] J. Ferrus, D. Cecchinato, E. B. Pjetursson, N. P. Lang, M. Sanz, and J. Lindhe, "Factors influencing ridge alterations following immediate implant placement into extraction sockets," *Clinical Oral Implants Research*, vol. 21, no. 1, pp. 22–29, 2010.

[9] L. F. Cooper, G. J. Reside, F. Raes et al., "Immediate provisionalization of dental implants placed in healed alveolar ridges and extraction sockets: a 5-year prospective evaluation," *The International Journal of Oral & Maxillofacial Implants*, vol. 29, no. 3, pp. 709–717, 2014.

[10] R. J. Lazzara, "Immediate implant placement into extraction sites: surgical and restorative advantages," *The International Journal of Periodontics & Restorative Dentistry*, vol. 9, no. 5, pp. 332–343, 1989.

[11] R. Cornelini, A. Scarano, U. Covani, G. Petrone, and A. Piattelli, "Immediate one-stage postextraction implant: A Human Clinical and Histologic Case Report," *International Journal of Oral and Maxillofacial Implants*, vol. 15, no. 3, pp. 432–437, 2000.

[12] J. A. Lindeboom, J. W. Frenken, L. Dubois, M. Frank, I. Abbink, and F. H. Kroon, "Immediate loading versus immediate provisionalization of maxillary single-tooth replacements: a prospective randomized study with biocomp implants," *Journal of Oral and Maxillofacial Surgery*, vol. 64, no. 6, pp. 936–942, 2006.

[13] M. Degidi and A. Piattelli, "Comparative analysis study of 702 dental implants subjected to immediate functional loading and immediate non-functional loading to traditional healing periods with a follow-up of up to 24 months," *The International Journal of Oral & Maxillofacial Implants*, vol. 20, no. 1, pp. 99–107, 2005.

[14] L. Schropp and F. Isidor, "Timing of implant placement relative to tooth extraction," *Journal of Oral Rehabilitation*, vol. 35, no. 1, pp. 33–43, 2008.

[15] D. Nisand and F. Renouard, "Short implant in limited bone volume," *Periodontology 2000*, vol. 66, no. 1, pp. 72–96, 2014.

[16] M. Davarpanah, H. Martinez, J.-F. Tecucianu, R. Celletti, and R. Lazzara, "Small-diameter implants: indications and contraindications," *Journal of Esthetic Dentistry*, vol. 12, no. 4, pp. 186–194, 2000.

[17] G. J. Christensen, "The increased use of small-diameter implants," *Journal of the American Dental Association*, vol. 140, no. 6, pp. 709–712, 2009.

[18] L. Malchiodi, P. Ghensi, A. Cucchi, and G. Corrocher, "A comparative retrospective study of immediately loaded implants in postextraction sites versus healed sites: results after 6 to 7 years in the maxilla.," *The International Journal of Oral & Maxillofacial Implants*, vol. 26, no. 2, pp. 373–384, 2011.

[19] E. Mijiritsky, O. Mardinger, Z. Mazor, and G. Chaushu, "Immediate provisionalization of single-tooth implants in fresh-extraction sites at the maxillary esthetic zone: up to 6 years of follow-Up," *Implant Dentistry*, vol. 18, no. 4, pp. 326–333, 2009.

[20] S. T. Chen, T. G. Wilson Jr., and C. H. F. Hämmerle, "Immediate or early placement of implants following tooth extraction: review of biologic basis, clinical procedures, and outcomes," *The International Journal of Oral & Maxillofacial Implants*, vol. 19, supplement, pp. 12–25, 2004.

[21] M. Esposito, M. G. Grusovin, I. P. Polyzos, P. Felice, and H. V. Worthington, "Timing of implant placement after tooth extraction: immediate, immediate-delayed or delayed implants? A Cochrane systematic review," *European Journal of Oral Implantology*, vol. 3, no. 3, pp. 189–205, 2010.

[22] A. Scarano, G. Iezzi, G. Petrone, V. C. Marinho, M. Corigliano, and A. Piattelli, "Immediate postextraction implants: a histologic and histometric analysis in monkeys," *The Journal of Oral Implantology*, vol. 26, no. 3, pp. 163–169, 2000.

[23] M. Paolantonio, M. Dolci, A. Scarano et al., "Immediate implantation in fresh extraction sockets. A controlled clinical and histological study in man," *Journal of Periodontology*, vol. 72, no. 11, pp. 1560–1571, 2001.

[24] M. Sanz, D. Cecchinato, J. Ferrus, E. B. Pjetursson, N. P. Lang, and J. Lindhe, "A prospective, randomized-controlled clinical trial to evaluate bone preservation using implants with different geometry placed into extraction sockets in the maxilla," *Clinical Oral Implants Research*, vol. 21, no. 1, pp. 13–21, 2010.

[25] R. Cornelini, A. Scarano, U. Covani, G. Petrone, and A. Piattelli, "Immediate One-Stage Postextraction Implant: A Human Clinical and Histologic Case Report," *International Journal of Oral and Maxillofacial Implants*, vol. 15, no. 3, pp. 432–437, 2000.

[26] D. Botticelli, T. Berglundh, and J. Lindhe, "Hard-tissue alterations following immediate implant placement in extraction sites," *Journal of Clinical Periodontology*, vol. 31, no. 10, pp. 820–828, 2004.

[27] G. E. Romanos, C. G. Toh, C. H. Siar, D. Swaminathan, and A. H. Ong, "Histologic and histomorphometric evaluation of peri-implant bone subjected to immediate loading: an experimental study with macaca fascicularis," *International Journal of Oral and Maxillofacial Implants*, vol. 17, no. 1, pp. 44–51, 2002.

[28] G. E. Romanos, C. G. Toh, C. H. Siar, H. Wicht, H. Yacoob, and G.-H. Nentwig, "Bone-implant interface around titanium implants under different loading conditions: a histomorphometrical analysis in the *Macaca fascicularis* monkey," *Journal of Periodontology*, vol. 74, no. 10, pp. 1483–1490, 2003.

[29] J. Blanco, A. Liñares, J. Pérez, and F. Muñoz, "Ridge alterations following flapless immediate implant placement with or without immediate loading—part II: a histometric study in the Beagle dog," *Journal of Clinical Periodontology*, vol. 38, no. 8, pp. 762–770, 2011.

[30] M. Caneva, D. Botticelli, F. Rossi, L. C. Cardoso, F. Pantani, and N. P. Lang, "Influence of implants with different sizes and configurations installed immediately into extraction sockets on peri-implant hard and soft tissues: an experimental study in dogs," *Clinical Oral Implants Research*, vol. 23, no. 4, pp. 396–401, 2012.

[31] S. Szmukler-Moncler, A. Piattelli, G. A. Favero, and J.-H. Dubruille, "Considerations preliminary to the application of early and immediate loading protocols in dental implantology," *Clinical Oral Implants Research*, vol. 11, no. 1, pp. 12–25, 2000.

[32] T. Grandi, G. Garuti, R. Samarani, P. Guazzi, and A. Forabosco, "Immediate loading of single post-extractive implants in the anterior maxilla: 12-month results from a multicenter clinical study," *Journal of Oral Implantology*, vol. 38, no. 1, pp. 477–484, 2012.

[33] S. Szmukler-Moncler, H. Salama, Y. Reingewirtz, and J.-H. Dubruille, "Timing of loading and effect of micromotion on bone-dental implant interface: review of experimental literature," *Journal of Biomedical Materials Research*, vol. 43, no. 2, pp. 192–203, 1998.

[34] R. Warkentin, "Immediate tooth replacement: strategies for success," *International Journal of Oral Implantology and Clinical Research*, vol. 1, no. 1, pp. 27–32, 2010.

[35] S. Job, V. Bhat, and E. Naidu, "In vivo evaluation of crestal bone heights following implant placement with 'flapless' and 'with-flap' techniques in sites of immediately loaded implants," *Indian Journal of Dental Research*, vol. 19, no. 4, pp. 320–325, 2008.

[36] M. Caneva, D. Botticelli, L. A. Salata, S. L. S. Souza, E. Bressan, and N. P. Lang, "Flap vs. 'flapless' surgical approach at immediate implants: a histomorphometric study in dogs," *Clinical Oral Implants Research*, vol. 21, no. 12, pp. 1314–1319, 2010.

[37] D. A. Garber, M. A. Salama, and H. Salama, "Immediate total tooth replacement," *Compendium of Continuing Education in Dentistry*, vol. 22, no. 3, pp. 210–218, 2001.

[38] R. Gangar, B. S Sadhwani, S. Anchlia, and S. Sadhwani, "Immediate placement implant in fresh extraction socket: a clinical study of seven cases," *International Journal of Oral Implantology & Clinical Research*, vol. 4, no. 1, pp. 7–15, 2013.

[39] A. Ferrara, C. Galli, G. Mauro, and G. M. Macaluso, "Immediate provisional restoration of postextraction implants for maxillary single-tooth replacement," *The International Journal of Periodontics and Restorative Dentistry*, vol. 26, no. 4, pp. 371–377, 2006.

[40] A. Funato, M. A. Salama, T. Ishikawa, D. A. Garber, and H. Salama, "Timing, positioning, and sequential staging in esthetic implant therapy: a four-dimensional perspective," *International Journal of Periodontics and Restorative Dentistry*, vol. 27, no. 4, pp. 313–323, 2007.

[41] T. G. Wilson Jr., J. Carnio, R. Schenk, and D. Cochran, "Immediate implants covered with connective tissue membranes: human biopsies," *Journal of Periodontology*, vol. 74, no. 3, pp. 402–409, 2003.

[42] T. G. Wilson Jr., R. Schenk, D. Buser, and D. Cochran, "Implants placed in immediate extraction sites: a report of histologic and histometric analyses of human biopsies," *The International Journal of Oral & Maxillofacial Implants*, vol. 13, no. 3, pp. 333–341, 1998.

[43] M. P. Cristalli, R. Marini, G. La Monaca, C. Sepe, F. Tonoli, and S. Annibali, "Immediate loading of post-extractive single-tooth implants: a 1-year prospective study," *Clinical Oral Implants Research*, vol. 26, no. 9, pp. 1070–1079, 2015.

[44] J. Y. K. Kan, K. Rungcharassaeng, and J. Lozada, "Immediate placement and provisionalization of maxillary anterior single implants: 1-year prospective study," *International Journal of Oral and Maxillofacial Implants*, vol. 18, no. 1, pp. 31–39, 2003.

[45] M. S. Block, D. E. Mercante, D. Lirette, W. Mohamed, M. Ryser, and P. Castellon, "Prospective evaluation of immediate and delayed provisional single tooth restorations," *Journal of Oral and Maxillofacial Surgery*, vol. 67, no. 11, supplement, pp. 89–107, 2009.

[46] J. M. P. Ottoni, Z. F. L. Oliveira, R. Mansini, and A. M. Cabral, "Correlation between placement torque and survival of single-tooth implants," *International Journal of Oral and Maxillofacial Implants*, vol. 20, no. 5, pp. 769–776, 2005.

[47] G. Cannizzaro, M. Leone, V. Ferri, P. Viola, G. Federico, and M. Esposito, "Immediate loading of single implants inserted flapless with medium or high insertion torque: a 6-month follow-up of a split-mouth randomised controlled trial," *The European Journal of Oral Implantology*, vol. 5, no. 4, pp. 333–342, 2012.

[48] A. Barone, L. Rispoli, I. Vozza, A. Quaranta, and U. Covani, "Immediate restoration of single implants placed immediately after tooth extraction," *Journal of Periodontology*, vol. 77, no. 11, pp. 1914–1920, 2006.

38

Ectopic Teeth in Ovarian Teratoma: A Rare Appearance

Yashwant Ingale,[1] Akhil A. Shankar,[2] Samapika Routray,[3] Manoj Agrawal,[4] Ajit Kadam,[5] and Tushar Patil[6]

[1] *Department of Dentistry, Yashwantrao Chavan Memorial Hospital, Pimpri, Pune 410018, India*
[2] *Department of Oral Pathology and Microbiology, YMT Dental College, Kharghar, Navi Mumbai, India*
[3] *Department of Oral Pathology and Microbiology, Institute of Dental Sciences, SOA University, Bhubaneswar, Odisha 751003, India*
[4] *Oral and Maxillofacial Surgeon, Talera Hospital, Pimpri, Pune 410018, India*
[5] *Department of Oral Pathology and Microbiology, Seema Dental College, Rishikesh, Uttarakhand, India*
[6] *Department of Pathology, Yashwantrao Chavan Memorial Hospital, Pimpri, Pune 410018, India*

Correspondence should be addressed to Samapika Routray; drroutray.samapika@gmail.com

Academic Editors: A. Epivatianos, A. Markopoulos, and M. H. K. Motamedi

Teratoma consists of tissues derived from all the three germ layers, and there may be presence of appendages as a representation of these germ layers as well. Teratomas of the ovary are known to occur in a fairly large number of women. These may be present clinically at a much later stage, permitting a limited treatment plan. Newer diagnostic techniques are always welcome in identifying these lesions. This case report discusses the case of a 40-year-old woman with a large teratoma in the right ovary and its diagnostic and surgical modalities.

1. Introduction

Teratoma is a true neoplasm arising from totipotential cells and made up of a variety of parenchymal cell types representative of more than one germ layer; usually all three [1]. It is defined as the proliferation of tissues from all the germ layers in a location which is not native for the tissues [2]. Although they are usually surgically removed as they may present a risk of functional incapacitance of the organ involved, they rarely represent the risk of being malignant. Mature cysts, that is, teratomas, of the ovary are found as the most common germ cell tumour comprising of 33% of the ovarian tumours [3]. 20% of all ovarian tumors in adults and 50% of all ovarian tumors in children are unilateral, and 8 to 15% are bilateral [4]. They are found primarily in the reproductive years or may be seen in the postmenopausal phase or in childhood. They also have a low rate of malignant transformation, which occurs more in the postmenopausal phase and is related to poor prognosis. Ovarian teratomas are equally common and are frequently found in two varieties, namely, solid and cystic.

Most of the tumours take up the features similar to dermoid cyst with ectodermal derivatives, and a majority of the malignant teratomas are squamous cell carcinomas with the other being carcinoids, adenocarcinoma, melanomas, and types of sarcomas [5]. The cystic variant is more consistent with dermoid cyst having hair as the commonest appendage. Microscopically 100% tumors have ectodermal derivatives, mesodermal structures in 93%, and endodermal derivatives in 71% [5]. Other appendages encountered in a teratoma may include teeth, fat, and sebaceous material. Robboy and Scully conducted an analysis of the contents of the teratomas and have presented the occurrence of all classes of teeth [6]. Wollin and Ozonoff also report the occurrence of teeth in developing teratomas which are readily identifiable at the radiographic level [7]. Teratomas often contain teeth, and sometime it may present in imperfect forms as mandible or human body like structures (homunculus) [8]. The benign cystic teratomas of the ovary had features ranging from skin to hair, teeth, sebaceous material, fat, and connective tissue [9].

Advancement in imaging techniques has aided in the diagnosis, as well as adequate planning prior to the surgery. CT and MR imaging of pelvic regions are usually diagnostic of ovarian teratomas, wherein a CT shows typically fat-attenuated within a cyst, and an MR usually reflects the identification of the sebaceous components [10]. Teeth may tend to be located in a well-defined nipple like structure covered with hair known as Rokitansky's protuberance. This exhibits a variety of tissues and hence must be selected for microscopy [11]. Dodd and Budzik suggested that the identification of teeth, a dermoid plug, or a fat/fluid level is diagnostic of a benign cystic ovarian teratoma [12]. The cut surface usually shows a mixed cystic space, with solid consistency with extensive deposits of calcium as well as cartilage and bone like material, and in some areas small, fine dark hairs and pale white structures resemble teeth [13], which may be recognized in 29% of ovarian tumours [14].

2. Case Report

This case reported here represents a benign teratoma of the right ovary in a 40-year-old female patient reporting to the outpatient department. The provisional diagnosis was given as a right complicated cyst with an indication for dermoid cyst. Family history was noncontributory. The patient gave a history of menopause two years prior to the checkup. Further investigations of an ultrasonography (USG) revealed a 51 mm × 47 mm well-defined lesion with calcification of 8 mm noted in the right ovary, suggestive of a complicated ovarian cyst or a probable dermoid cyst offered as USG diagnosis. Commonly used marker for ovarian cancers, CA-125, was assessed, and normal levels of which suggested the absence of malignancy. An access to the lesion was established by a transverse incision over the abdomen, and the cystic tumour was obtained in toto. A cut section showed the presence of derivatives of all three layers, namely, teeth, sebaceous material, connective tissue, and fat. Grossing revealed the presence of mucinous material and few molariform teeth (Figure 1). The patient was followed up with ultrasound for a period of up to 2 years, wherein there were no signs of recurrence, and the patient was asymptomatic. The specimen was subjected to routine histopathological examination which revealed the presence of multiple glandular structures lined by low cuboidal to tall columnar cells and at places showing the presence of pseudostratification (Figure 2). Odontogenic remnants showing blastemal cells with peripheral palisading were evident amidst a loose spindle cell stroma with collagen (Figures 3 and 4). Ectodermal derivatives such as skin, hair, sebaceous glands, neural tissues, and keratin material are also seen.

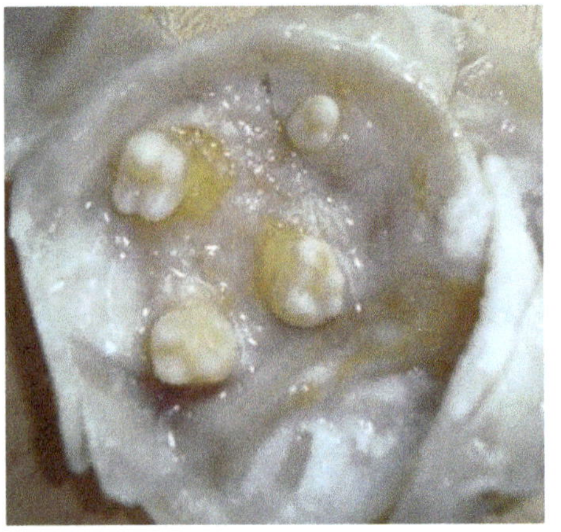

Figure 1: Gross specimen revealing the presence of molariform teeth.

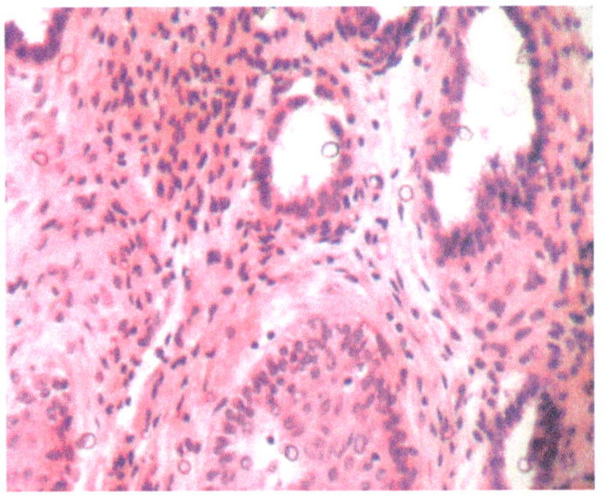

Figure 2: Low power photomicrograph (×100) exhibiting glandular structures with pseudostratification.

3. Discussion

A teratoma is defined as a benign tumour derived from all three germ layers, showing evidence of tissue formation from ectoderm, mesoderm, and endoderm and not being native to the tissue [2]. Ovarian teratomas are known to show a diverse variety of tissues such as hair, teeth, fat, sebaceous material, and teeth formed that resemble all the classes [7]. These tumors form around 33% of all the ovarian tumours, and hence, accurate diagnosis is of prime importance [3]. Origin of teratomas has been a matter of fascination for centuries. Some common beliefs have also blamed witches, nightmares, or adultery with devil. Scully [15] has suggested a histologic classification of ovarian tumours too.

The malignant transformation of an ovarian teratoma has an incidence of less than 1% [3]. This prompted the study of the origin of benign cystic teratomas of the ovary, which was attempted by performing chromosome-banding studies on normal tissues as compared to teratomas, wherein they concluded that the normal tissues are heterozygous for 17 chromosome polymorphisms at or near the centromere, whereas the teratomas are uniformly homozygous [16]. These findings and those employing electrophoretic variants indicate that ovarian teratomas are parthenogenetic tumors that arise from an ovum [16] or a single germ cell after the first meiotic division [17].

Various diagnostic modalities have been included to avoid misdiagnosis at the time of surgery initiating a dilemma in the surgeons mind. Radiographs may provide clues but only if there are calcified masses seen. Ultrasound is an important diagnostic tool which may aid the clinician in diagnosis, and a simple classification suggested on the echo patterns by Caspi et al. has made it possible to diagnose ovarian teratomas in more than 97% of the cases [17]. Although CT and MRI shall always provide the most accurate

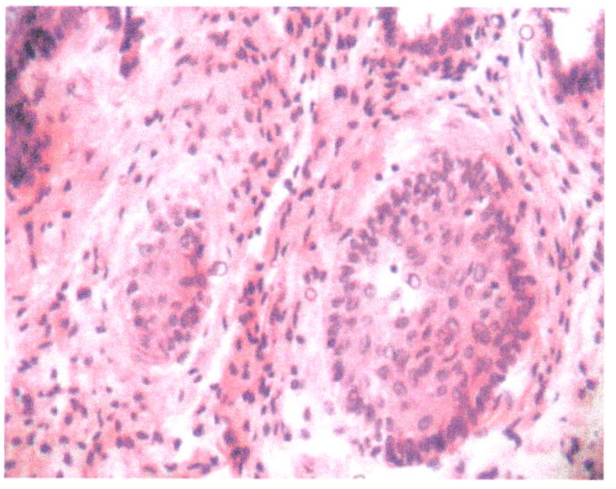

FIGURE 3: High power photomicrograph (×400) showing islands of odontogenic rests.

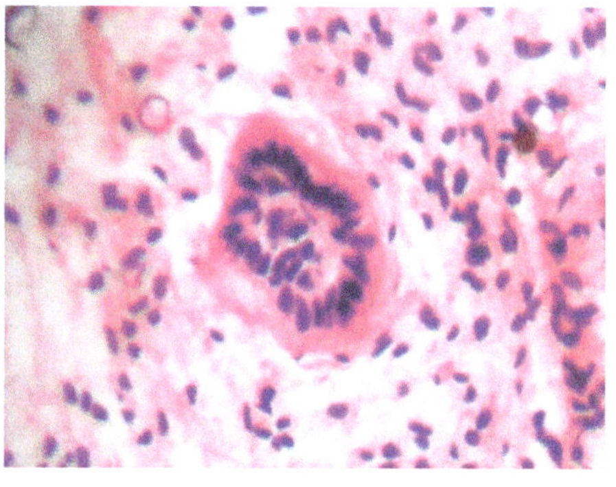

FIGURE 4: High power photomicrograph (×400) of odontogenic remnants showing blastemal cells with peripheral palisading.

diagnosis, routine screening by ultrasound may still provide a beneficial and cost effective method and also make the possible diagnosis at a much earlier stage.

Our case presents a 40-year-old woman with a history of menopause 2 years prior to the admission. The lesion in the right ovary was evident on the ultrasound and also presented calcified masses, which were indicative of teeth. Following surgery, the gross specimen revealed a cystic lesion and the presence of molariform teeth making it an obvious diagnosis. The histopathological examination revealed the presence of odontogenic like epithelium and developing teeth, which indicated that the lesion may have formed more teeth or a mandible if it would have been left undisturbed. Hence, an accurate diagnosis of such lesions with appropriate methods holds great importance in providing a correct view to the surgeon and aiding in complete removal of the lesion.

Conflict of Interests

The authors declared that they have no conflict of interests, and no competing financial interests exist.

References

[1] V. Kumar, A. K. Abbas, and N. Fausto, "Neoplasia," in *Pathological Basis of Diseases*, pp. 269–342, Elsevier, 7th edition, 2005.

[2] D. R. Gnepp, *Diagnostic Surgical Pathology of the Head and Neck*, Elsievier, 2nd edition, 2009.

[3] R. T. Wu, P. L. Torng, D. Y. Chang et al., "Mature cystic teratoma of the ovary: a clinicopathologic study of 283 cases," *Chinese Medical Journal*, vol. 58, no. 4, pp. 269–274, 1996.

[4] S. H. Ein, J. M. M. Darte, and C. A. Stephens, "Cystic and solid ovarian tumors in children: a 44-year review," *Journal of Pediatric Surgery*, vol. 5, no. 2, pp. 148–156, 1970.

[5] W. J. Blackwell, M. B. Dockerty, J. C. Masson, and R. D. Mussey, "Dermoid cyst of the ovary, their clinical and pathologic significance," *American Journal of Obstetrics & Gynecology*, vol. 51, pp. 151–172, 1946.

[6] S. J. Robboy and R. E. Scully, "Ovarian teratoma with glial implants on the peritoneum: an Analysis of 12 Cases," *Human Pathology*, vol. 1, no. 4, pp. 643–653, 1970.

[7] E. Wollin and M. B. Ozonoff, "Serial development of teeth in an ovarian teratoma: a thirteen-year," *The New England journal of medicine*, vol. 265, pp. 897–898, 1961.

[8] J. Miyake and K. Ireland, "Ovarian mature teratoma with homunculus coexisting with an intrauterine pregnancy," *Archives of Pathology and Laboratory Medicine*, vol. 110, no. 12, pp. 1192–1194, 1986.

[9] G. W. H. Stamp and E. M. McConnell, "Malignancy arising in cystic ovarian teratomas: a report of 24 cases," *British Journal of Obstetrics and Gynaecology*, vol. 90, no. 7, pp. 671–675, 1983.

[10] E. K. Outwater, E. S. Siegelman, and J. L. Hunt, "Ovarian teratomas: tumor types and imaging characteristics," *Radiographics*, vol. 21, no. 2, pp. 475–490, 2001.

[11] H. M. Dick and L. H. Honore, "Dental structures in benign ovarian cystic teratomas (dermoid cysts). A study of ten cases with a review of the literature," *Oral Surgery Oral Medicine and Oral Pathology*, vol. 60, no. 3, pp. 299–307, 1985.

[12] G. D. Dodd III and R. F. Budzik Jr., "Lipomatous tumors of the pelvis in women: spectrum of imaging findings," *American Journal of Roentgenology*, vol. 155, no. 2, pp. 317–322, 1990.

[13] M. El Shafie, R. W. Furay, and L. V. Chablani, "Ovarian teratoma with peritoneal and lymph node metastases of mature glial tissue: a benign condition," *Journal of Surgical Oncology*, vol. 27, no. 1, pp. 18–22, 1984.

[14] M. J. Siegel, W. H. McAlister, and G. D. Shackelford, "Radiographic findings in ovarian teratomas in children," *American Journal of Roentgenology*, vol. 131, no. 4, pp. 613–615, 1978.

[15] R. E. Scully, "Ovarian Tumours," *American Journal of Pathology*, vol. 87, pp. 686–720, 1977.

[16] D. Linder, B. K. McCaw, and F. Hecht, "Parthenogenic origin of benign ovarian teratomas," *New England Journal of Medicine*, vol. 292, no. 2, pp. 63–66, 1975.

[17] B. Caspi, Z. Appelman, D. Rabinerson, U. Elchalal, Y. Zalel, and Z. Katz, "Pathognomonic echo patterns of benign cystic teratomas of the ovary: classification, incidence and accuracy rate of sonographic diagnosis," *Ultrasound in Obstetrics and Gynecology*, vol. 7, no. 4, pp. 275–279, 1996.

39

Treatment of Class III with Facemask Therapy

Snigdha Pattanaik and Sumita Mishra

Department of Orthodontics and Dentofacial Orthopaedics, Institute of Dental Sciences, Siksha 'O' Anusandhan University, Bhubaneswar, Odisha 751003, India

Correspondence should be addressed to Sumita Mishra; sumita.mitali@gmail.com

Academic Editor: Hüsamettin Oktay

Class III malocclusion is one of the most difficult problems to treat in the mixed dentition. It has a multifactorial etiology involving both genetic and environmental causes. The dental and skeletal effects of maxillary protraction with a facemask are well documented in several studies. Although treatment in the late mixed or early permanent dentition can be successful, results are generally better in the deciduous or early mixed dentition. The following case shows early treatment of a young patient with severe sagittal and transverse discrepancy of the maxilla and mandible, using a facemask.

1. Introduction

Class III malocclusion is one of the most difficult problems to treat in the mixed dentition [1]. It occurs in about 1% of North American population and is prevalent particularly in Asiatic countries. Class III malocclusion has a multifactorial etiology involving both genetic and environmental causes [2–4]. The dental and skeletal effects of maxillary protraction with a facemask are well documented in several studies [5–9]. Although treatment in the late mixed or early permanent dentition can be successful, results are generally better in the deciduous or early mixed dentition [10, 11]. The following case shows early treatment of a young patient with severe sagittal and transverse discrepancy of the maxilla and mandible using a facemask.

2. Incidence

Various combinations exist for occurrence of such malocclusions:

Mandibular prognathism: 20%.

Maxillary retrusion: 25%.

Combination: 22%.

Remainder: no anteroposterior skeletal imbalances.

3. Diagnosis and Etiology

A 12-year-old female in the mixed dentition presented with Class III skeletal and dental malocclusion, a prognathic mandible, retrognathic maxilla, and proclined lower incisors (Figure 1). She had symmetrical maxillary and asymmetrical mandibular arch forms with the molars and canines in Class III relationships. All permanent teeth were present except upper, lower second deciduous molars and lower left first deciduous molar.

Centric relation, as determined by mandibular manipulation, was coincident with centric occlusion, suggesting a true mandibular-prognathic Class III malocclusion rather than a pseudo-Class III.

Cephalometric measurements indicated a prognathic mandible and a retrognathic maxillary position.

Our diagnosis was a true Class III due to a prognathic mandible and retrognathic maxilla.

The etiology was genetic with a history of consanguineous marriage and both her brother and sister had similar malocclusion.

4. Treatment Objectives

The purpose of treatment was to correct the sagittal and transverse arch discrepancies through stimulation of maxillary

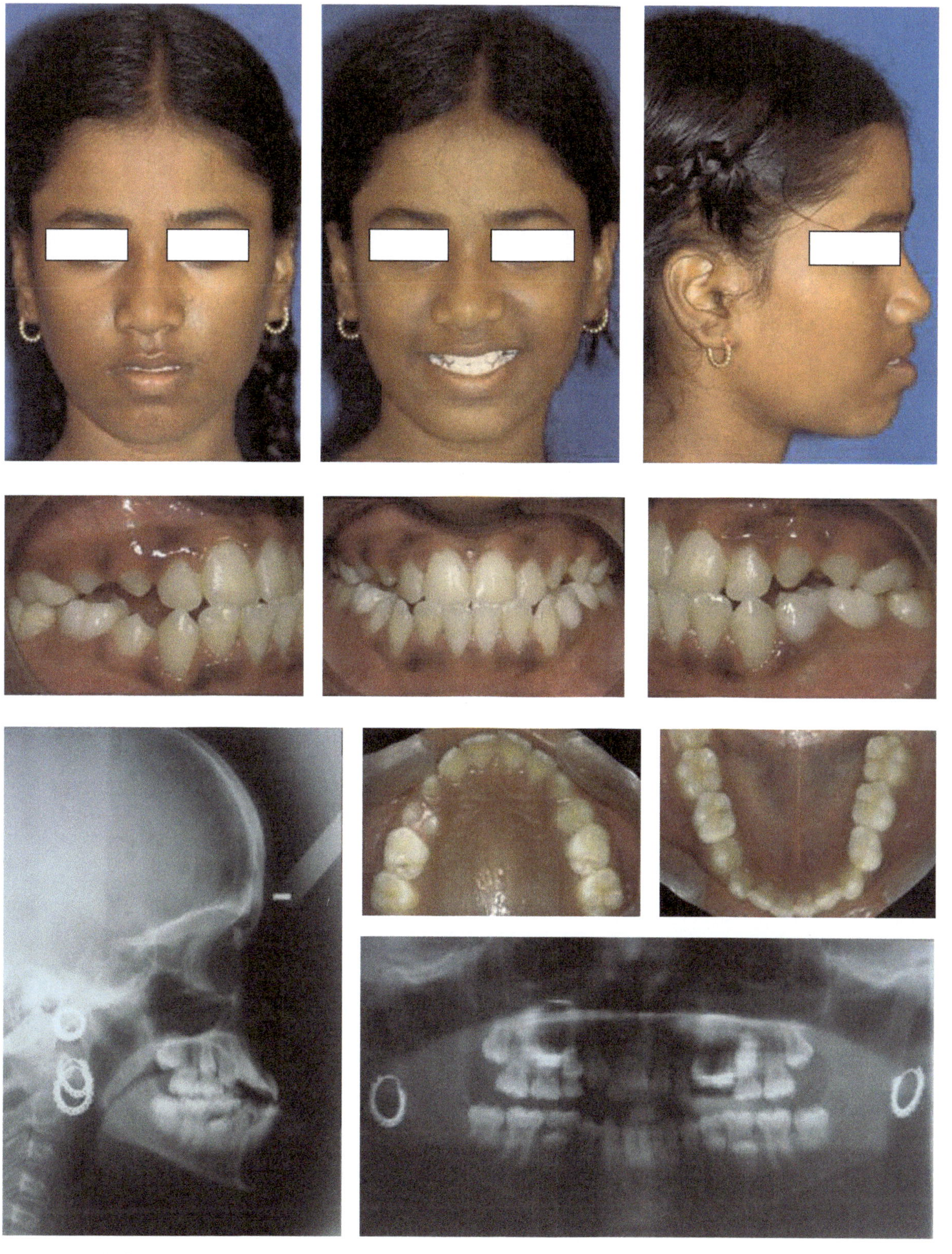

FIGURE 1: 12-year-old female patient with Class III dental and skeletal malocclusion, prognathic mandible, proclined lower incisors, and reverse overjet.

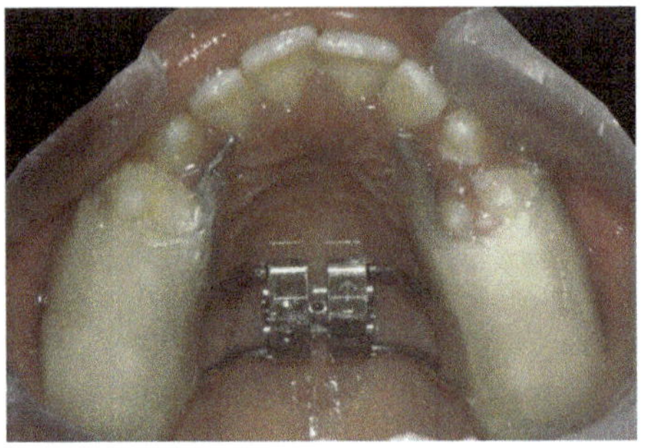

FIGURE 2: RME with Hyrax Expansion.

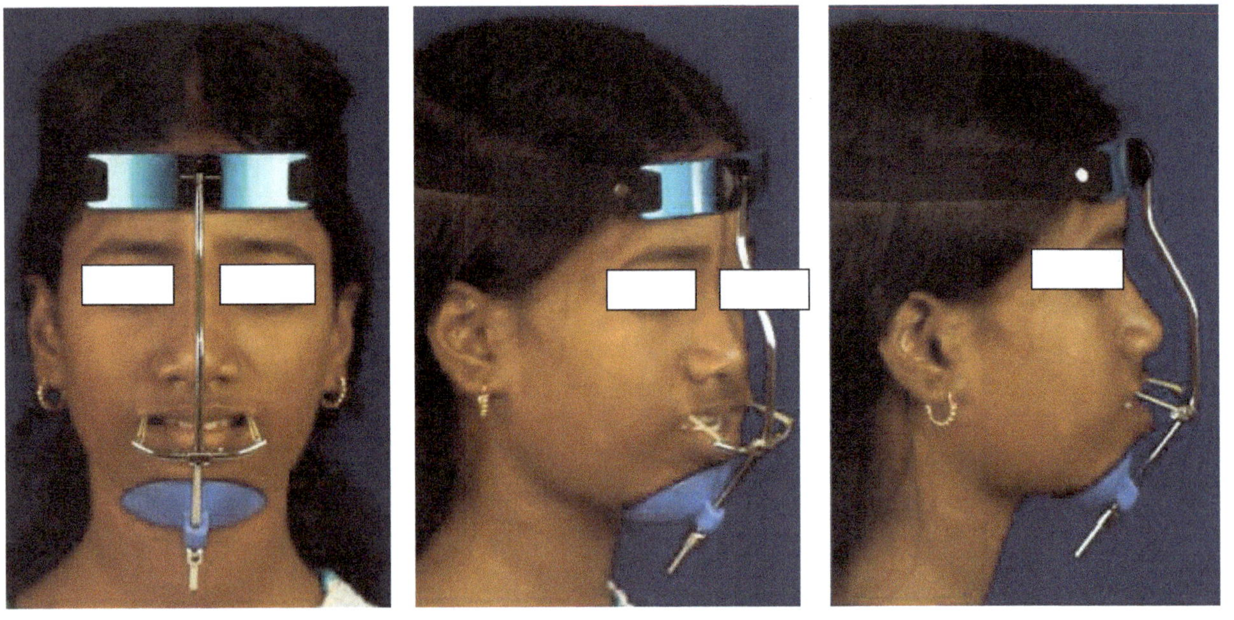

FIGURE 3: Facemask therapy.

growth and redirection of mandibular growth; correct the anterior and posterior crossbites; and obtain Class I molar and canine relationships with correct overbite and overjet along with coincident midlines [12–14]. An alternative to early treatment was to delay fixed-appliance therapy until the permanent dentition had erupted and the growth spurt had ended. This plan, however, would have required extractions and camouflage treatment.

On the other hand, early protraction facemask therapy could effectively reduce the skeletal discrepancy, simplifying orthodontic treatment and reducing the tendency to relapse. The patient was young enough that good cooperation could be expected. The treatment objectives were as follows.

(i) Leveling and Aligning Both the Arches. Leveling and alignment are important to achieve proper occlusion.

(ii) Correction of Overjet. With the expansion, positive overjet can be achieved.

(iii) Correction of Molar Relation on Both Sides. Molar relation needs correction from Class II to Class I occlusion.

(iv) Correction of Canine Relation. Canine relation needs to be stable Class I canine.

(v) Achieving Lip Competency. With the correction of overjet, lip competency can be achieved.

5. Treatment Plan

The treatment planning included the following:

(1) Assessment of growth potential:

  (i) Average growth pattern with 65–85% growth remaining.

(2) Assessment of etiologic factors:

  (i) Hereditary.

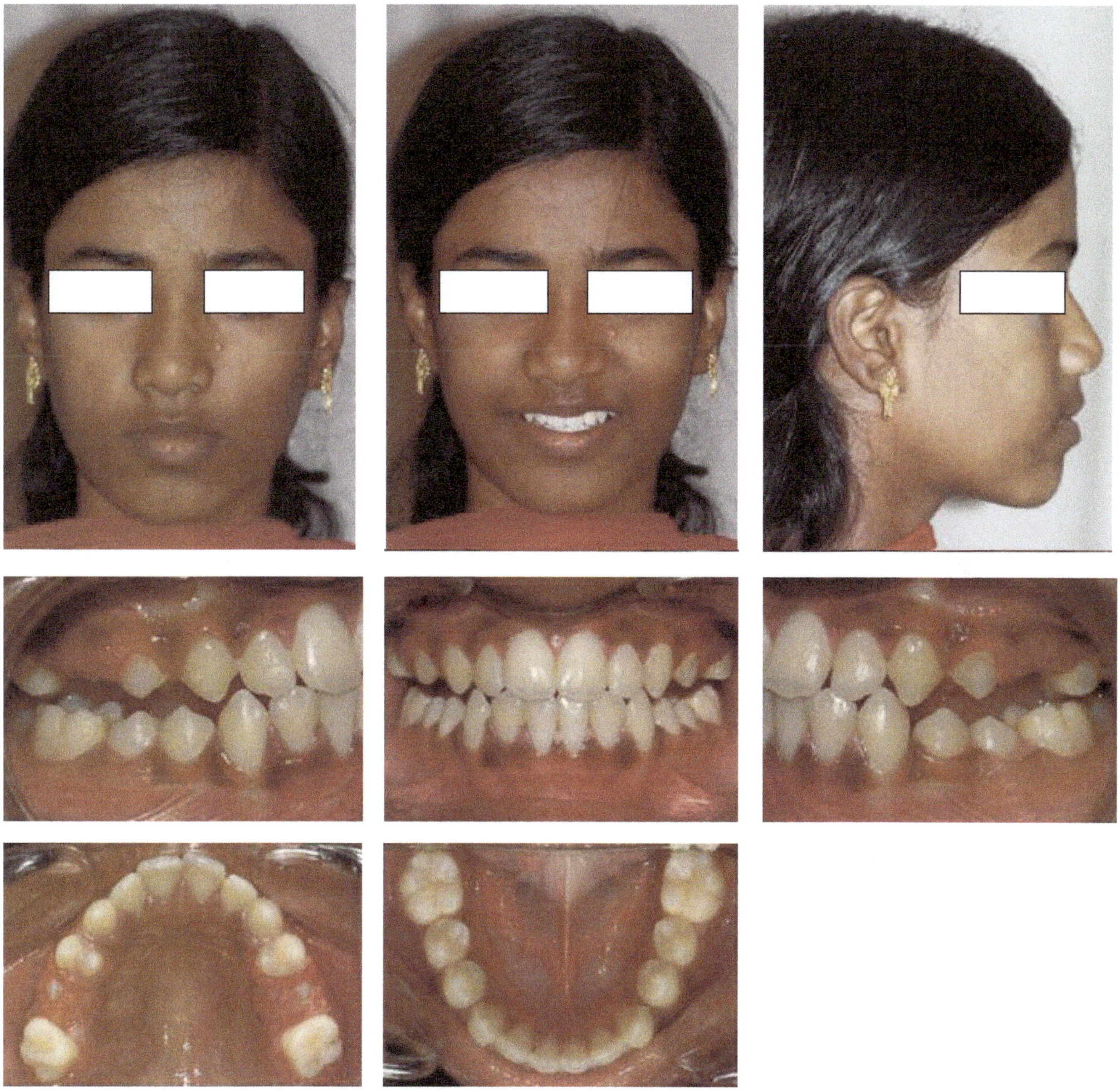

FIGURE 4: After facemask therapy.

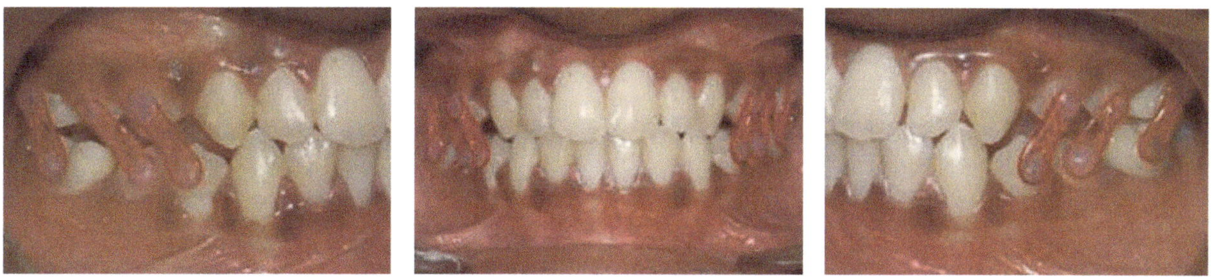

FIGURE 5: Occlusal settling.

TABLE 1: Comprehensive cephalometric evaluation (sagittal and dentoalveolar).

S. number	Measurements	Normal values	Before treatment	After treatment
1	SNA	80° ± 2°	80°	84°
2	SNB	80° ± 2°	84°	82°
3	ANB	2° ± 2°	−4°	2°
4	Co-Gn-Mandibular length		111 mm	113 mm
5	Co-point A		80 mm	85 mm
6	Na I to Pog	Small −8 to −6	−2 mm	+1 mm
7	I to SN	102°	104°	105°
8	I to PP	720	56°	55°
9	I to MP (IMPA)	90	97°	96°
10	I to NB	25°	34°	33°
11	Interincisal angle	132°	115°	115°
12	I to NA	4 mm	8 mm	6 mm
13	I to Apog	2–4 mm	10 mm	5 mm
14	I to NB	4 mm	9 mm	6 mm

TABLE 2: Comprehensive cephalometric evaluation (vertical).

S. number	Measurements	Normal values	Before treatment	After treatment
		Angular measurements		
1	Facial axis (Ricketts)	90° ± 3	95°	91°
2	*y*-axis	66°	60°	61°
3	Sn-Go-Gn	32°	26°	29°
4	FH-M.P. (F.M.A.)	25°	24°	25°
5	Angle of inclination	85°	87°	85°
6	Basal-plane angle Pal-MP	25°	21°	24°
7	OCC - Pal	11°	8°	4°
8	OCC - Man	14°	16°	18°
9	Gonial angle Ar-G0-Gn (Bjork)	130° ± 7°	124°	124°
10	Upper Gonial angle	50°–55°	54°	54°
11	Lower Gonial angle	70°–75°	70°	70°

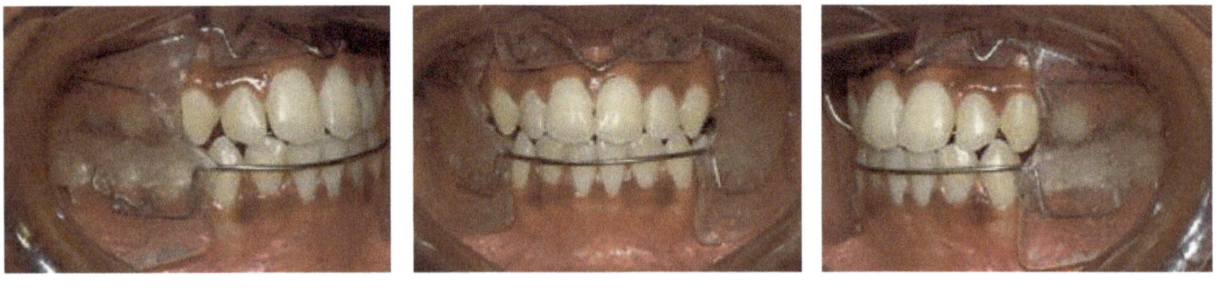

FIGURE 6: Retention with Fr-3.

(3) Planning for final interincisal relationship:

(i) Ideal overjet and bite.

The appliance included protraction facemask with bonded RME to correct the skeletal relation and the retention plan included Frankel-III. RME with Hyrax Expansion screw was activated once per day until we achieved the desired increase in transverse dimension (Figure 2). After the patient is accustomed to wearing, facemask treatment is initiated (Figure 3). A force of 14 OZ/side is delivered to the maxillary complex. The appliance is worn full time (about 20 hours/day) for 6 months. After facemask therapy (Figure 4), occlusal settling was done (Figure 5) and the patient was retained using a Frankel-3 appliance (Figure 6), 20 hours per day, with the patient removing the appliance only during activities such as eating and playing sports.

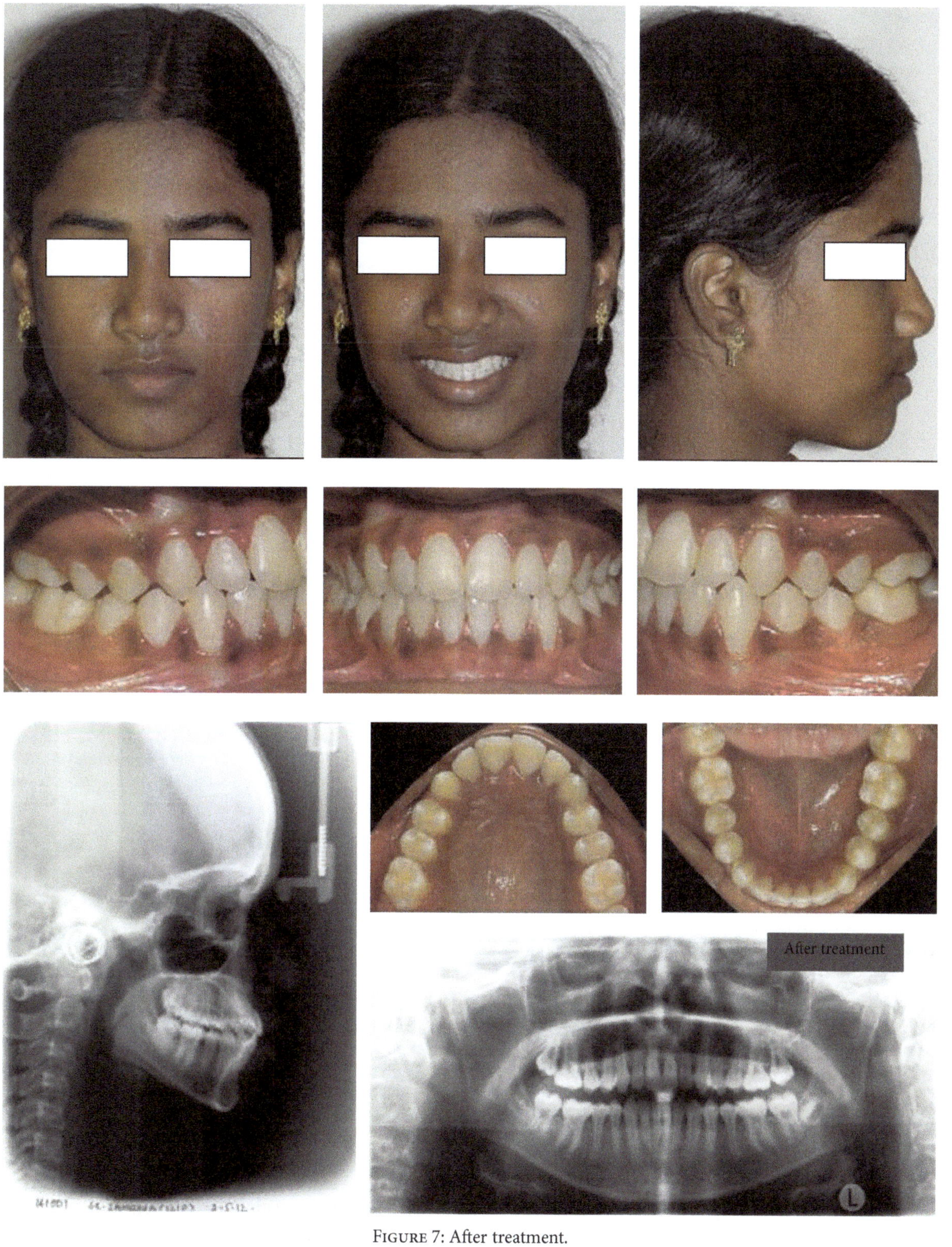

FIGURE 7: After treatment.

6. Treatment Results

Patient compliance was excellent with both the facemask and the elastics. The patient displayed a bilateral Class I canine occlusion and a Class I molar relationship (Figure 7). The arch forms were symmetrical and well aligned. The SNA angle had increased while SNB decreased resulting in a normal jaw relationship (ANB = 2°). Normal overbite (1 mm) and overjet (3 mm) were achieved, and the midlines were centered. Vertical skeletal measurements remained near-constant with

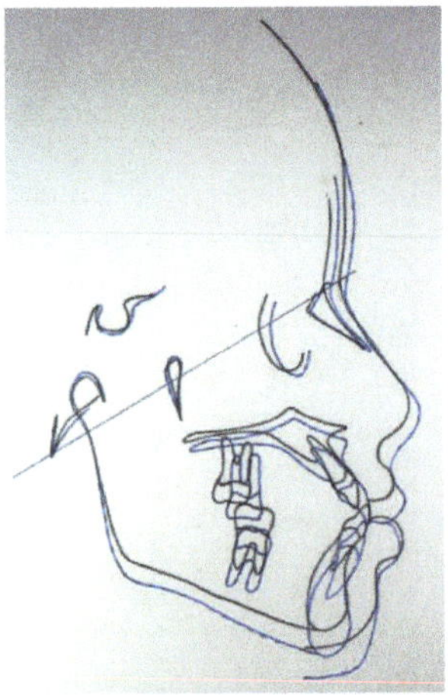

FIGURE 8: Superimposition.

an increase in Sn-Go-Gn angle by 3 degrees. The buccal crossbite was corrected. Canine rise and incisal guidance were established; lateral and jaw-opening excursions were smooth and straight. The patient's face appeared symmetrical with competent lips. The esthetic balance was significantly improved in the lateral view and the lips were in a normal relationship. Intraoral radiographs showed good root parallelism.

Cephalometric analysis confirmed that the concave profile had been straightened (Figure 8). Results are demonstrated in Tables 1 and 2.

7. Discussion

Numerous studies have demonstrated the importance of early treatment in Class III patients. We have chosen Facemask RME therapy for achieving maxillary skeletal protraction, redirecting mandibular growth in downward and backward direction. Maxillary protraction is recommended for patients with skeletal Class III malocclusion and maxillary deficiency. For most patients with Class III malocclusion seen in the early mixed dentition or late deciduous dentition, Facemask is the customary choice [15]. Skeletal correction can also be corrected by using miniplates anchored with intermaxillary elastics followed by fixed mechanotherapy [16].

Most of the studies on the effects of posteroanterior traction of the maxillary complex in Class III patients have demonstrated that improvement in intermaxillary sagittal skeletal relationships was associated with an increase in vertical skeletal relationships which can be particularly unfavorable in hyperdivergent Class III patients. But, in recent studies, the vertical skeletal features do not influence the short term outcomes of RME/FM therapy [17]. As in our case, vertical measurements did not show any marked difference. Lingual tipping of the lower incisors has been achieved. After the facial mask and the RME appliance have been removed, the patient is retained using FR-3 appliance [18].

It is used since it is easiest to manage clinically because no substantial postural change is produced in the maxillo-mandibular relationship. The effects produced are similar to that of facemask therapy.

Conflict of Interests

The authors declare that there is no conflict of interests regarding the publication of this paper.

References

[1] T. M. Graber, R. L. Van, and K. W. L. Vig, "Treatment of patients in the mixed dentition," in *Orthodontics: Current Principles and Techniques*, T. M. Graber and R. L. Vanarsdall, Eds., pp. 565–569, Mosby, St. Louis, Mo, USA, 2009.

[2] G. Cozzani, "Extraoral traction and class III treatment," *American Journal of Orthodontics*, vol. 80, no. 6, pp. 638–650, 1981.

[3] L. De Toffol, C. Pavoni, T. Baccetti, L. Franchi, and P. Cozza, "Orthopedic treatment outcomes in Class III malocclusion: a systematic review," *Angle Orthodontist*, vol. 78, no. 3, pp. 561–573, 2008.

[4] J. A. McNamara Jr., "An orthopedic approach to the treatment of Class III malocclusion in young patients.," *Journal of Clinical Orthodontics*, vol. 21, no. 9, pp. 598–608, 1987.

[5] P. Ngan, "Early timely treatment of class III malocclusion," *Seminars in Orthodontics*, vol. 11, no. 3, pp. 140–145, 2005.

[6] J. Delaire, "Confection dur masque orthopedique," *Revue de Stomatologie et de Chirurgie Maxillo-Faciale*, vol. 72, pp. 579–584, 1971.

[7] P. Ngan, "Early treatment of Class III malocclusion: is it worth the burden?" *American Journal of Orthodontics & Dentofacial Orthopedics*, vol. 129, no. 4, supplement, pp. S82–S85, 2006.

[8] P. V. Westwood, J. A. McNamara Jr., T. Baccetti, L. Franchi, and D. M. Sarver, "Long-term effects of class III treatment with rapid maxillary expansion and facemask therapy followed by fixed appliances," *American Journal of Orthodontics and Dentofacial Orthopedics*, vol. 123, no. 3, pp. 306–320, 2003.

[9] P. Ngan, S. H. Wei, U. Hagg, K. Y. Yiu, D. Merwin, and B. Stickel, "Effect of protraction headgear on class III malocclusion," *Quintessence International*, vol. 23, no. 3, pp. 197–207, 1992.

[10] P. K. Turley, "Managing the developing Class III malocclusion with palatal expansion and facemask therapy," *American Journal of Orthodontics & Dentofacial Orthopedics*, vol. 122, no. 4, pp. 349–352, 2002.

[11] S. J. Sung and H. S. Baik, "Assessment of skeletal and dental changes by maxillary protraction," *American Journal of Orthodontics and Dentofacial Orthopedics*, vol. 114, no. 5, pp. 492–502, 1998.

[12] J. S. McGill and J. A. McNamara Jr., "Treatment and post-treatment effects of rapid maxillary expansion and facial mask therapy," in *Growth Modification: What Works What Doesn't and Why*, J. A. McNamara, Ed., vol. 36 of *Monograph, Craniofacial Growth Series*, Center for Human Growth and Development, Ann Arbor, Mich, USA, 1999.

[13] M. D. Williams, D. M. Sarver, P. L. Sadowsky, and E. Bradley, "Combined rapid maxillary expansion and protraction facemask in the treatment of class III malocclusions in growing children: a prospective long-term study," *Seminars in orthodontics*, vol. 3, no. 4, pp. 265–274, 1997.

[14] J. S. McGill, *Orthopedic alterations induced by rapid maxillary expansion and face mask therapy [M.S. thesis]*, University of Michigan, Ann Arbor, Mich, USA, 1995.

[15] D. Gencer, E. Kaygisiz, S. Yüksel, and T. Tortop, "Comparison of double-plate appliance/facemask combination and facemask therapy in treating Class III malocclusions," *Angle Orthodontist*, vol. 85, no. 2, pp. 278–283, 2015.

[16] E. Esenlik, C. Ağlarcı, G. E. Albayrak, and Y. Fındık, "Maxillary protraction using skeletal anchorage and intermaxillary elastics in Skeletal Class III patients," *Korean Journal of Orthodontics*, vol. 45, no. 2, pp. 95–101, 2015.

[17] C. Pavoni, C. Masucci, S. Cerroni, L. Franchi, and P. Cozza, "Short-term effects produced by rapid maxillary expansion and facemask therapy in class III patients with different vertical skeletal relationships," *The Angle Orthodontist*, vol. 85, no. 6, pp. 927–933, 2015.

[18] J. A. McNamara Jr. and S. A. Huge, "The functional regulator (FR-3) of Fränkel," *American Journal of Orthodontics*, vol. 88, no. 5, pp. 409–424, 1985.

Direct Midline Diastema Closure with Composite Layering Technique: A One-Year Follow-Up

Bora Korkut, Funda Yanikoglu, and Dilek Tagtekin

Department of Restorative Dentistry, Faculty of Dentistry, Marmara University, 34746 Istanbul, Turkey

Correspondence should be addressed to Bora Korkut; bora.korkut@marmara.edu.tr

Academic Editor: Tatiana Pereira-Cenci

Objective. Maxillary anterior spacing is a common aesthetic complaint of patients. Midline diastema has a multifactorial etiology such as labial frenulum, microdontia, mesiodens, peg-shaped lateral incisors, agenesis, cysts, habits such as finger sucking, tongue thrusting, or lip sucking, dental malformations, genetics, proclinations, dental-skeletal discrepancies, and imperfect coalescence of interdental septum. Appropriate technique and material for effective treatment are based on time, physical, psychological, and economical limitations. Direct composite resins in diastema cases allow dentist and patient complete control of these limitations and formation of natural smile. *Clinical Considerations.* In this case report a maxillary midline diastema was closed with direct composite resin restorations in one appointment without any preparation. One bottle total etch adhesive was used and translucent/opaque composite resin shades were layered on mesial surfaces of the teeth that were isolated with rubber dam and Teflon bands. Finishing and polishing procedures were achieved by using polishing discs. Patient was informed for recalls for every 6 months. *Conclusions.* At one-year recall no sensitivities, discolorations, or fractures were detected on teeth and restorations. Direct composite resins seemed to be highly aesthetic and durable restorations that can satisfy patients as under the conditions of case presented.

1. Introduction

Maxillary anterior spacing or diastema is a common aesthetic complaint of patients [1]. Keene described midline diastema as anterior midline spacing greater than 0.5 mm between the proximal surfaces of adjacent teeth [2]. It was reported that maxilla has a higher prevalence of midline diastema than mandible [3]. The midline diastema has a multifactorial etiology. In addition to the labial frenulum, microdontia, mesiodens, peg-shaped lateral incisors, lateral incisor agenesis, cysts in the midline region, habits such as finger sucking, tongue thrusting, and/or lip sucking, dental malformations, genetics, maxillary incisor proclination, dental-skeletal discrepancies, and imperfect coalescence of the interdental septum should be considered factors that can cause diastema [4, 5]. The width to length ratio of the central incisors for aesthetic rehabilitation in complex midline diastema closure cases determines the treatment plan. Decisions such as the amount of distal proximal reduction, the number of teeth to be treated, the placement and location of prominences and concavities to create the illusion, and the decision for full-veneers or just adding to the interproximal are decided according to that ratio [6]. The appropriate technique and material for a patient are also based on time, physical, psychological, and economic limitations [7, 8]. Direct composite resins in diastema closure cases allow dentist and patient complete control in formation of natural smile [9]. Improved materials and techniques are often introduced leading professionals to endless improvement while fulfilling their patients' aesthetic demands [10]. Recent aesthetic composite resin materials have similar physical and mechanical properties to that of the natural tooth and possess an appearance like natural dentin and enamel [11]. They offer an expanded range of shades and varying opacities designed specifically for layering technique whereas early brands of composite resins offered only "body" shades and appeared dull and dense [11–13].

This case report describes direct aesthetic midline diastema closure with composite layering technique.

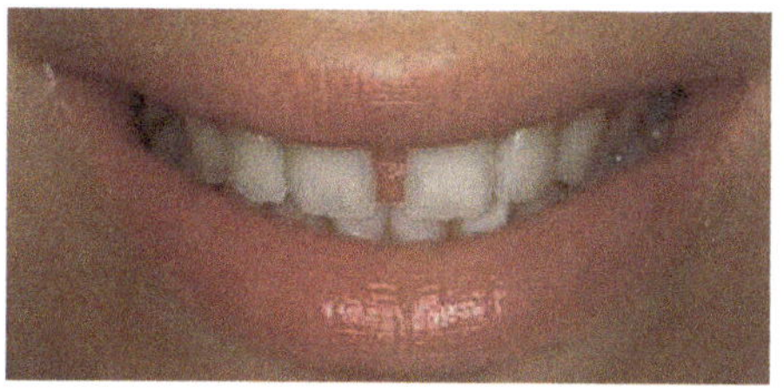

FIGURE 1: Preoperative extraoral view of the patient with aesthetic problems due to the tongue thrust.

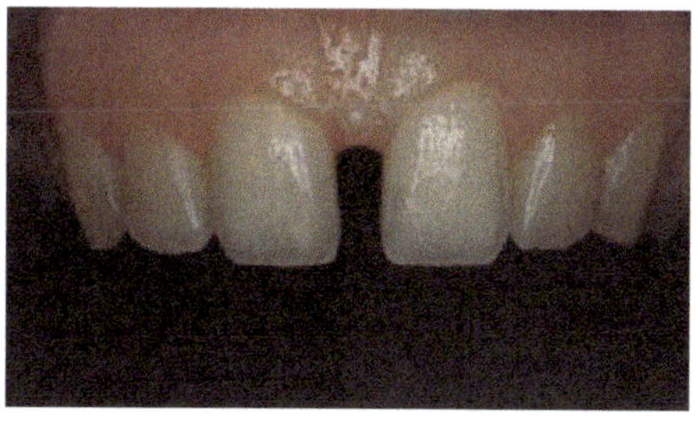

FIGURE 2: Preoperative intraoral view of the patient and the midline diastema.

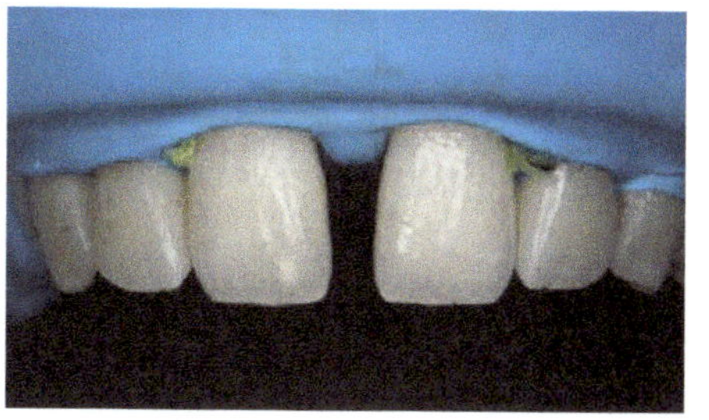

FIGURE 3: Maxillary anterior teeth were isolated with rubber dam and the central incisors were retracted with retraction cord. No preparations were achieved.

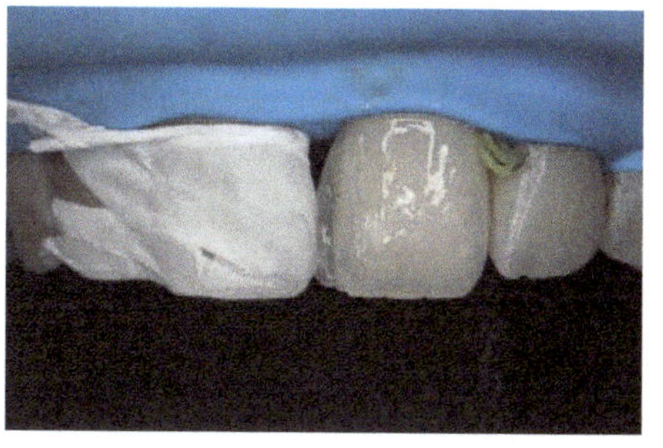

FIGURE 4: The adjacent central incisor was covered with Teflon band while the other was restored. A thin layer of JE shade transparent composite resin was used palatinally as enamel.

2. Case Report

A 32-year-old male patient reported to the Department of Restorative Dentistry, Faculty of Dentistry, Marmara University, with the chief complaint of spacing in the upper front tooth region. Patient's medical history did not reveal any systemic diseases and intraoral examination revealed presence of midline spacing between maxillary central incisors (~4 mm) due to tongue thrust parafunction (Figure 1). No dental caries were observed in both clinical and radiographical examinations. As a more conservative, economical, aesthetic, and quicker option, direct aesthetic partial composite laminate veneers as build-ups for both maxillary central incisors were considered.

Firstly, shade selection was considered A1 shade of Vita guide for the teeth to be restored. In order to simulate a natural A1 shade outlook, the shades BW, A1, and JE (Gaenial, GC, Japan) were decided to be used together as layers. No preparations were performed before the restoration procedure (Figure 2). All maxillary incisors were isolated with rubber dam (Kerr, USA) and the central incisors were retracted by using retraction cord (Figure 3). The adjacent central incisor was covered with Teflon band while the other was restored. 37% phosphoric acid (Etching Gel, Kerr, USA) was applied on the mesial surface to be restored for 15 seconds, rinsed for 20 seconds, and dried with air slightly. Then a single bottle bonding agent (Adper Single Bond, 3M ESPE, USA) was applied and polymerized for 20 seconds with a LED light generator (Demi Led Light Curing System, Kerr, USA). A thin layer of JE shade transparent composite resin was used palatinally as enamel (Figure 4). A thin layer of BW shade opaque composite resin was placed roughly as second layer (Figure 5). A1 shade composite resin was used as dentin layer and a thin layer JE shade was used as the top enamel layer. Labial surfaces of the restorations were flattened by using a red banded knife-edge tip diamond bur (Acurata, Germany) (Figure 6). Polishing discs (Ultra Gloss Composite Polishing System, Axis, USA) were used for detailed polishing from rough to fine grains by using a low speed handpiece (DURAtec 2068D, Germany) (Figures 7 and 8).

The patient was motivated for oral hygiene and informed for recalls. At the 6-month recall the restorations were just polished with polishing discs. At one-year recall no sensitivities, discolorations, or fractures were detected on the teeth and the restorations (Figure 9).

3. Discussion

The direct composite resin restorations can be placed in a single visit, often do not require preliminary models or wax-ups, and do not involve laboratory fees that escalate costs. In terms of aesthetic dentistry, these restorations offer numerous advantages that other possible treatment options such as ceramic veneers and orthodontic treatment do not have. They are kinder to the opposing dentition compared to ceramic materials [14] and, in the event of an unforeseen fracture, they can be repaired easily compared to costly and time-consuming repairs or remakes for porcelain alternatives [15]. There are also some disadvantages of direct composite resin restorations compared to some indirect porcelain alternatives. Most composite materials possess less fractural toughness, shear, and compressive strength and are not ideally suited for ultra-high-stress areas found in

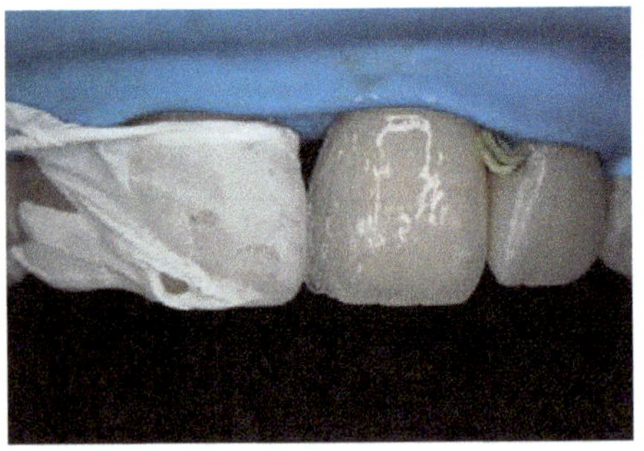

FIGURE 5: A thin layer of BW shade opaque composite resin was placed roughly as the second layer.

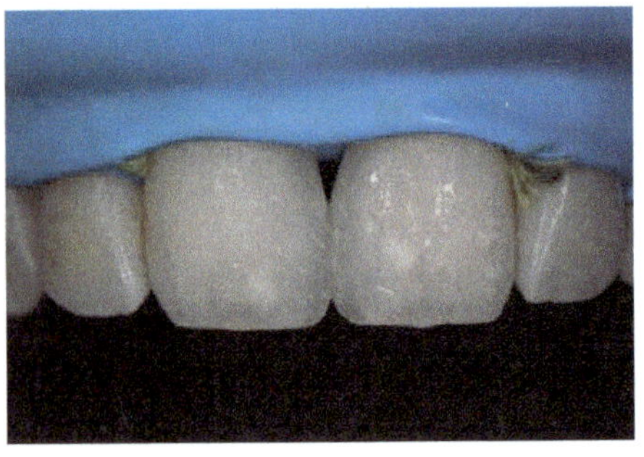

FIGURE 6: A1 shade composite resin was used as dentin layer and a thin layer of JE shade was used as the top enamel layer. Labial surfaces of the restorations were flattened by using a red banded knife-edge tip diamond bur.

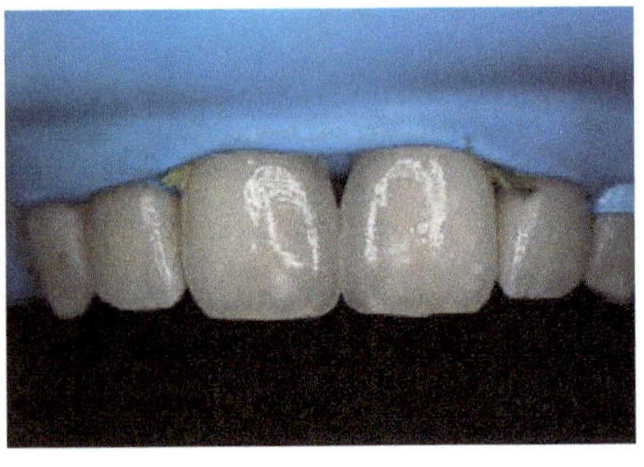

FIGURE 7: Polishing discs were used for detailed polishing from rough to fine grit.

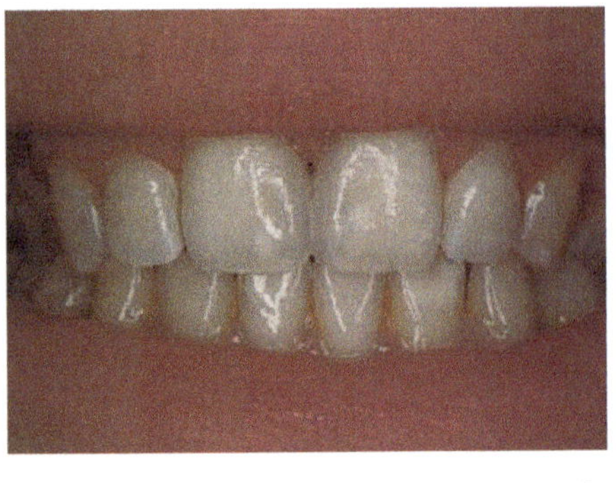

FIGURE 8: Postoperative view of the restorations just after removal of the rubber dam and the retraction cords.

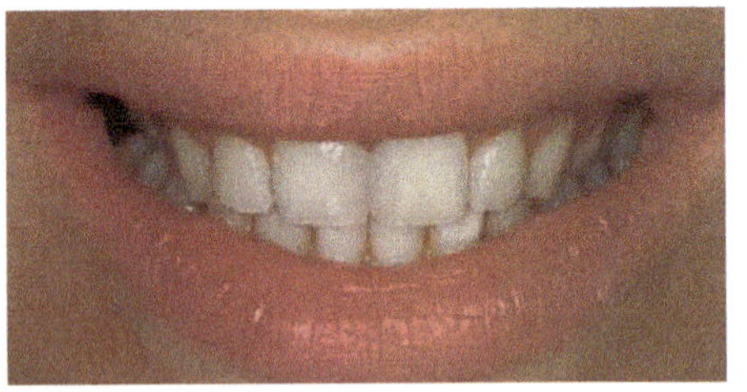

FIGURE 9: The view of the restorations at one-year recall.

certain clinical situations [16, 17]. Presence of unmanaged parafunctional forces such as bruxism, Class III end-to-end occlusal schemes, or noxious oral habits such as nail biting can potentially jeopardize the longevity of direct composite resin restorations [12, 18]. Moreover, the color stability of direct composite resin restorations is not as inert as glazed ceramics; however, this depends on the quality of finishing and polishing procedures and can be prevented with recalls [19, 20]. Regardless of the fact that direct composite resin restorations have these disadvantages, the developing adhesive techniques and better quality resin materials give dentists the chance to create more conservative, functional, aesthetic, economic, and long lasting restorations also in a very short chair time [21, 22].

In this case report, one-year recall of a midline diastema closure treatment by using direct composite resins was assessed. Creating a wax-up restoration previously to simulate the diastema closure and building a silicon matrix to guide final composite resin restoration are a common method for this kind of cases [8, 22]. However, in this case report, another technique was used without creating a silicon matrix. The midline diastema was closed by building up the mesial surfaces of central incisors one by one. The teeth were isolated with rubber dam, retraction cords, and the central incisor adjacent to the one to be restored was covered with Teflon band. Teflon band is a very thin band that gives the opportunity to create very close contact and perfect isolation where resin based restoration materials do not adhere. There was no need for using transparent matrix bands or wedges in this technique. This isolation technique allowed us to create two separate restorations having a really close natural alike contact without creating a dark triangle because of not using wedge which are important advantages compared with the silicon matrix technique [8]. The teeth were restored one by one by layering technique that can also be used in silicon matrix technique [13]. The treatments without creating previous wax-up restorations and a silicon matrix were performed in a very short period of time which is another advantage. In this technique the positioning of the midline and the location of the contact area were decided by the dentist allowing him/her to simulate a natural outlook. However, these decisions and restorations without a guide such as silicon matrix are not easy to perform. The dentist should be well experienced about this technique in order to create a correct midline as well as a natural smile design which can be calculated as a disadvantage compared with the other technique.

Restoration using ceramic fragment is another treatment option for these cases. It is an indirect ceramic restoration that is prepared in a laboratory and attached to previously prepared area of tooth. This technique needs at least two appointments which can be defined as a disadvantage compared with direct techniques. According to the manipulation of the technician, the restorations by using ceramic fragments can be functional and simulate natural esthetics [11]. On the other hand recent studies also showed that direct composite resin restorations are considered functional, stable, aesthetical, and cheaper restorations completed in less chair time by using appropriate techniques for patients with appropriate occlusion [8, 13]. Capability of being repaired easily in case of fractures is another important advantage of direct composite resin restorations. Although direct resin restorations are considered to be stable, the color stability of ceramic restorations is still much better. The best solution for this problem is the perfection in finishing and polishing procedures and frequent recalls [8, 21]. In this case report direct composite resin restorations were decided as the treatment method due to aesthetical demands of the patient having restricted time and money.

At six-month and one-year recalls the general outlook of the maxillary anterior teeth was considered natural and aesthetical. Clinically, both restorations have no fractures and also the restoration margins on both maxillary central incisors demonstrated no discolorations. Although one-year follow-up does not seem long enough and further long term follow-ups are required, restoration problems such as marginal leakage, discolorations, fractures, and debonding for composite resins generally merge within 6 months after the treatment. By taking this into consideration and according to the positive results, an experienced dentist with proper case selection, using an appropriate technique and modern materials, can perform highly aesthetic and durable direct composite resin restorations that can satisfy patients as under the conditions of the case presented.

Conflict of Interests

The authors of this paper declare that there is no conflict of interests regarding the publication of this paper.

References

[1] K. Koora, M. S. Muthu, and P. V. Rathna, "Spontaneous closure of midline diastema following frenectomy," *Journal of Indian Society of Pedodontics and Preventive Dentistry*, vol. 25, no. 1, pp. 23–26, 2007.

[2] H. J. Keene, "Distribution of diastemas in the dentition of man," *American Journal of Physical Anthropology*, vol. 21, no. 4, pp. 437–441, 1963.

[3] J. T. Kaimenyi, "Occurrence of midline diastema and frenum attachments amongst school children in Nairobi, Kenya," *Indian Journal of Dental Research*, vol. 9, no. 2, pp. 67–71, 1998.

[4] Weber, *Quoted in: Orthodontic Principles and Practice*, edited by: T. M. Graber, W.B. Saunders Company, 3rd edition, 1972.

[5] O. M. Tanaka, A. Y. K. Morino, O. F. Machuca, and N. Á. Schneider, "When the midline diastema is not characteristic of the 'ugly duckling' stage," *Case Reports in Dentistry*, vol. 2015, Article ID 924743, 5 pages, 2015.

[6] N. Blitz, "Direct bonding in diastema closure—high drama, immediate resolution," *Oral Health*, vol. 86, no. 7, pp. 23–29, 1996.

[7] P. R. Chalifoux, "Perception esthetics: factors that affect smile design," *Journal of Esthetic and Restorative Dentistry*, vol. 8, no. 4, pp. 189–192, 1996.

[8] R. Prabhu, S. Bhaskaran, K. G. Prabhu, M. Eswaran, G. Phanikrishna, and B. Deepthi, "Clinical evaluation of direct composite restoration done for midline diastema closure-long-term study," *Journal of Pharmacy and Bioallied Sciences*, vol. 7, no. 6, article 559, 2015.

[9] B. G. Dale and K. W. Aschheim, Eds., *Esthetic Dentistry: A Clinical Approach to Techniques and Materials*, vol. 11, Lea and Febiger, Philadelphia, Pa, USA, 1993.

[10] Y.-K. Lee, B.-S. Lim, and C.-W. Kim, "Effect of surface conditions on the color of dental resin composites," *Journal of Biomedical Materials Research*, vol. 63, no. 5, pp. 657–663, 2002.

[11] B. Bağış and H. Y. Bağış, "Porselen laminate veneerlerin klinik uygulama aşamaları: klinik bir olgu sunumu," *Ankara Üniversitesi Diş Hekimliği Fakültesi Dergisi*, vol. 33, no. 1, pp. 49–57, 2006.

[12] R. Hickel, D. Heidemann, H. J. Staehle, P. Minnig, and N. H. Wilson, "Direct composite restorations: extended use in anterior and posterior situations," *Clinical Oral Investigations*, vol. 8, no. 2, pp. 43–44, 2004.

[13] G. Khashayar, A. Dozic, C. J. Kleverlaan, A. J. Feilzer, and J. Roeters, "The influence of varying layer thicknesses on the color predictability of two different composite layering concepts," *Dental Materials*, vol. 30, no. 5, pp. 493–498, 2014.

[14] P. Magne and U. C. Belser, "Porcelain versus composite inlays/onlays: effects of mechanical loads on stress distribution, adhesion, and crown flexure," *The International Journal of Periodontics & Restorative Dentistry*, vol. 23, no. 6, pp. 543–555, 2003.

[15] S. Berksun, P. S. Kedici, and S. Saglam, "Repair of fractured porcelain restorations with composite bonded porcelain laminate contours," *The Journal of Prosthetic Dentistry*, vol. 69, no. 5, pp. 457–458, 1993.

[16] R. E. Jordan, *Esthetic Composite Bonding Techniques and Materials*, Mosby-Year Book, St. Louis, Mo, USA, 2nd edition, 1993.

[17] C. F. J. Stappert, U. Ozden, T. Gerds, and J. R. Strub, "Longevity and failure load of ceramic veneers with different preparation designs after exposure to masticatory simulation," *Journal of Prosthetic Dentistry*, vol. 94, no. 2, pp. 132–139, 2005.

[18] K. W. Hemmings, U. R. Darbar, and S. Vaughan, "Tooth wear treated with direct composite restorations at an increased vertical dimension: results at 30 months," *The Journal of Prosthetic Dentistry*, vol. 83, no. 3, pp. 287–293, 2000.

[19] D. A. Garber, R. E. Goldstein, and R. A. Feinman, *Porcelain Laminate Veneers*, Quintessence Publishing, Chicago, Ill, USA, 1988.

[20] B. Bağış and H. Y. Bağış, "Porselen laminate veneerlerin klinik Uygulama aşamaları: Klinik bir olgu sunumu," *Ankara Üniversitesi Diş Hekimliği Fakültesi Dergisi*, vol. 33, pp. 49–57, 2006.

[21] A. Azzaldeen and A. H. Muhamad, "Diastema closure with direct composite: architectural gingival contouring," *Journal of Advanced Medical and Dental Sciences Research*, vol. 3, no. 1, pp. 134–139, 2015.

[22] M. Demirci, S. Tuncer, E. Öztaş, N. Tekçe, and Ö. Uysal, "A 4-year clinical evaluation of direct composite build-ups for space closure after orthodontic treatment," *Clinical Oral Investigations*, vol. 19, no. 9, pp. 2187–2199, 2015.

41

A Case of Brain Abscess Caused by Medication-Related Osteonecrosis of the Jaw

Kenji Yamagata, Hiroki Nagai, Osamu Baba, Fumihiko Uchida, Naomi Kanno, Shogo Hasegawa, Toru Yanagawa, and Hiroki Bukawa

Department of Oral and Maxillofacial Surgery, Institute of Clinical Medicine, Faculty of Medicine, University of Tsukuba, 1-1-1 Tennodai, Tsukuba, Ibaraki 305-8575, Japan

Correspondence should be addressed to Kenji Yamagata; y-kenji@md.tsukuba.ac.jp

Academic Editor: Paolo Giacomo Arduino

Reports of brain abscesses caused by medication-related osteonecrosis of the jaw (MRONJ) are very rare. We here present the case of a 76-year-old man with terminal-stage prostatic carcinoma and a brain abscess caused by MRONJ at the maxilla. The patient had been treated with zoledronic acid and denosumab for bone metastasis. For the brain abscess, an antibiotic regimen based on ceftriaxone and metronidazole and a sequestrectomy contributed to a successful outcome. In the case of maxillary MRONJ extending to the maxillary sinus, active resection of the infected bone should be considered to prevent the spread of the infection beyond the maxillary sinus, into the ethmoid sinus, and into the brain.

1. Introduction

A brain abscess is a rare, life-threatening infection. It appears as a localized area of suppuration within the brain. Although brain abscesses have historically been resistant to antimicrobial chemotherapy, recent advances in neuroscanning techniques such as CT and MR imaging and the introduction of more effective antibiotics have reduced the mortality rate to 0–25% [1, 2]. Brain abscesses spreading from the pericranial contiguous focus of the paranasal sinuses, the middle ear, or a dental infection are reported to account for 25–50% of the cases [2]. There are very few reports of a brain abscess secondary to odontogenic infection [3].

Osteonecrosis of the jaw is a common side effect of antiresorptive drugs [4], which are administered to cancer patients to treat bone metastasis, multiple myeloma, and osteoporosis. However, reports of a brain abscess resulting from medication-related osteonecrosis of the jaw (MRONJ) are very rare. We here describe the case of a brain abscess caused by a maxillary MRONJ that extended to the maxillary sinus and ethmoid sinus.

2. Case Report

A 76-year-old man came to the Department of Oral and Maxillofacial Surgery, University of Tsukuba Hospital, with a three-month history of swelling of the left mandible. He had been diagnosed with stage IV prostatic carcinoma and multiple distant metastases and had been treated with zoledronic acid 4 mg for 22 times and denosumab 120 mg for 4 times. His face was symmetrical, with a fistula and pus discharge on the skin of the left mandible. The regional lymph nodes were normal, and there was no trismus. Examination of the oral cavity showed gingival swelling, redness, pus discharge, and loosening of teeth 35 and 36. Tooth 17 was lost naturally 2 months after the first visit, which revealed a sequestrum in the mouth; the sequestrum expanded over the next 8 months (Figure 1). A panoramic radiograph revealed separated sequestra of the right maxilla and the left mandible (Figure 2). Computed tomography (CT) revealed maxillary osteitis and sinusitis (Figure 3). An abscess had formed in the right maxillary sinus, and the patient complained of mild ophthalmalgia. Therefore, we performed a sequestrectomy of the right maxilla and drained the maxillary sinus under local

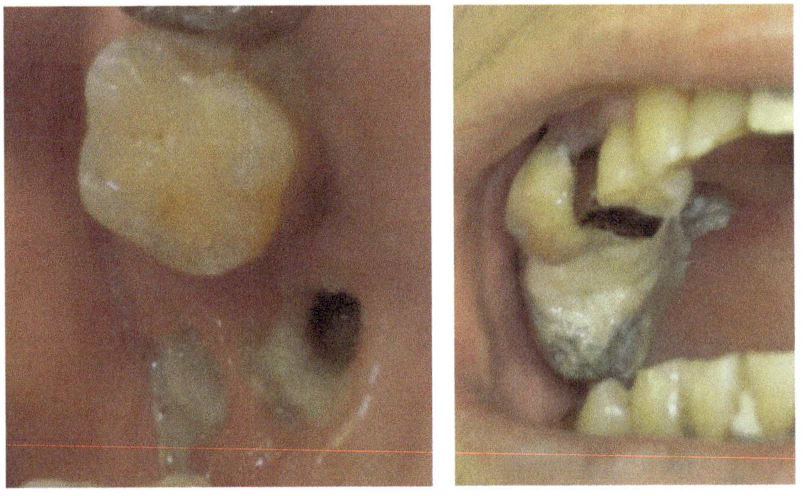

Figure 1: Intraoral examination.

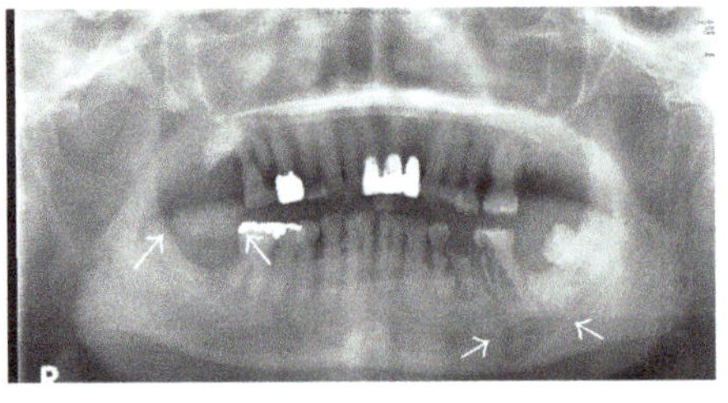

Figure 2: Preoperative panoramic radiograph.

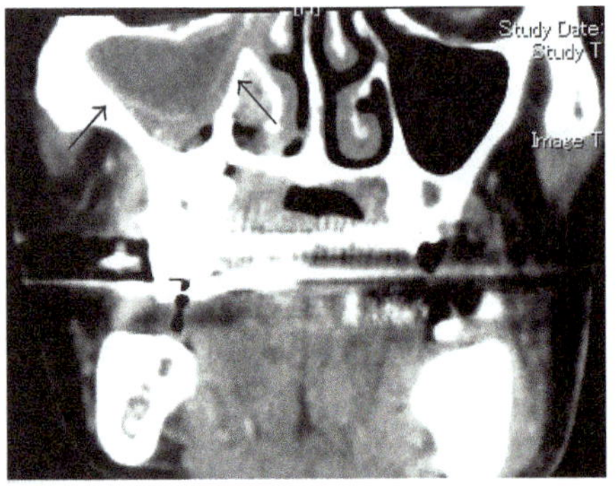

Figure 3: Preoperative CT revealing an abscess formation.

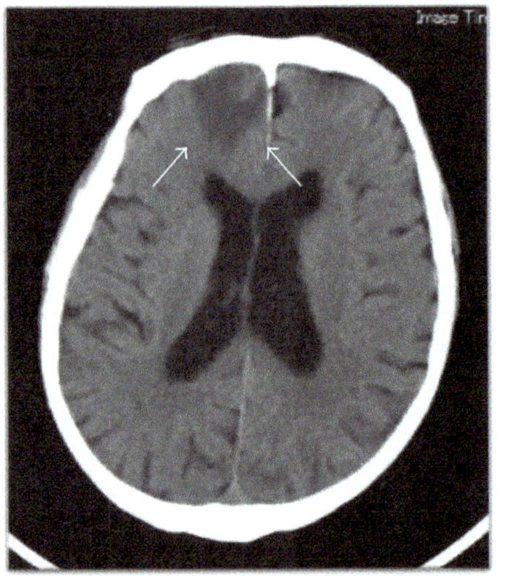

Figure 4: A CT showing a hypodense image in the right frontal lobe.

anesthesia. The postsurgical course on day 0 was uneventful, and the patient was discharged from the hospital; however, he was found unconscious in his house on the day after surgery and was brought by ambulance to the emergency room (ER) at our hospital. The patient's consciousness level was 13 in the Glasgow Coma Scale (eye opening 4, verbal response 4, motor response 5), and he had left conjugate deviation and left hemiparesis. General convulsions occurred continuous to the left upper and lower limb convulsions. The convulsions were resolved by administering diazepam (5 mg) twice and fosphenytoin (900 mg) once. Laboratory results showed elevated WBC (10,300/μL) and CRP (2.08 mg/dL). A brain CT revealed a hypodense lesion in the right frontal lobe (Figure 4). A T2-weighted MRI revealed a right frontal-lobe abscess and ethmoid sinusitis. The maxillary sinus was connected to the oral cavity, and the abscess in the maxillary sinus had disappeared (Figure 5). Diffusion-weighted imaging (DWI) MR imaging showed a low apparent diffusion coefficient (ADC) (Figure 6). A fall in the ADC in the fluid-filled lesion was highly suggestive of abscess.

The infection was suspected to have originated from the maxillary sequestrum and spread through the maxillary sinus, ethmoid sinus, and frontal sinus, and, by contiguity, to the frontal lobe. Although a bacterial culture of the maxillary sinus revealed only gram-positive and gram-negative bacilli and gram-positive cocci, these species were not found.

The patient was treated with ceftriaxone 2 g q12h and metronidazole 500 mg q8h for 50 days, with valproate Na 800 mg for convulsions. The enhanced area of brain infection disappeared in follow-up MR images (Figure 7). This case was

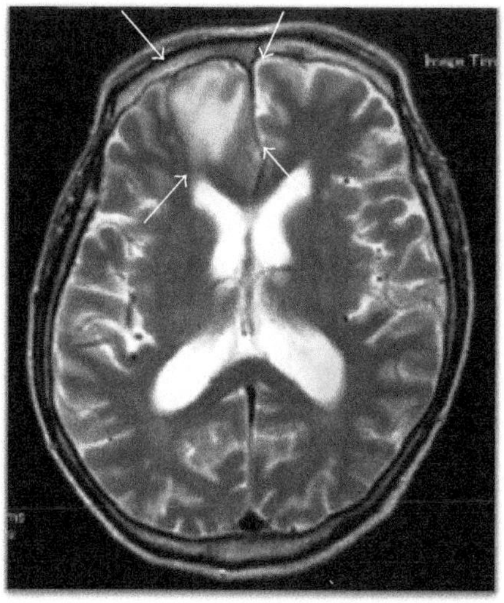

Figure 5: MR images (T2WI) showing hypointensity lesion in the right frontal lobe.

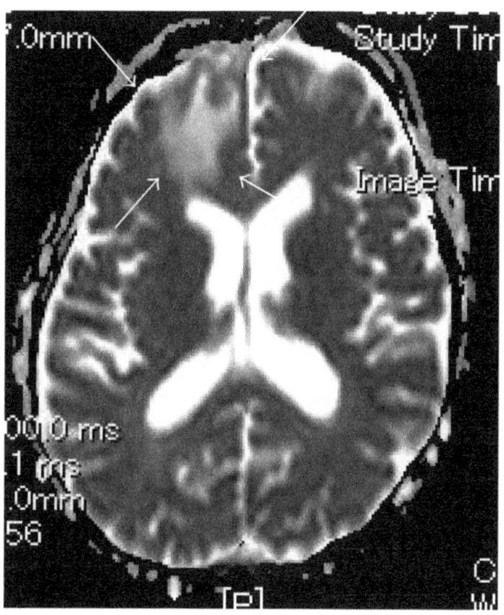

Figure 6: MR imaging (DWI) showing low apparent diffusion coefficient (ADC).

treated conservatively, without surgery, because the patient had terminal-stage cancer. The patient was discharged from the hospital after 2 months, without any left-limb paralysis.

3. Discussion

Brain abscess can originate exogenously, as when lesions are caused by skull trauma or surgery or, endogenously, from infections of continuous structures (e.g., otitis media sinusitis, mastoiditis, dental infections), from meningitis, or from the hematogenous spread of a remote infection (e.g., infective endocarditis, cyanotic congenital heart disease, pulmonary infections) [5]. A brain abscess caused by MRONJ is very rare.

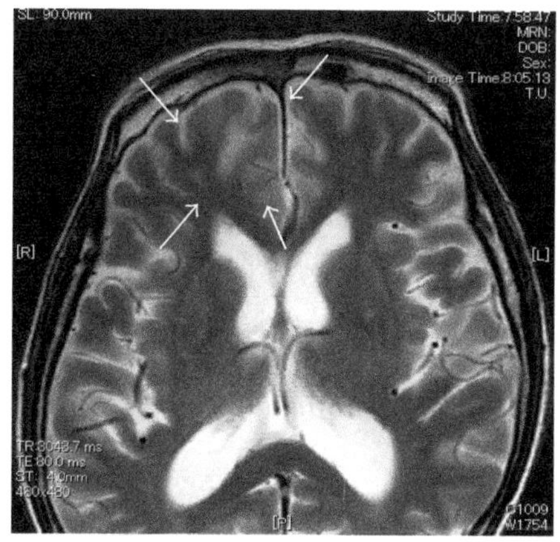

Figure 7: MR image (T2WI) obtained one month after beginning treatment.

The number of patients with MRONJ has grown recently. MRONJ is defined by the following characteristics: current or previous treatment with antiresorptive or antiangiogenic agents, exposed bone or bone that can be probed through an intraoral or extraoral fistula in the maxillofacial region that has persisted for more than 8 weeks, and no history of radiotherapy to the jaw or any obvious metastatic disease in the jaw [4].

A dental infection or ethmoid or frontal sinusitis that spreads to the brain generally causes a solitary brain abscess in the frontal lobe. Poor prognostic indicators include delayed diagnosis, a disease with rapid progression, coma, multiple lesions, intraventricular rupture, and fungal etiology, all of which are indicators seen in immunocompromised patients. Our patient was immunocompromised due to terminal prostate cancer. In the past, the overall mortality due to brain abscess was as high as 60%. Fortunately, new antibacterial approaches and new imaging technologies have decreased this mortality, and recent large case series have reported a mortality of 0%–25% [1, 2].

For a brain abscess originating from the paranasal sinuses, middle ear, or a dental infection, Arlotti et al. [5] recommend treatment with metronidazole 500 mg q8h and cefotaxime 2 g q6h or piperacillin/tazobactam 4.5 g q6h [5]. Accordingly, our patient was treated with ceftriaxone 2 g q12h and metronidazole 500 mg q8h for 50 days (ceftriaxone, like cefotaxime, is a third-generation cephalosporin). The pathogens related to this clinical scenario are the microaerophilic and anaerobic streptococci *Haemophilus* sp., *Bacteroides* sp., and *Fusobacterium* sp. in the paranasal sinusitis and streptococci, gram-negative bacilli, and *B. fragilis* in the dental infection [2]. In the present case, a bacterial culture of the brain abscess revealed only gram-positive and gram-negative bacilli and gram-positive cocci.

The treatment of cerebral abscess includes the immediate administration of high-dose intravenous antibiotics, followed by surgical craniotomy and resection of the abscess cavity with the removal of possible septic foci [3, 6]. Our patient was immediately treated with high-dose intravenous antibiotics. However, we did not perform a craniotomy or resection of the frontal-lobe abscess because of the patient's poor general condition. The point of origin of the infection, the necrotic maxillary bone, was removed under anesthesia prior to the patient's loss of consciousness.

The clinical symptoms and signs are nonspecific for brain abscesses, which present differently depending on the origin, size, and location of the abscess [5]; the virulence of the infecting organisms; and the underlying systemic conditions. The most common symptoms are headache, nausea, vomiting, fever, focal neurological deficits, and an alteration of mental status [7]. Our patient presented postoperatively with loss of consciousness and general convulsions following convulsions of the left upper and lower limbs. The patient complained of mild ophthalmalgia before surgery; in retrospect, we suspected that the ophthalmalgia was a symptom of the brain abscess. The patient's early diagnosis, supported by imaging, was important for the successful outcome.

In conclusion, when maxillary MRONJ extends to the maxillary sinus, active resection of the infected bone should be considered to prevent the spread of the infection beyond the maxillary sinus, to the ethmoid sinus, and into the brain.

Conflict of Interests

The authors declare that there is no conflict of interests regarding the publication of this paper.

References

[1] G. E. Mathisen and J. P. Johnson, "Brain abscess," *Clinical Infectious Diseases*, vol. 25, no. 4, pp. 763–781, 1997.

[2] H. Alvis-Miranda, S. M. Castellar-Leones, M. A. Elzain, and L. R. Moscote-Salazar, "Brain abscess: current management," *Journal of Neurosciences in Rural Practice*, vol. 4, no. 5, supplement 1, pp. S67–S81, 2013.

[3] J. Yang, S. Y. Liu, M. Hossaini-Zadeh, and M. A. Pogrel, "Brain abscess potentially secondary to odontogenic infection: case report," *Oral Surgery, Oral Medicine, Oral Pathology and Oral Radiology*, vol. 117, no. 2, pp. e108–e111, 2014.

[4] S. L. Ruggiero, T. B. Dodson, J. Fantasia et al., "American Association of Oral and Maxillofacial Surgeons position paper on medication-related osteonecrosis of the jaw—2014 update," *Journal of Oral and Maxillofacial Surgery*, vol. 72, no. 10, pp. 1938–1956, 2014.

[5] M. Arlotti, P. Grossi, F. Pea et al., "Consensus document on controversial issues for the treatment of infections of the central nervous system: bacterial brain abscesses," *International Journal of Infectious Diseases*, vol. 14, supplement 4, pp. S79–S92, 2010.

[6] A. I. Mylonas, F. H. Tzerbos, M. Mihalaki, D. Rologis, and I. Boutsikakis, "Cerebral abscess of odontogenic origin," *Journal of Cranio-Maxillo-Facial Surgery*, vol. 35, no. 1, pp. 63–67, 2007.

[7] M. Ben Hadj Hassine, L. Oualha, A. Derbel, and N. Douki, "Cerebral abscess potentially of odontogenic origin," *Case Reports in Dentistry*, vol. 2015, Article ID 267625, 4 pages, 2015.

New Parameter for In-Office Dental Bleaching

Cristina Dupim Presoto,[1] Janaina Freitas Bortolatto,[1] Priscila Petrucelli Freire de Carvalho,[1] Tamara Carolina Trevisan,[1] Michael Christopher Floros,[2] and Osmir Batista de Oliveira Junior[1]

[1]*Department of Restorative Dentistry, Araraquara Dental School, Universidade Estadual Paulista (UNESP), 1680 Humaitá Street, 14801-903 Araraquara, SP, Brazil*
[2]*Departments of Physics & Astronomy and Chemistry, Trent Centre for Biomaterials Research, Trent University, Peterborough, ON, Canada K9J 7B8*

Correspondence should be addressed to Cristina Dupim Presoto; crispresoto@hotmail.com

Academic Editor: Michelle A. Chinelatti

Dental bleaching is considered a conservative and biologically safe treatment for discolored teeth. Despite this, one of the major undesirable effects of bleaching is dentin sensitivity which may occur during and after treatment. To address these sensitivity issues, new dental bleaching preparations with lower concentrations of hydrogen peroxide (H_2O_2) have recently been introduced to the market. This paper presents a clinical case report of a 20-year-old female patient admitted to the Araraquara Dental School, UNESP, Brazil. The patient underwent dental bleaching using one of the new products with reduced hydrogen peroxide concentration, Lase Peroxide Lite 6%, a 6% H_2O_2 gel containing titanium oxide nanoparticles doped with nitrogen (6% H_2O_2/N-doped TiO_2).

1. Introduction

The demand for aesthetic dentistry has increased continuously [1–4], and the smile's appearance has become an important part of the social attractiveness of a person and their interactive communication skill [1, 2, 4, 5].

Currently, dental bleaching has been recognized as an effective method for the treatment of discolored teeth, being considered a conservative and biologically safe type of treatment [4, 6–9].

Hydrogen peroxide (H_2O_2) is a chemical substance with high oxidative power and is the most widely used agent for in-office teeth whitening at concentrations ranging mainly from 25 to 35% [10–13]. Peroxide agents are highly unstable and when in contact with the tissue, they dissociate into water, oxygen, and free radicals, the latter accounting for the observed bleaching effect due to their ability to oxidize organic pigments [9]. It is known that the diffusion of H_2O_2 through the dentin depends on the concentration of the gel, the period of time that the agent is in contact with the tooth [13], and the thickness of the dental structure [8, 14].

One of the major undesirable effects of bleaching is tooth sensitivity [4, 7, 9, 12, 13, 15–18] that occurs during and after the treatment and may represent a degree of biological damage to the dentin-pulp complex [4, 7, 9, 13, 15–17]. There are many factors that are known to increase sensitivity, such as high concentrations of H_2O_2, high enamel permeability, prolonged use of bleaching agents, heat during application through accelerator lamps, and differences in the structural morphology of enamel and dentin with pores which facilitate the infiltration of bleaching [8, 12, 15, 16]. Sensitivity issues have led some manufacturers to release bleaching gels with lower concentrations of H_2O_2 in order to minimize the side effects produced by peroxide radicals [9, 13, 17].

Aiming to increase both efficacy and safety, new bleaching agents with lower concentrations of H_2O_2 based on the catalytic action of a nanoparticle semiconductor additive such as titanium dioxide (TiO_2) activated by light sources [9, 16–20] are now entering the market [4, 9, 13, 16–20]. A significant reduction in the sensitivity of bleaching treatments which use nitrogen doped titanium dioxide and 15% H_2O_2 concentration has been reported in the literature

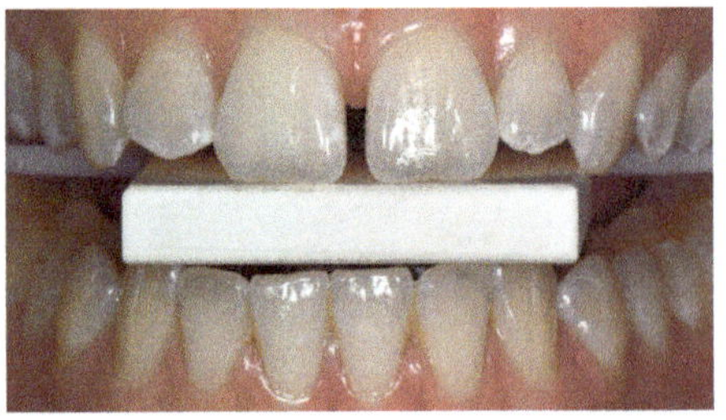

FIGURE 1: Initial picture taken with calibration block.

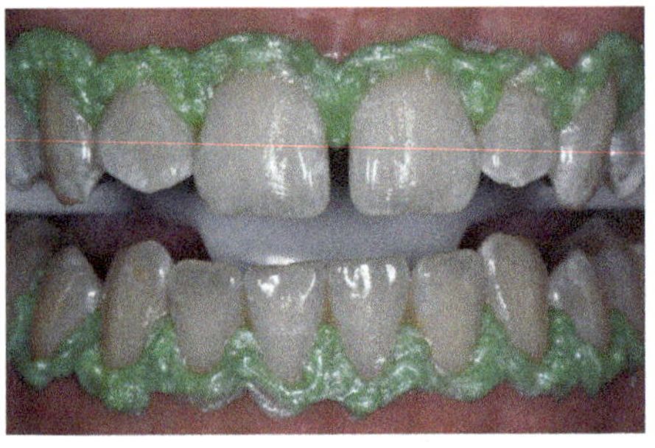

FIGURE 2: Gingival barrier properly applied and light-cured.

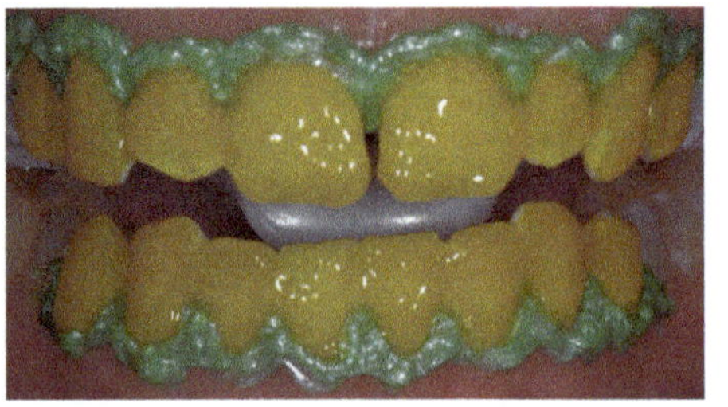

FIGURE 3: Bleaching gel applied to the buccal surface of the upper and lower teeth.

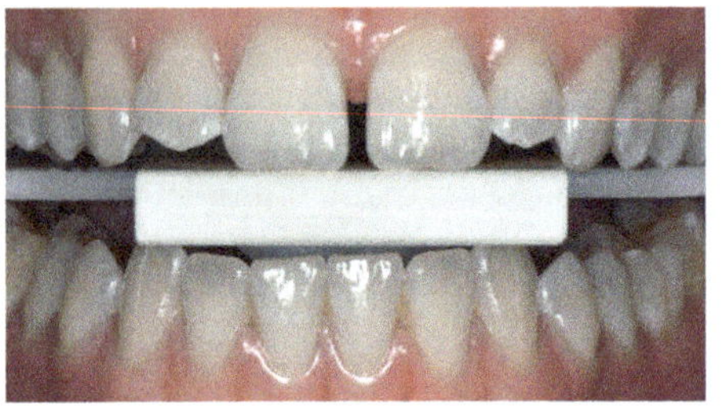

FIGURE 4: Final picture taken with calibration block.

[8, 9, 16–18]. Nevertheless, bleaching agents with 6% H_2O_2/N-doped TiO_2 are innovative and significantly lower in peroxide concentration and, to our knowledge, there are few clinical studies evaluating in-office tooth bleaching with agents at this concentration [17, 18]. Thus, this study aims to present a case report using this new product.

2. Case Presentation

A female patient, PPFC, 20 years old, attended the Operative Dentistry Clinic at Araraquara Dental School, UNESP, Brazil, and reported dissatisfaction with the aesthetics of her anterior teeth. Despite the midline diastema between central incisors, the factor that most bothered her was the color of her teeth. During the clinical exam, there were no factors observed which would contraindicate the use of tooth bleaching. As the patient was young, we decided to use a bleaching agent with a minimal H_2O_2 concentration. We used a new product, Lase Peroxide Lite 6% (6% H_2O_2/N-doped TiO_2) (DMC Equipment, São Carlos, SP, Brazil), which is activated by a light source. The light source used was a Whitening Lase II (DMC Equipment, São Carlos, SP, Brazil), a new type of in-office photocatalytic equipment composed of six violet LEDs (405 nm wavelength) and three infrared lasers (808 nm).

Before beginning the treatment, initial photography with a ceramic block for calibration was performed and retained for subsequent analysis using ScanWhite, a specific software program for the objective assessment of tooth bleaching levels based on computational processing of digital images (Figure 1). Subsequently, professional dental prophylaxis was performed with a Robinson brush with a pumice and water paste. A gingival barrier (Lase Protect, DMC, São Carlos, SP, Brazil) was then applied and light-cured for 10 seconds for each dental element (Figure 2).

The bleaching agent was mixed and applied in homogeneous layers on the buccal surfaces of the upper and lower anterior teeth (Figure 3). The 6% H_2O_2/N-doped TiO_2 gel is provided in two phases, a peroxide and a thickener, which should be mixed in proportions of 3 drops of peroxide for 1 drop of thickener. In this case, for whitening the upper and lower arches until the premolars region, we used a total of 18 drops of peroxide and 6 drops of thickener. After the gel's application, it was kept in contact with dental surface for 12 minutes and photocatalyzed by LED/laser light, alternating the irradiation between the upper and lower arches every minute. Afterwards, the bleaching gel was removed and a new application sequence was performed. Three clinical sessions were held with two application cycles of the bleaching agent in each of them and a 7-day interval between the sessions.

One week following the end of the bleaching treatment, a new photography session was performed with the same calibration block (Figure 4). The initial and final images were compared in ScanWhite to determine how much the teeth responded to the whitening procedure. The images were first transmitted to the software and a calibration was performed. Next, for each picture, an area was selected in the middle third of labial surface of the anterior teeth. The result showed 22 tones of whitening for the upper right central incisor and 50 tones for the right canine (Figure 5). The patient reported that she was very satisfied with the final color of her teeth.

Tooth sensitivity was measured by a visual analogue scale (VAS), which provides a range of scores from 0 to 100, where 0 represents no pain and 100 represents extreme pain. At the end of each clinic session, the patient was asked to mark on the scale their perceived sensitivity both during and after the session. She reported sensitivity only during the first application in the second session and this was classified as

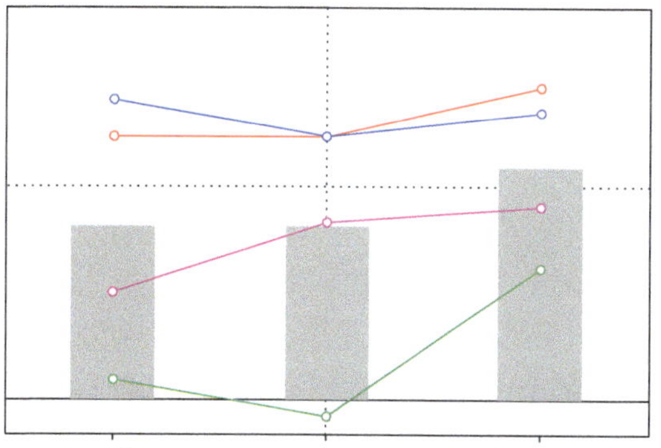

FIGURE 5: Overall result of bleaching.

low, with an intensity of 20% in a shock sensation and with a 1-second duration.

3. Discussion

The presence of sensitivity to bleaching treatments with high concentration gels and the search for an alternative with both efficacy and safety were the main reasons why bleaching agents with lower concentrations of H_2O_2 were introduced to the market [4, 8, 13, 17, 18]. Initially, it was believed that a high concentration gel and long contact time with dental structure would be required to obtain greater efficacy with bleaching procedures [9, 21]. Nonetheless, the use of 15% H_2O_2/TiO_2 photocatalyzed by LED was recently reported and demonstrated that, besides having lower sensitivity compared to products with 35% concentration, this preparation also provided greater bleaching efficacy [8, 9, 16, 17, 20]. We also observed this finding in the clinical case presented here using a preparation with only 6% H_2O_2.

The presence of N-doped TiO_2 semiconductor allows a reduction in the required concentration of H_2O_2, which improves the biocompatibility of the final product by significantly reducing dental sensitivity during and after the procedure, directly increasing the safety of the whitening procedure [9, 17–19]. By incorporating N-doped TiO_2 nanoparticles, it is necessary to photocatalyze the gel with a light source in order to improve its action. This new class of bleaching agents is safer and effective for promoting bleaching with a reduced concentration of free radical peroxides, thereby minimizing damage to the tooth structure [22].

In a clinical study using a 6% H_2O_2 varnish system for in-office whitening, da Mata and Marques [10] reported that none of the patients showed any sensitivity, which was a common side effect upon using gels with high peroxide concentrations. By using a 6% H_2O_2 varnish, Calatayud et al. [23] also demonstrated that the application of the gel showed significant clinical efficacy when applied to in-office bleaching and also when applied by patients themselves at home.

In the clinical case described in this paper, upon comparing the results before and after the bleaching procedure, the choice for central incisors and canines teeth was done to ensure a more homogeneous sample, as central and lateral incisors usually have the same color and, together, could distort the results of the hemiarch's mean score [23–25]. In Figure 5, a major color alteration is observed for the canines when compared to central incisors. The results showed that the use of these new bleaching gels provides color alteration needed for patient satisfaction in addition to lowering dental sensitivity. Therefore, this case reported a successful bleaching treatment for young patients, combining the great aesthetic results, as desired by patients, and also improved biocompatibility and safety from a lower concentration of bleaching gel.

Consent

The authors declare that the patient gave her informed consent for the case report to be published.

Competing Interests

The authors declare that there is no conflict of interests regarding the publication of this paper.

References

[1] F. N. Hattab, M. A. Qudeimat, and H. S. Al-Rimawi, "Dental discoloration: an overview," *Journal of Esthetic Dentistry*, vol. 11, no. 6, pp. 291–310, 1999.

[2] A. Joiner, "Tooth colour: a review of the literature," *Journal of Dentistry*, vol. 32, no. 1, pp. 3–12, 2004.

[3] S. B. Mehta, S. Banerji, and R. Aulakh, "Patient assessment: preparing for a predictable aesthetic outcome," *Dental Update*, vol. 42, no. 1, pp. 78–86, 2015.

[4] C. Kose, A. Calixto, J. Bauer, A. Reis, and A. Loguercio, "Comparison of the effects of in-office bleaching times on whitening and tooth sensitivity: a single blind, randomized clinical trial," *Operative Dentistry*, vol. 41, no. 2, pp. 138–145, 2016.

[5] S. T. Henson, S. J. Lindauer, W. G. Gardner, B. Shroff, E. Tufekci, and A. M. Best, "Influence of dental esthetics on social perceptions of adolescents judged by peers," *American Journal of Orthodontics and Dentofacial Orthopedics*, vol. 140, no. 3, pp. 389–395, 2011.

[6] B. A. Matis, Y. Wang, T. Jiang, and G. J. Eckert, "Extended at-home bleaching of tetracycline-stained teeth with different concentrations of carbamide peroxide," *Quintessence International*, vol. 33, no. 9, pp. 645–655, 2002.

[7] J. E. Dahl and U. Pallesen, "Tooth bleaching—a critical review of the biological aspects," *Critical Reviews in Oral Biology and Medicine*, vol. 14, no. 4, pp. 292–304, 2003.

[8] G. Moncada, D. Sepúlveda, K. Elphick et al., "Effects of light activation, agent concentration, and tooth thickness on dental sensitivity after bleaching," *Operative Dentistry*, vol. 38, no. 5, pp. 467–476, 2013.

[9] J. F. Bortolatto, H. Pretel, M. C. Floros et al., "Low concentration H_2O_2/TiO_N in office bleaching: a randomized clinical trial," *Journal of Dental Research*, vol. 93, no. 7, pp. 66S–71S, 2014.

[10] A. D. da Mata and D. N. Marques, "A novel technique for in-office bleaching with a 6% hydrogen peroxide paint-on varnish,"

The European Journal of Esthetic Dentistry, vol. 1, no. 1, pp. 70–77, 2006.

[11] A. Joiner, "The bleaching of teeth: a review of the literature," *Journal of Dentistry*, vol. 34, no. 7, pp. 412–419, 2006.

[12] W. Buchalla and T. Attin, "External bleaching therapy with activation by heat, light or laser—a systematic review," *Dental Materials*, vol. 23, no. 5, pp. 586–596, 2007.

[13] A. Reis, S. Kossatz, G. C. Martins, and A. D. Loguercio, "Efficacy of and effect on tooth sensitivity of in-office bleaching gel concentrations: a randomized clinical trial," *Operative Dentistry*, vol. 38, no. 4, pp. 386–393, 2013.

[14] S. E. A. Camargo, M. C. Valera, C. H. R. Camargo, M. N. Gasparoto Mancini, and M. M. Menezes, "Penetration of 38% hydrogen peroxide into the pulp chamber in bovine and human teeth submitted to office bleach technique," *Journal of Endodontics*, vol. 33, no. 9, pp. 1074–1077, 2007.

[15] C. A. S. Costa, H. Riehl, J. F. Kina, N. T. Sacono, and J. Hebling, "Human pulp responses to in-office tooth bleaching," *Oral Surgery, Oral Medicine, Oral Pathology, Oral Radiology and Endodontology*, vol. 109, no. 4, pp. e59–e64, 2010.

[16] J. Martin, E. Fernandez, V. Bahamondes et al., "Dentin hypersensitivity after teeth bleaching with in-office systems. randomized clinical trial," *American Journal of Dentistry*, vol. 26, no. 1, pp. 10–14, 2013.

[17] J. F. Bortolatto, T. C. Trevisan, P. S. Bernardi et al., "A novel approach for in-office tooth bleaching with 6 % H_2O_2/TiO_N and LED/laser system—a controlled, triple-blinded, randomized clinical trial," *Lasers in Medical Science*, vol. 31, no. 3, pp. 437–444, 2016.

[18] H. B. Dias, E. T. Carrera, J. F. Bortolatto, M. F. de Andrade, and A. N. de Souza Rastelli, "LED and low level laser therapy association in tooth bleaching using a novel low concentration H_2O_2/N-doped TiO_2 bleaching agent," *Laser Physics*, vol. 26, no. 1, Article ID 015602, 2016.

[19] K. Sakai, J. Kato, H. Kurata et al., "The amounts of hydroxyl radicals generated by titanium dioxide and 3.5% hydrogen peroxide under 405-nm diode laser irradiation," *Laser Physics*, vol. 17, no. 8, pp. 1062–1066, 2007.

[20] T. Suemori, J. Kato, T. Nakazawa et al., "Effects of light irradiation on bleaching by a 3.5% hydrogen peroxide solution containing titanium dioxide," *Laser Physics Letters*, vol. 5, no. 5, pp. 379–383, 2008.

[21] H. O. Heymann, "Tooth whitening: facts and fallacies," *British Dental Journal*, vol. 198, no. 8, p. 514, 2005.

[22] T. Maetani, F. Yoshino, A. Yoshida et al., "An investigation of application of novel tooth bleaching using low concentration of hydrogen peroxide—dental application of electron spin resonance (ESR) technique for detecting reactive oxygen species," *Oral Therapeutics and Pharmacology*, vol. 27, no. 2, pp. 109–115, 2008.

[23] J. Oteo Calatayud, P. Mateos de la Varga, C. Oteo Calatayud, and M. J. Calvo Box, "Comparative clinical study of two tooth bleaching protocols with 6% hydrogen peroxide," *International Journal of Dentistry*, vol. 2009, Article ID 928306, 5 pages, 2009.

[24] C. Zantner, F. Derdilopoulou, P. Martus, and A. M. Kielbassa, "Randomized clinical trial on the efficacy of 2 over-the-counter whitening systems," *Quintessence International*, vol. 37, no. 9, pp. 695–706, 2006.

[25] N. U. Wetter, E. P. Branco, A. M. Deana, and J. E. P. Pelino, "Color differences of canines and incisors in a comparative long-term clinical trial of three bleaching systems," *Lasers in Medical Science*, vol. 24, no. 6, pp. 941–947, 2009.

43

Late Developing Supernumerary Premolars: Reports of Two Cases

Soghra Yassaei,[1] Mahdjoube Goldani Moghadam,[1] and S. M. Ali Tabatabaei[2]

[1] *Department of Orthodontics, Faculty of Dentistry, Shahid Sadoughi University of Medical Sciences, Yazd 89195/165, Iran*
[2] *Private Practice, Yazd 89195/165, Iran*

Correspondence should be addressed to Mahdjoube Goldani Moghadam; mahdjoube.gm@gmail.com

Academic Editors: A. Epivatianos and A. Markopoulos

This paper presents two cases of late developing supernumerary premolars. Case 1 is a female patient with nonsyndromic multiple supernumerary teeth located in the maxillary right premolar-molar region, maxillary left premolar region, and the mandibular right and left premolar regions. In this patient surgical removal of all supernumerary teeth was carried out to avoid complications during orthodontic treatment. Case 2 is a female aged 19 years in whom formation of a mandibular supernumerary premolar was observed which was not present at age 13. The patient was made aware of the supernumerary tooth presence, and periodic radiographic assessment was planned.

1. Introduction

Excess in the number of teeth which is often referred to as supernumerary is a developmental anomaly [1]. Etiologically, the occurrence of supernumerary teeth has not been yet completely determined. In attempts to explain the condition several theories have been proposed including the phylogenetic theory [2], the dichotomy theory (splitting of the tooth germ) [3, 4], the hyperactivity theory (hyperactive dental lamina) [1], and occurrence due to combined genetic and environmental effects [5]. Supernumerary teeth can occur anywhere in the dental arch, but they are mostly found in the maxilla [6]. The prevalence of supernumerary teeth varies between 0.1% and 3.8%, and they are more common in the permanent dentition [7]. Supernumerary teeth can be categorized in terms of chronology, topography, and morphology. Chronologically, they can develop before deciduous teeth (predeciduous), simultaneous to permanent teeth or after them (postpermanent dentition). Based on the morphology, supernumerary teeth can be defined as supplemental (eumorphic) or rudimentary (including conic shape, tuberculate, molariform, and odontome). Mesiodens, paramolar, distomolar, and parapremolar, are words to describe the topography (location) of the supernumeraries [7].

Supernumerary premolars represent between 8 and 9.1 percent of all supernumerary teeth [8, 9]. They are more likely to develop in the mandible than in the maxilla and often resemble the normal premolars in shape and size [10].

The majority of supernumeraries in the permanent dentition develop later than normal teeth of that region and are supposed to form postpermanent dentition developing from hyperactivity of dental lamina [11]. The presence of supernumeraries is associated with complications including delayed eruption of the permanent teeth, displacement of them, cyst formation, and resorption of neighboring structures such as root resorption [6]. They can also interfere in orthodontic space closure and implant placement [7]. When supernumeraries are diagnosed, a decision whether to monitor or remove them is needed to be made. In special situations removal of supernumeraries is preferred such as when the teeth need to be aligned orthodontically. Occasionally, supernumerary teeth are detected incidentally during radiographic examination. Regarding surgical risks, when complications associated with supernumeraries seem unlikely, periodic radiographic assessment would be recommended. Radiographic assessment is of great importance in diagnosis and management of supernumeraries. Advances in radiographic techniques and introduction of three-dimensional computed tomography (3D CT) and cone beam computed tomography (CBCT) have allowed undistorted view and better evaluation of supernumeraries especially in cases of multiple supernumeraries [12].

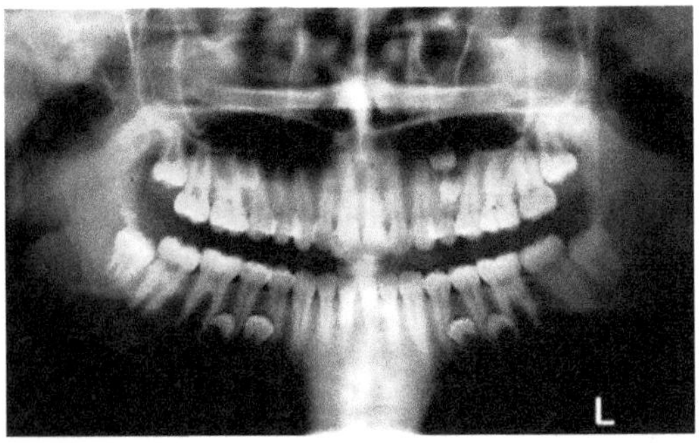

FIGURE 1: Panoramic radiograph of the patient showing the presence of seven supernumerary premolars.

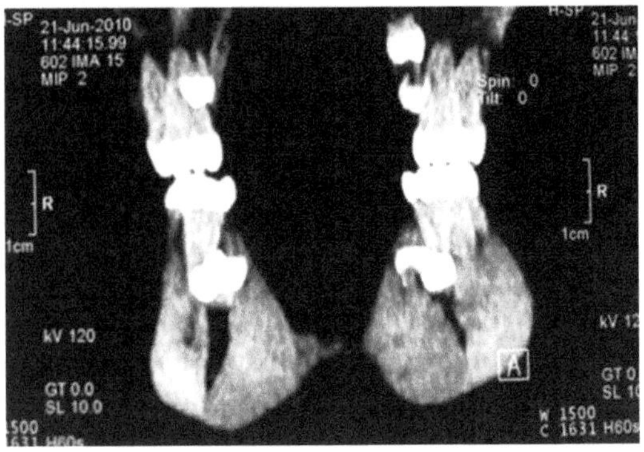

FIGURE 2: CT scan to evaluate the position of supernumeraries.

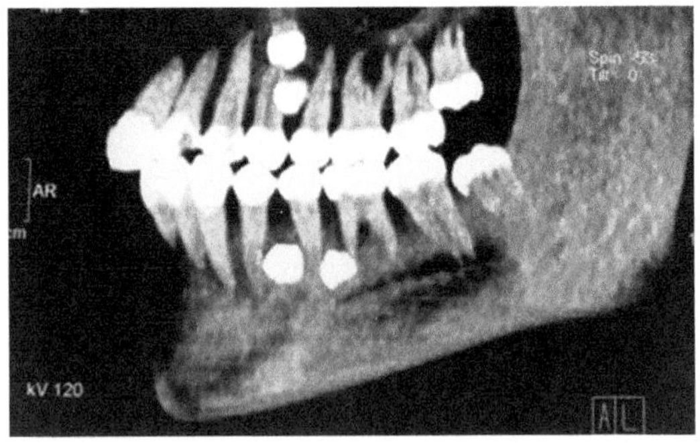

FIGURE 3: CT scan view of the left side to locate exact position of four supernumeraries.

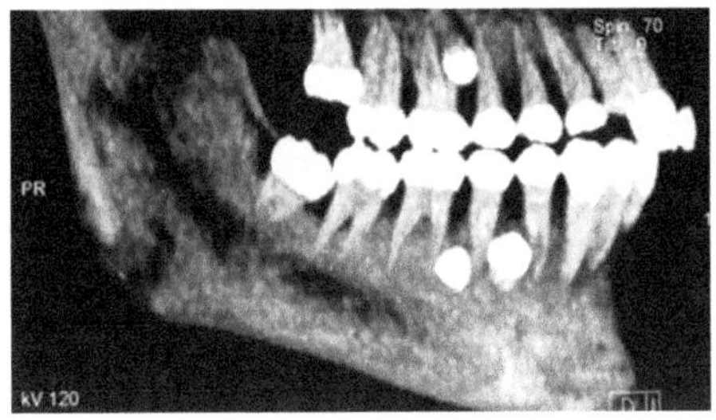

FIGURE 4: CT scan view of the right side showing three supernumeraries.

There have been reports of late developing supernumeraries in the literature [13–16]. Two further cases of late developing supernumerary premolars and two different approaches for their management are described in this paper.

2. Case Presentation

2.1. Case 1. The patient was a 15-year-old Iranian girl who was referred to the orthodontic clinic for treatment of Class II malocclusion. Family medical history was noncontributory and extraoral examination did not show any abnormality. In the panoramic view, the presence of seven supernumerary teeth resembling premolars which were located in the maxillary right premolar-molar region, maxillary left premolar region, and the mandibular right and left premolar regions was detected (Figure 1).

A general physician was consulted who confirmed there was no associated syndrome. The situation was explained to the patient and her parents. Further CT scans were taken to evaluate the position of the supernumeraries (Figures 2, 3, and 4).

The orthodontic treatment plan included extraction of upper second premolars, banding of first molars and bracket bonding on the remaining teeth, aligning, leveling, canine retraction, and anterior retraction. In order to prevent root resorption during initial phase of aligning and leveling and also to avoid incomplete space closure during canine retraction, a decision was made to surgically remove all supernumerary teeth.

2.2. Case 2. A 19-year-old Iranian female visited a general dental practitioner to asses her third molars. A panoramic radiograph was taken to evaluate the third molar teeth which revealed the presence of a supernumerary premolar in early stage of crown formation between the roots of mandibular right second premolar and first molar (Figure 5). The patient had been treated for her mild crowding at the age of 13 with nonextraction approach (the mandibular left first premolar had been extracted before referring the patient for orthodontic treatment), and her preorthodontic treatment panoramic radiograph was available. The old panoramic radiograph showed normal dentition, and there was no sign of supernumerary tooth (Figure 6). In this case the patient became aware of the condition and periodic monitoring of the supernumerary tooth and the third molar teeth by radiographic examination was planned.

3. Discussion

Supernumerary teeth may appear as a single tooth or multiple teeth. Multiple supernumeraries are not common finding, and occurrence of five or more supernumeraries has been estimated less than 1 percent [17]. Multiple supernumeraries are more likely to occur as part of a syndrome such as Cleidocranial dysplasia, Gardner's syndrome, orodigitofacial dystosis, Down's syndrome, Crouzon's disease, and Hallermann Streiff syndrome but can also occur without such an association [7, 17].

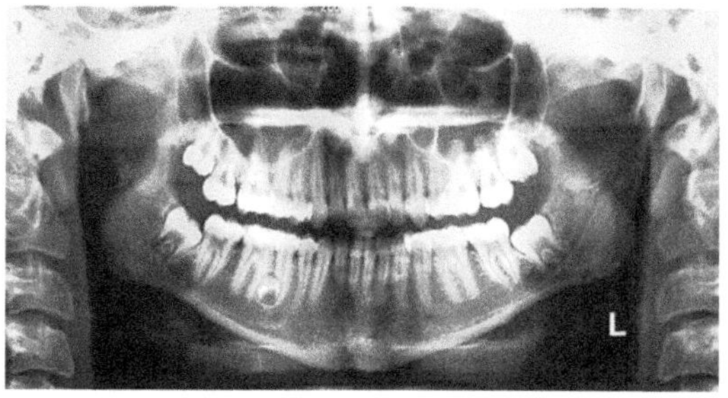

FIGURE 5: Panoramic radiograph taken at 19 years of age showing development of a supernumerary premolar.

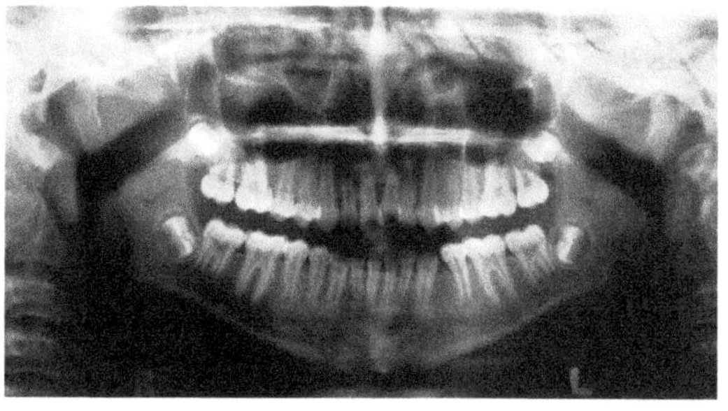

FIGURE 6: Panoramic radiograph of the same patient as in Figure 5 at 13 years of age showing no sign of the supernumerary tooth.

As stated earlier about 8–9.1 percent of all supernumerary teeth are supernumerary premolars [8, 9]. Unlike other supernumeraries, supernumerary premolars are more prevalent in the mandible and usually resemble normal premolars in shape and size [6]. These supernumeraries have tendency to begin their development later than the normal for teeth of that area [7]. It has been shown that calcification of premolars initiates between 1.5 and 2.5 years of age while it may not be evident until 3-4 years of age in radiographic views [18]. It has been reported that supernumerary premolars commence their formation 7–11 years after normal premolars [19, 20].

The patient in Case 1 was a nonsyndromic female with multiple supplemental supernumerary teeth in four quadrants of her mouth. The panoramic radiograph taken prior to orthodontic treatment revealed seven supernumeraries which could interfere in space closing during orthodontic treatment and might cause complications such as resorption of adjacent roots. Therefore it was decided to remove all supernumerary teeth to prevent potential problems in orthodontic treatment. Surgical removal of supernumeraries should be performed with great caution to avoid damaging adjacent permanent teeth, which may cause ankylosis of these teeth and consequently may create difficulty in the course of orthodontic treatment. Moreover the possibility of supernumeraries' fusion to the neighboring teeth should be kept in mind [21, 22].

In Case 2 a supernumerary premolar was found by chance in the panoramic radiograph taken for assessment of third molar teeth. Patient had undergone a course of orthodontic treatment at age 13, and there was no sign of a supernumerary tooth in the available preorthodontic panoramic radiograph. In this case it was unlikely that the supernumerary premolar caused any interference in terms of function or esthetic. It has been reported that pathological changes occur in merely 2 percent of supernumerary premolars [23]. Based on these facts it was decided to leave the supernumerary teeth and to keep the condition under periodic radiographic observation.

4. Conclusion

Orthodontists should be aware that late development of supernumeraries can occur any time in the course of orthodontic treatment or after its completion. Although it is not a routine practice to screen for the late development of teeth during or after orthodontic treatment, possibility of their complications should always be taken into consideration.

References

[1] R. E. Primosch, "Anterior supernumerary teeth—assessment and surgical intervention in children," *Pediatric Dentistry*, vol. 3, no. 2, pp. 204–215, 1981.

[2] J. D. Smith, "Hyperdontia: report of case," *The Journal of the American Dental Association*, vol. 79, no. 5, pp. 1191–1192, 1969.

[3] J. F. Liu, "Characteristics of premaxillary supernumerary teeth: a survey of 112 cases," *ASDC Journal of Dentistry for Children*, vol. 62, no. 4, pp. 262–265, 1995.

[4] G. S. Taylor, "Characteristics of supernumerary teeth in the primary and permanent dentition," *The Dental Practitioner and Dental Record*, vol. 22, no. 5, pp. 203–208, 1972.

[5] A. H. Brook, "A unifying aetiological explanation for anomalies of human tooth number and size," *Archives of Oral Biology*, vol. 29, no. 5, pp. 373–378, 1984.

[6] E. C. Stafne, "Supernumerary teeth," *Dental Cosmos*, vol. 74, pp. 653–659, 1932.

[7] P. Abhishek, M. Kundabala, D. Marisha, M. Mandakini, and S. Manuel, "Management of supernumerary teeth," *Journal of Conservative Dentistry*, vol. 14, no. 3, pp. 221–224, 2011.

[8] M. M. Nazif, R. C. Ruffalo, and T. Zullo, "Impacted supernumerary teeth: a survey of 50 cases," *The Journal of the American Dental Association*, vol. 106, no. 2, pp. 201–204, 1983.

[9] H. Grahnen and B. Lindahl, "Supernumerary teeth in the permanent dentition: a frequency study," *Odontologisk Revy*, vol. 12, pp. 290–294, 1961.

[10] S. Masih, H. S. Sethi, N. Singh, and A. M. Thomas, "Differential expressions of bilaterally unerupted supernumerary teeth," *Journal of the Indian Society of Pedodontics and Preventive Dentistry*, vol. 29, no. 4, pp. 320–322, 2011.

[11] M. I. Leco-Berrocal, J. F. Martín-Morales, and J. M. Martínez-González, "An observational study of the frequency of supernumerary teeth in a population of 2000 patients," *Medicina Oral, Patología Oral y Cirugía Bucal*, vol. 12, no. 2, pp. 134–138, 2007.

[12] H. U. Brauer, "Case report: non-syndromic multiple supernumerary teeth localized by cone beam computed tomography," *European Archives of Paediatric Dentistry*, vol. 11, no. 1, pp. 41–43, 2010.

[13] G. A. Morgan, P. R. Morgan, and S. A. Crouch, "Recurring mandibular supplemental premolars," *Oral Surgery, Oral Medicine, Oral Pathology, Oral Radiology, and Endodontology*, vol. 30, no. 4, pp. 501–504, 1970.

[14] J. J. Breckon and S. P. Jones, "Late forming supernumeraries in the mandibular premolar region," *British Journal of Orthodontics*, vol. 20, no. 4, p. 375, 1993.

[15] S. M. Cochrane, J. R. Clark, and N. P. Hunt, "Late developing supernumerary teeth in the mandible," *British Journal of Orthodontics*, vol. 24, no. 4, pp. 293–296, 1997.

[16] N. Gibson, "A late developing mandibular premolar supernumerary tooth," *Australian Dental Journal*, vol. 46, no. 1, pp. 51–52, 2001.

[17] K. Gunduz and M. Muglali, "Non-syndrome multiple supernumerary teeth: a case report," *Journal of Contemporary Dental Practice*, vol. 8, no. 4, pp. 81–87, 2007.

[18] J. H. Scott and N. B. B. Symons, *Introduction to Dental Anomaly*, Churchill Livingstone, London, UK, 5th edition, 1967.

[19] M. L. Kantor, C. S. Bailey, and E. J. J. Burkes, "Duplication of the premolar dentition," *Oral Surgery, Oral Medicine, Oral Pathology, Oral Radiology, and Endodontology*, vol. 66, no. 1, pp. 62–64, 1988.

[20] L. K. Rubenstein, S. J. Lindauer, R. J. Isaacson, and N. Germane, "Development of supernumerary premolars in an orthodontic population," *Oral Surgery, Oral Medicine, Oral Pathology, Oral Radiology, and Endodontology*, vol. 71, no. 3, pp. 392–395, 1991.

[21] F. C. Loh and J. F. Yeo, "Paramolar with bifid crown," *Oral Surgery, Oral Medicine, Oral Pathology, Oral Radiology, and Endodontology*, vol. 76, no. 2, pp. 257–258, 1993.

[22] E. Nunes, I. G. de Moraes, P. M. de Novaes, and S. M. de Sousa, "Bilateral fusion of mandibular second molars with supernumerary teeth: case report," *Brazilian Dental Journal*, vol. 13, no. 2, pp. 137–141, 2002.

[23] I. Bodin, P. Julin, and M. Thomsson, "Hyperodontia. I. Frequency and distribution of supernumerary teeth among 21,609 patients," *Dentomaxillofacial Radiology*, vol. 7, no. 1, pp. 15–17, 1978.

Vestibular Schwannoma Presenting as Oral Dysgeusia: An Easily Missed Diagnosis

Emma Brown[1] and Konrad Staines[2]

[1] *Oral Medicine Department, Bristol Dental Hospital, Lower Maudlin Street, Bristol BS1 2LY, UK*
[2] *Oral Medicine Department, University of Bristol Dental School, Lower Maudlin Street, Bristol BS1 2LY, UK*

Correspondence should be addressed to Emma Brown; elbrown7@hotmail.co.uk

Academic Editor: Miguel Peñarrocha

We present a case of a fifty-year-old male patient who was referred to the Oral Medicine Department with a complaint of a salty taste. History taking subsequently revealed that the patient was also experiencing intermittent numbness of his left lower lip, tinnitus, and a feeling of fullness in the left ear. Magnetic resonance imaging was performed which revealed a large vestibular schwannoma affecting the left vestibulocochlear nerve, which was treated surgically. This case shows the importance of taking a detailed history in a patient presenting with an initial complaint of oral dysgeusia. It also highlights the possibility of significant underlying pathology, presenting with initial low level, nonspecific complaints such as an altered taste, and the rationale for imaging patients who report unilateral facial hypoesthesia.

1. Introduction

Oral dysgeusia is defined as a gustatory disturbance relating to a distorted taste perception, or to a persistent taste sensation in the absence of stimulation [1], and can be very distressing for the patient. Patients with taste disturbances are commonly referred to and investigated within Oral Medicine Departments in the UK. Identifiable causes of dysgeusia can include local factors, drugs, systemic disease, and peripheral or central neurological conditions; see Table 1 [1–5].

Local factors influencing taste include infections of the oral cavity, such as candidiasis or dental abscess, trauma, or hyposalivation [1–3]. Over 250 drugs have been associated with oral dysgeusia, of which the most common are outlined in Table 1 [3–5]. Dysgeusia can also be a manifestation of a systemic disease such as an underlying haematinic deficiency, diabetes mellitus, Crohn's disease, or Sjögren's syndrome [1, 3]. Rarely, damage to the peripheral or central nervous system can be the cause. Tumours affecting the cerebellopontine angle, such as a schwannoma or meningioma, can cause taste disturbances. Central neurological causes such as ischaemia, haemorrhage, or demyelination affecting the gustatory pathway in the brain, or temporal lobe epilepsy, also require exclusion [1].

In a significant number of cases, the taste disturbance cannot be attributed to an identifiable cause and therefore a diagnosis of idiopathic oral dysgeusia is made. Although altered taste is a rare symptom of vestibular schwannoma, this case illustrates the need for a high index of clinical suspicion when assessing patients with seemingly low level symptoms, such as oral dysgeusia.

2. Case Presentation

2.1. History. A fifty-year-old male patient was referred to the Oral Medicine Department by his General Dental Practitioner with a primary complaint of an altered taste. The taste disturbance had been affecting the patient for six months and manifested as a constant salty taste. His General Medical Practitioner had empirically prescribed omeprazole to exclude gastric oesophageal reflux disease as a potential cause. However, this was ineffective and therefore the patient had discontinued the treatment.

Additionally, the patient also complained of a cracked tongue surface and intermittent numbness of his lower left lip and chin. He had experienced three episodes of facial hypoesthesia affecting the mandibular division of the left

Table 1: Possible causes of oral dysgeusia [1–5].

Local factors	Dental abscess, candida infection, trauma to the oral cavity, hyposalivation, removable prostheses, and gastric oesophageal reflux disease
Drugs	Antimicrobials Antibacterials: cephalosporins, ciprofloxacin, clarithromycin, clindamycin, co-trimoxazole, doxycycline, imipenem with cilastatin, metronidazole, ofloxacin, penicillins, trimethoprim, tetracycline, and vancomycin Antivirals: aciclovir, ganciclovir, indinavir, ritonavir, and zidovudine Antifungals: fluconazole and griseofulvin Central nervous system Antiparkinsonians: bromocriptine, levodopa, and pergolide Migraine medications: naratriptan and sumatriptan Muscle relaxants: baclofen and methocarbamol Tricyclic antidepressants: amitriptyline, clomipramine, desipramine, doxepin, imipramine, nortriptyline, and trimipramine Selective serotonin reuptake inhibitors: citalopram, fluoxetine, fluvoxamine, and sertraline Antipsychotics: clozapine, olanzapine, and risperidone Benzodiazepines: alprazolam, clonazepam, flurazepam, and midazolam Mood stabilisers: lithium Cardiovascular Angiotensin-converting enzyme inhibitors: captopril, enalapril, lisinopril, and perindopril Beta-adrenoreceptor blockers: labetalol, metoprolol, propranolol, and timolol Calcium-channel blockers: amlodipine, diltiazem, and nifedipine Potassium-sparing diuretics: amiloride and triamterene Statins: atorvastatin, fluvastatin, and simvastatin Antiarrhythmics: amiodarone, flecainide, and procainamide Endocrine Diabetic medications: glibenclamide, metformin, and tolbutamide Other Antineoplastics: busulfan, dacarbazine, vinblastine, and vincristine Antimalarials: hydroxychloroquine, pyrimethamine, and quinine Bisphosphonates: alendronic acid, etidronic acid, and pamidronic acid Bronchodilators: salbutamol and terbutaline Nonsteroidal anti-inflammatories: celecoxib, diclofenac, ketoprofen, and ketorolac
Systemic disease	Diabetes mellitus, haematinic deficiency (ferritin, folate, or vitamin B12), Sjögren's syndrome, Crohn's disease, and chronic kidney disease
Peripheral nervous system	Syndromes affecting the facial, glossopharyngeal, or vagal nerves (e.g., Bell's palsy) and tumours of the skull base or cerebellopontine angle (meningioma, schwannoma, epidermoid tumour, and brain metastasis)
Central nervous system	Ischaemia, haemorrhage, or demyelination affecting the brainstem, thalamus or cortical components of the gustatory pathway, and temporal lobe epilepsy

trigeminal nerve, which had all been self-limiting and resolved spontaneously.

Medical history was clear except for tinnitus and a feeling of fullness affecting the left ear for the past three years. This had been diagnosed by the General Medical Practitioner as Eustachian tube dysfunction and treated with fluticasone nasal spray. This had no benefit in relieving the symptoms and was discontinued. The patient therefore took no regular medication.

Socially, the patient was a semiretired office based worker. He was a nonsmoker and had a low alcohol intake.

2.2. Examination. Cranial nerve examination at the initial clinic appointment did not reveal any sensory disturbance along the trigeminal nerves or motor deficit of the facial nerves. The eyes were unaffected, with no lacrimation abnormalities identified. Swallow and phonation were not affected. The uvula was not deviated, and the movement of the palate and tongue was normal. Extra oral examination of the head and neck showed normal anatomy, with no facial swelling and no cervical lymphadenopathy. Intraorally the soft tissues of the mouth were healthy with no mucosal lesions detected and no obvious source of infection that could cause the oral dysgeusia. The cracked tongue surface was deemed to be a variation of normal anatomy termed a fissured tongue.

2.3. Investigations. An orthopantomogram radiograph was completed, which confirmed the absence of dental or bony pathology. Blood investigations, including a full blood count, blood glucose, serum ferritin, folate, and vitamin B12 levels, all resulted as normal.

Due to the reported facial hypoesthesia, magnetic resonance imaging of the head was performed. This identified a large vestibular schwannoma of the left vestibulocochlear nerve (eighth cranial nerve). This measured 2.7 cm by 2.4 cm by 2.3 cm and was located in the left cerebellopontine angle, involving the left internal auditory meatus. There was associated compression of the brainstem and distortion of the fourth ventricle, without hydrocephalus (see Figures 1–4).

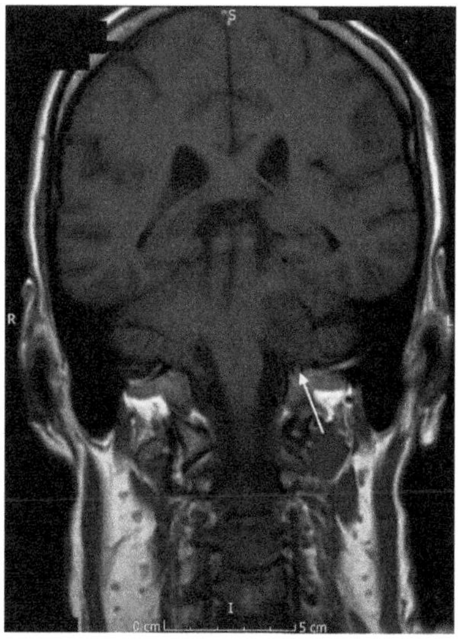

FIGURE 1: Coronal MR image (T1 weighted) showing the vestibular schwannoma affecting the left vestibulocochlear nerve.

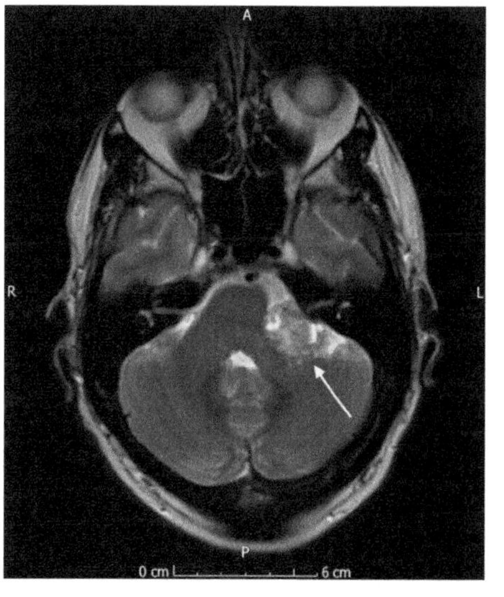

FIGURE 2: Axial MR image (T2 weighted, fat saturated) showing the vestibular schwannoma affecting the left vestibulocochlear nerve.

2.4. Treatment. The patient was referred to the Ear, Nose, and Throat Team for further management. They identified 45 to 50 decibels of sensorineural hearing loss in the left ear on audiogram. There was also some instability on standing, particularly when the patient's eyes were closed. The hypoesthesia of the left trigeminal nerve had worsened, with a constant tingling affecting the maxillary and mandibular divisions and reduced pin prick sensation in these regions.

Treatment options for vestibular schwannoma include monitoring with serial scanning to determine extent of tumour growth, microsurgery to remove or debulk the tumour, or stereotactic radiosurgery [6]. Following discussion at the Skull Base Multidisciplinary Team Meeting, which included a Clinical Oncologist, Neuroradiologist, Ear, Nose, and Throat Surgeon, and Neurosurgeon, a decision was made that microsurgery would be the best treatment option. This was due to the large size of the vestibular schwannoma, the neurological symptoms, and the associated compression of the brain stem. Therefore, the patient underwent surgical excision to remove the tumour and decompress the brainstem. This was undertaken in a joint case with the Ear, Nose, and Throat and Neurosurgery Teams. A translabyrinthine approach was used, which leads to complete hearing loss on the affected side but aims to preserve the facial nerve.

2.5. Outcome. Surgical treatment was successful and the histology showed a schwannoma comprising densely cellular Antoni A areas with less densely cellular Antoni B areas. There was no significant mitotic activity or necrosis. Immunohistochemistry showed that it was strongly positive for S100. The conclusion was that it was a benign schwannoma of the left cerebellopontine angle, WHO Grade I. These results were discussed postoperatively at the Skull Base

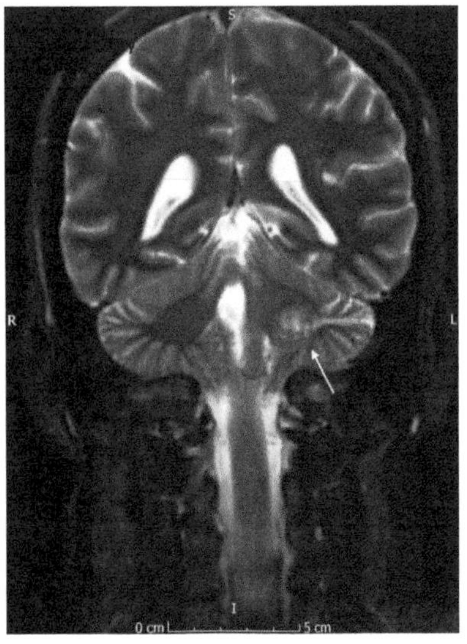

FIGURE 3: Coronal MR image (T2 weighted, fat saturated) showing the vestibular schwannoma affecting the left vestibulocochlear nerve.

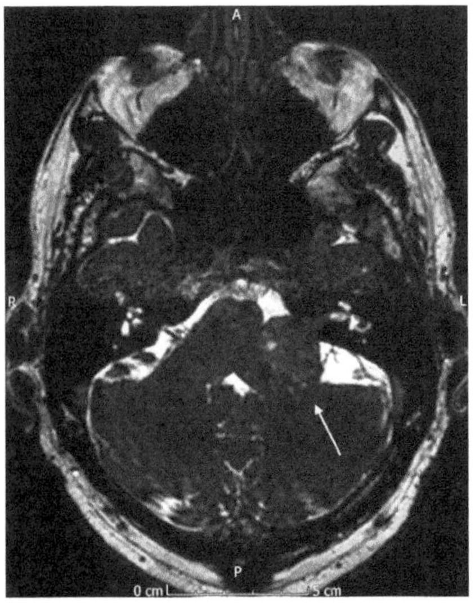

FIGURE 4: Axial MR image (T2 diffusion-weighted image) showing the vestibular schwannoma affecting the left vestibulocochlear nerve.

Multidisciplinary Team Meeting and it was agreed that the patient would be followed up by the Neurosurgery Team.

The patient is doing well postoperatively. The aural fullness in the left ear has now completely resolved, and the tinnitus is barely noticeable. The facial hypoesthesia that affected the maxillary and mandibular divisions of the left trigeminal nerve preoperatively has also completely resolved. There was some minor facial weakness, House-Brackmann Grade II, which was present immediately after surgery and has now returned to normal. Furthermore, the oral dysgeusia has improved since the surgery, with an occasional salty taste still noticed. The patient is now awaiting CROS hearing aids to help with his hearing loss on the left side. His balance

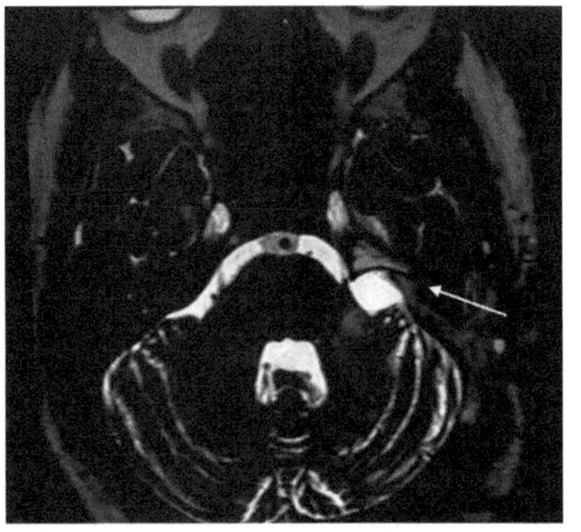

FIGURE 5: Axial MR image (T2 weighted, 3D DRIVE CLEAR) showing the postoperative changes.

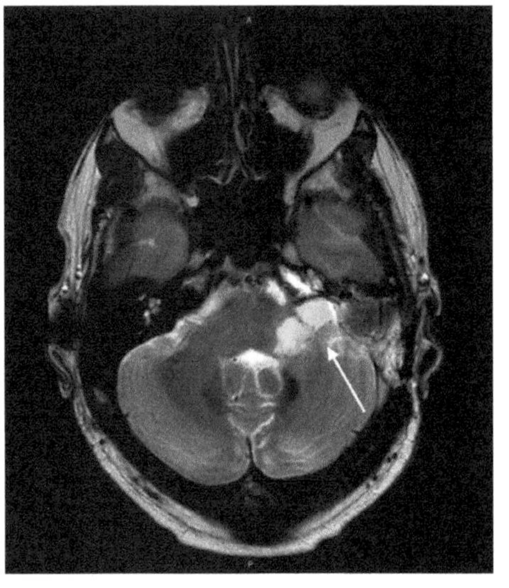

FIGURE 6: Axial MR image (T2 weighted) showing the postoperative changes.

was severely affected from the surgery but this has now significantly improved.

Postoperative magnetic resonance imaging was performed at six months postoperatively (see Figures 5–7). The figures show normal postsurgical changes involving the petrous bone and cerebellopontine angle. The left sided vestibular schwannoma has been resected. There is a cavity in the left middle cerebellar peduncle which is likely to represent an area of perioperative ischaemia. There is a thin cuff of residual tissue anterior to the site of the cerebellopontine angle tumour. The remnant of the schwannoma will be monitored by the Neurosurgery Team with a further magnetic resonance imaging in one year.

3. Discussion

Vestibular schwannomas, also termed acoustic neuromas, are benign tumours of the vestibulocochlear nerve [7–14]. They arise from the Schwann cells which comprise the myelin

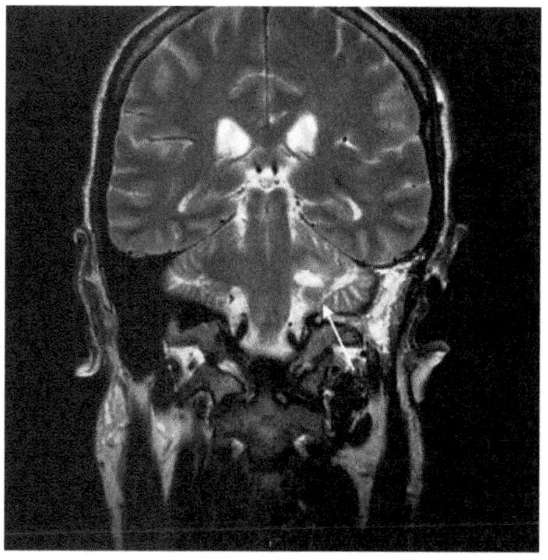

FIGURE 7: Coronal MR image (T2 weighted) showing the postoperative changes.

sheath surrounding the vestibular branch of the eighth cranial nerve [14] and account for 80–90% of cerebellopontine angle tumours [7, 8, 11, 12]. The aetiology of vestibular schwannoma is unknown. The most common symptoms are unilateral hearing loss, tinnitus, or unsteadiness [7–13]. As the tumour grows it compresses surrounding intracranial structures. Compression of the trigeminal nerve can lead to facial hypoesthesia, which is found in 7–26% of patients with vestibular schwannoma [9, 15], and usually begins in the region of the anterior mandible [9]. In 2.2–17% of patients the facial nerve is affected, due to the close anatomical relationship of the facial nerve to the vestibulocochlear nerve in the region of the cerebellopontine angle [9, 11, 15]. Pressure on the motor fibres can lead to facial weakness; and involvement of the sensory branch, the nervus intermedius which receives special sensory taste information from the anterior two-thirds of the tongue, via the chorda tympani, can have an impact on taste [15, 16]. There are a number of studies reporting facial numbness as the presenting feature of a vestibular schwannoma [7, 8, 12]. In another case, the patient presented with a burning sensation of the tongue [14], but no other report has described oral dysgeusia as the symptom prompting referral to secondary care.

Facial nerve dysfunction is rarely the presenting symptom of vestibular schwannoma [13]. However, literature shows that, in up to 17% of patients, the facial nerve is affected [15]. When the facial nerve is compressed by the tumour, taste disturbances appear earlier than facial palsy. This is because sensory nerves are more sensitive to compression than motor fibres [16]. A study by Watanabe et al. [17] found that preoperative taste disturbances were found in 28.7% of patients undergoing surgery for a vestibular schwannoma. Another study by Sahu et al. [16] tested 142 patients with vestibular schwannoma and found taste disturbances present in 40.8% of patients preoperatively. Matthies and Samii [15] found that taste disturbances were only reported in 1.8% of 1000 patients diagnosed with vestibular schwannoma, although they did not formally test this and assumed that the actual incidence would be higher. They also established that preoperative taste disturbance was a reliable indicator of facial nerve compromise and impending paresis.

Although oral dysgeusia is rarely the presenting symptom, it is clear that a significant proportion of patients with vestibular schwannoma do experience taste disturbances. It is therefore imperative that for patients presenting with altered taste a detailed history is taken. The history should specifically include questions relating to sensory loss, and the appropriate investigations should be performed to rule out any significant underlying pathology.

Conflict of Interests

The authors declare that there is no conflict of interests regarding the publication of this paper.

References

[1] J. G. Heckmann, S. M. Heckmann, C. J. G. Lang, and T. Hummel, "Neurological aspects of taste disorders," *Archives of Neurology*, vol. 60, no. 5, pp. 667–671, 2003.

[2] N. Su, V. Ching, and M. Grushka, "Taste disorders: a review," *Journal of the Canadian Dental Association*, vol. 79, article d86, 2013.

[3] T. Maheswaran, P. Abikshyeet, G. Sitra, S. Gokulanathan, V. Vaithiyanadane, and S. Jeelani, "Gustatory dysfunction," *Journal of Pharmacy and Bioallied Sciences*, vol. 6, no. 5, pp. 30–33, 2014.

[4] R. Douglass and D. Heckman, "Drug-related taste disturbance—a contributing factor in geriatric syndromes," *Canadian Family Physician*, vol. 56, no. 11, pp. 1142–1147, 2010.

[5] M. Abdollahi and M. Radfar, "A review of drug-induced oral reactions," *Journal of Contemporary Dental Practice*, vol. 4, no. 1, pp. 10–31, 2003.

[6] E. Myrseth, P.-H. Pedersen, P. Møller, and M. Lund-Johansen, "Treatment of vestibular schwannomas. Why, when and how?" *Acta Neurochirurgica*, vol. 149, no. 7, pp. 647–660, 2007.

[7] D. J. Holt, P. M. Foy, and E. A. Field, "Orofacial paraesthesia: an unusual presentation of acoustic neuroma," *Dental Update*, vol. 29, no. 3, pp. 141–142, 2002.

[8] R. Pérusse, "Acoustic neuroma presenting as orofacial anesthesia," *International Journal of Oral and Maxillofacial Surgery*, vol. 23, no. 3, pp. 156–160, 1994.

[9] S. G. Harner and E. R. Laws Jr., "Clinical findings in patients with acoustic neurinoma," *Mayo Clinic Proceedings*, vol. 58, no. 11, pp. 721–728, 1983.

[10] S. Berrettini, F. Ravecca, F. Russo, P. Bruschini, and S. Sellari-Franceschini, "Some uncharacteristic clinical signs and symptoms of acoustic neuroma," *Journal of Otolaryngology*, vol. 26, no. 2, pp. 97–103, 1997.

[11] R. F. Bento, M. H. Pinna, and R. V. De Brito Neto, "Vestibular schwannoma: 825 cases from a 25-year experience," *International Archives of Otorhinolaryngology*, vol. 16, no. 4, pp. 466–475, 2012.

[12] R. C. Swensson, R. P. Swensson, F. E. C. Pizzini, P. R. Boldorini, and J. J. Jorge Jr., "An uncommon presentation of an VIII nerve tumor," *Brazilian Journal of Otorhinolaryngology*, vol. 74, no. 4, pp. 628–631, 2008.

[13] T. D. Erson, L. A. Loevner, D. C. Bigelow, and N. Mirza, "Prevalence of unsuspected acoustic neuroma found by magnetic resonance imaging," *Otolaryngology—Head and Neck Surgery*, vol. 122, no. 5, pp. 643–646, 2000.

[14] J. W. Ferguson and J. F. Burton, "Clinical presentation of acoustic nerve neuroma in the oral and maxillofacial region," *Oral Surgery, Oral Medicine, Oral Pathology*, vol. 69, no. 6, pp. 672–675, 1990.

[15] C. Matthies and M. Samii, "Management of 1000 vestibular schwannomas (acoustic neuromas): clinical presentation," *Neurosurgery*, vol. 40, no. 1, pp. 1–9, 1997.

[16] R. N. Sahu, S. Behari, V. K. Agarwal, P. Giri, and V. Jain, "Taste dysfunction in vestibular schwannomas," *Neurology India*, vol. 56, no. 1, pp. 42–46, 2008.

[17] K. Watanabe, N. Saito, M. Taniguchi, T. Kirino, and T. Sasaki, "Analysis of taste disturbance before and after surgery in patients with vestibular schwannoma," *Journal of Neurosurgery*, vol. 99, no. 6, pp. 999–1003, 2003.

45

Seven-Year Follow-Up of Peutz-Jeghers Syndrome

Hamid Reza Mozaffari,[1] **Fetemeh Rezaei,**[1] **Roohollah Sharifi,**[2] **and S. Ghasem Mirbahari**[3]

[1]*Department of Oral Medicine, School of Dentistry, Kermanshah University of Medical Sciences, Kermanshah, Iran*
[2]*Department of Endodontics, School of Dentistry, Kermanshah University of Medical Sciences, Kermanshah, Iran*
[3]*Department of Pathology, School of Medicine, Kermanshah University of Medical Sciences, Kermanshah, Iran*

Correspondence should be addressed to Fetemeh Rezaei; f.rezaei@kums.ac.ir

Academic Editor: Yousef S. Khader

One of the clinicopathological criteria for diagnosing Peutz-Jeghers syndrome (PJS) is mucocutaneous pigmentation. We present a 57-year-old Iranian female patient with diffuse pigmentation in buccal and labial mucosa. The first colonoscopy revealed one 0.5 cm rectal polyp. However surveillance colonoscopies over a 7-year polyp showed over 100 colorectal polyps.

1. Introduction

Peutz-Jeghers syndrome (PJS) is a rare inherited autosomal dominant disease with an incidence of 1 in 12–30,000 live births, characterized by mucocutaneous pigmentation and multiple hamartomatous polyps in the gastrointestinal tract. PJS patients have a marked increase of risk of developing cancer [1].

A germline mutation in *STK11*, a tumour suppressor gene localized to chromosome 19p13.2–13.3, is an underlying abnormality [2].

The clinicopathological criteria of World Health Organisation (WHO) for diagnosing PJS are as follows:

(1) Three or more polyps, with histological features of PJS.

(2) A family history of PJS with any number of polyps.

(3) A family history of PJS with characteristic mucocutaneous pigmentation.

(4) Characteristic mucocutaneous pigmentation with any number of polyps [3].

To improve the understanding, diagnosis, and treatment of PJS, we now report a case of PJS.

2. Case Present

A 57-year-old Iranian female patient was referred to us (oral medicine specialist), with a chief complaint of pigmentation in oral cavity for more than 15 years.

The patient had scattered dark brown to black macules, most of them measuring <0.5 cm on the buccal and labial mucosa. These pigmentations were asymptomatic and well circumscribed and did not fade under pressure (Figure 1).

There were not any similar macules on the tongue, lips, perioral skin, nostril, hands, and feet. She was previously healthy and took no regular medications. She had no abdominal pain, nausea, vomiting, diarrhea, or history of changing in bowel habits or any significant loss of weight or appetite. In family survey, just her brother had PJS with perioral pigmentation and intestinal polyps compatible with Peutz-Jeghers polyp on histology and without any signs and symptoms of GI diseases, but unfortunately he died in car accident many years ago. Her children (two daughters and one boy) do not have any sign or symptom of this syndrome.

Biopsy of pigmentation on buccal mucosa was performed. Histopathologically there is evidence of increased basilar melanin with melanin incontinence into the submucosa (Figure 2).

The patient with primary diagnosis of PJS was referred to gastroenterologists for more diagnostic assessments.

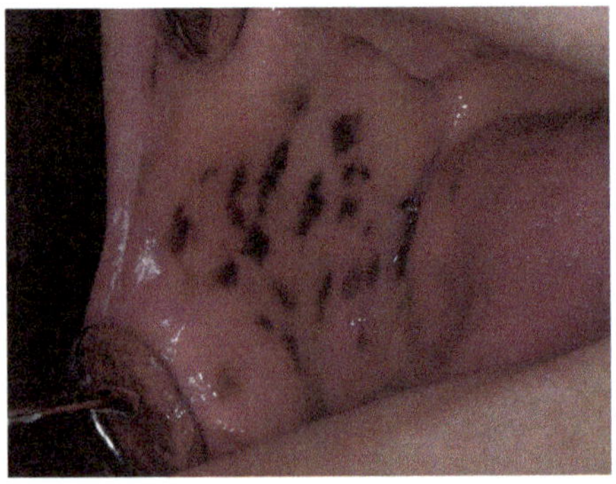

FIGURE 1: Mucocutaneous pigmentation on the buccal mucosa.

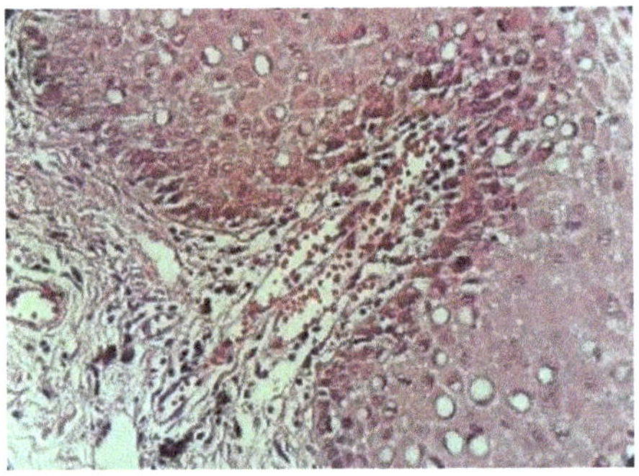

FIGURE 2: Biopsy of pigmentation on buccal mucosa indicates increased basilar melanin with melanin incontinence into the submucosa (H&E staining).

In the first colonoscopy, there was only one polyp in the rectum measuring 0.5 cm in diameter, without any features of invasions or intussusceptions.

In the past 7 years the patient was examined for oral pigmentations and intestinal polyps every year. We did not observe any significant change in oral pigmentations during these years. She also did not have any sign or symptom of GI diseases except mild constipation, but endoscopy of GI showed the increase of the number of polyps every year. In the last colonoscopy there were more than 100 polyps with the size of <1 cm in the large bowel and rectum; no features of invasion and intussusceptions were noticed. Pathological examination of the polyps confirmed adenomatous and hamartomatous polyps (tubular type), with low grade dysplasia (Figure 3).

3. Discussion

In 1921, Dutch physician Peutz noted the combination of gastrointestinal polyps and mucocutaneous melanotic spots in three young children [4].

The presented case in this report was of particular interest since there are few reported cases of PJS with long-term follow-up [5]. We were able to visit the patient annually and trace her medical findings. Another important issue in this report was a different course of the disease. Her pigmentation

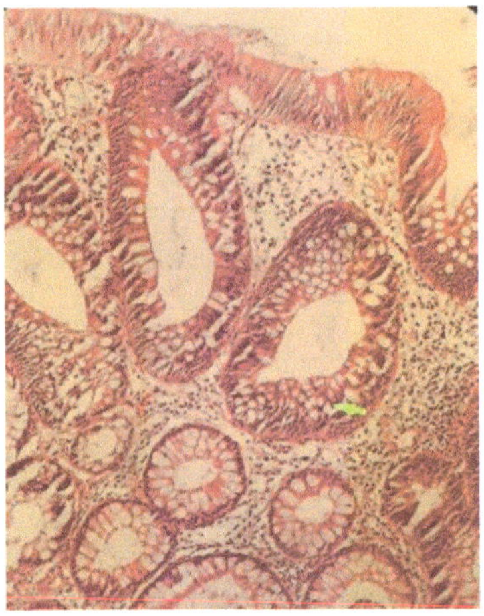

FIGURE 3: Pathological examination of the polyps confirmed adenomatous and hamartomatous polyps (tubular type), with low grade dysplasia (H&E staining).

showed little change but there was a dramatic increase in the development of colorectal polyps over 7 years.

Male-to-female ratio of PJS is 1 : 1. The average age at the time of diagnosis is 23 years in men and 26 years in women [6], but our patient was in sixth decade of her life.

Although most of pigmentations of PJS are located around of mouth cheek, nostril, periorbital, ears, and overall orifices of body [3], these pigmentations of our patient were located intraorally in buccal and labial mucosa. Also Mozaffar et al. reported a PJS without mucocutaneous pigmentation [6]. So PJS may have a variable spectrum of manifestations in mucocutaneous pigmentation. The probable explanation is novel mutations in contributing genes [7].

Hamartomatous polyps commonly involve the jejunum and patients usually have complained of GI diseases like abdominal pain, diarrhea or bleeding, and bowel obstruction including intussusception [8]. In our patient the colon was the most common site of these polyps and she did not have any sign and symptom of GI disturbance even after 7 years (with 100 polyps). Also Matini reported three cases of PJS without clinical symptoms like abdominal pain and acute or chronic rectal blood loss and with no evidence of gastrointestinal or extragastrointestinal malignancy during 14 years of follow-up [5].

The treatment for mucocutaneous pigmentations of PJS was usually considered unnecessary; but in some patients, the appearance of brown discoloration, especially on the skin, can be bothersome, so laser therapy can be a choice treatment [9]. The pigmentations of our patient were intraoral and the face skin was not involved so we did not treat them.

The opinions for treatment of polyps are different. Some consider these polyps as premalignant lesions, which should be paid considerable attention and removed by surgery or endoscopy. However, others found out that rate of cancer in these polyps is very low, so periodic endoscopic surveillance is enough [5, 10, 11]. As a limitation in this case report, there was not mutation analysis to find out a defect in the *STK11* gene is responsible for the PJS phenotype in this patient.

In the case we reported that our patient even with diffuse gastrointestinal polyposis does not have any complaint of abdomen pain, bloody stool, or other symptoms. So no particular medication or surgery was administrated while in periodic follow-up.

In conclusion clinical manifestations of PJS may be varied and the clinical course of this disease is not predictable.

4. Conclusion

In conclusion, it is recommended that any patient presenting with multiple pigmentation or incomprehensible discoloration in oral cavity should be investigated for systemic diseases like Peutz-Jeghers syndrome.

Consent

Written informed consent was obtained from the patient for publication and presenting of this case and any accompanying images.

Competing Interests

The authors declare that they have no competing interests.

References

[1] M. Kopacova, I. Tacheci, S. Rejchrt, and J. Bures, "Peutz-Jeghers syndrome: diagnostic and therapeutic approach," *World Journal of Gastroenterology*, vol. 15, no. 43, pp. 5397–5408, 2009.

[2] I. R. Schreibman, M. Baker, C. Amos, and T. J. McGarrity, "The hamartomatous polyposis syndromes: a clinical and molecular review," *American Journal of Gastroenterology*, vol. 100, no. 2, pp. 476–490, 2005.

[3] S. Bhattacharya, S. R. Mahapatra, R. Nangalia et al., "Melaena with peutz-jeghers syndrome: a case report," *Journal of Medical Case Reports*, vol. 4, article 44, 2010.

[4] F. Girvin, S. Glancy, and M. Dunlop, "Peutz-Jeghers syndrome: a case report and discussion of surveillance recommendations," *European Journal of Radiology Extra*, vol. 62, no. 3, pp. 81–84, 2007.

[5] E. Matini, H. Houshangi, E. Jangholi, F. P. Azad, R. Najipour, and A. Farshad, "Three cases in a family with different manifestations and no evidence of malignancy during 14 years follow up," *Iranian Red Crescent Medical Journal*, vol. 17, no. 12, Article ID e19271, 2015.

[6] M. Mozaffar, M. R. Sobhiyeh, M. Hasani, and M. Fallah, "Peutz-Jeghers syndrome without mucocutaneous pigmentation: a case report," *Gastroenterology and Hepatology from Bed to Bench*, vol. 5, no. 3, pp. 169–173, 2012.

[7] K. Shinmura, M. Gota, H. Tao et al., "A novel STK11 germline mutation in two siblings with Peutz-Jeghers syndrome complicated by primary gastric cancer," *Clinical Genetics*, vol. 67, no. 1, pp. 81–86, 2005.

[8] N. Sinha, U. Chatterjee, and S. Sarkar, "Jejunal carcinoma in a patient with Peutz-Jeghers syndrome," *Canadian Journal of Surgery*, vol. 52, no. 6, pp. E299–E300, 2009.

[9] Y. Li, Q. Zeng, Z. Liao, G. Zhang, R. Xiao, and H. Wen, "Peutz-Jeghers syndrome and family survey: a case report," *International Journal of Clinical and Experimental Pathology*, vol. 6, no. 5, pp. 982–984, 2013.

[10] S. Sung Kwan and R. C. Boland, "Endoscopic management in Juvenile Polyposis, Peutz-Jeghers syndrome, and other hamartomatous polyposis syndromes," *Techniques in Gastrointestinal Endoscopy*, vol. 8, no. 3, pp. 119–125, 2006.

[11] K. Akimaru, S. Katoh, S. Ishiguro, K. Miyake, K. Shimanuki, and T. Tajiri, "Resection of over 290 polyps during emergency surgery for four intussusceptions with Peutz-Jeghers syndrome: report of a case," *Surgery Today*, vol. 36, no. 11, pp. 997–1002, 2006.

Healing of an Extensive Periradicular Lesion Subsequent to a Proper Endodontic Treatment of a Mandibular First Premolar with Complex Anatomy

Hengameh Ashraf,[1] Payam Paymanpour,[1] Maryam Mojtahed Bidabadi,[1] and Reihaneh Hajrezai[2]

[1] *Department of Endodontics, Shahid Beheshti University of Medical Science, Tehran, Iran*
[2] *Department of Orthodontics, Dental Branch, Islamic Azad University, Tehran, Iran*

Correspondence should be addressed to Maryam Mojtahed Bidabadi; maryam.mojtahed@yahoo.com

Academic Editors: D. W. Boston, S.-I. Stratul, and E. F. Wright

Long-term success of endodontic treatment is strictly dependent on proper shaping and cleaning of the root canal system followed by obturation of entire prepared space. Anatomical variations should be considered during radiographic and clinical evaluation as parts of endodontic treatment. A mandibular premolar with three canals is quite rare and such a tooth requires special canal preparation and obturation techniques. An astute clinician should identify different canal configurations and treat them endodontically well, because presence of an untreated canal could be a reason for failure of endodontic treatment. This paper describes the conventional orthograde endodontic therapy on an unusual mandibular first premolar with three root canals.

1. Introduction

A thorough knowledge of anatomy and morphology of root canal system is essential for a successful root canal treatment. Bear in mind that parallel buccolingual radiographs may not always determine correct morphology of tooth. A two-dimensional radiographic view of a three-dimensional tooth, poses serious problems for anatomical assessment of a root canal system that need to be treated. Different horizontal angulations of X-ray cone are considered worthwhile adjuncts to clarify hidden aspects of root canal system. Because of anatomical variations, mandibular premolars are difficult for endodontic treatment and a higher failure rate is expected. As we know, main purpose of endodontic therapy is to prevent or resolve periradicular periodontitis. Periradicular radiolucencies develop depending on the balance between microbial virulence factors and host defenses [1]. A primary aim of all endodontic procedures, specially cleaning and shaping, is to remove infective microorganisms and necrotic tissues [2]. Considering that canals are often underprepared in apical one-third [3] and root canal systems cannot be completely disinfected [4–7], obturation of the prepared root canal space is necessary. Obturation reduces coronal leakage and bacterial recontamination, seals the apex from periapical tissue fluids, and entombs remaining irritants within canal [8]. Division of canals into two or more is a challenging situation for both cleaning shaping and obturation of root canal system that could result in periradicular periodontitis. Clinical exploration is essential to detect division of canal. During formation of the root, the apical foramen of each root has a wide opening limited by the epithelial diaphragm and the shape of the pulp canal is like a wide-open tube [9]. Differentiation of a root into separate canals occurs by continued deposition of dentin [10]. A higher number of extra canals in mandibular premolars of African descent have been reported compared with Caucasian patients [11]. International studies have shown the existence of second or third canal was noted in only 23.1 per cent of first mandibular premolars and in only 12.1 per cent of second mandibular premolars [12]. Table 1 describes some studies and case reports which reported mandibular first premolar with three canals.

TABLE 1: Trifurcated canals for the mandibular first premolar (%).

Zillich and Dowson [12]	4.3
Yoshioka et al. [13]	0
Sert and Byirli [14]	2.2
Al-Qudah and Awawdeh [15]	Case report
Nallapti [16]	Case report

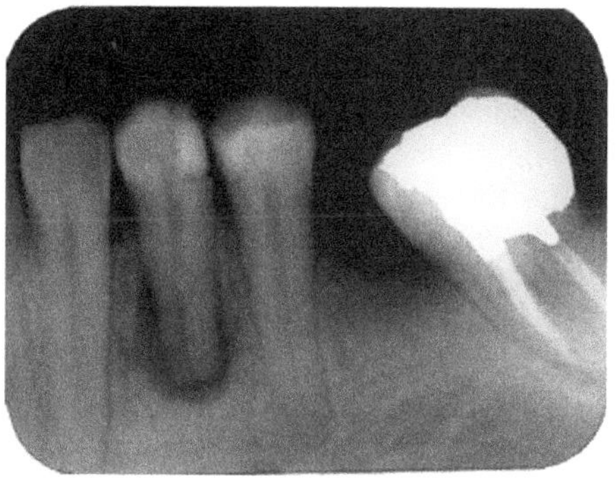

FIGURE 1: Periapical radiograph of mandibular left first premolar revealing complex root canal system.

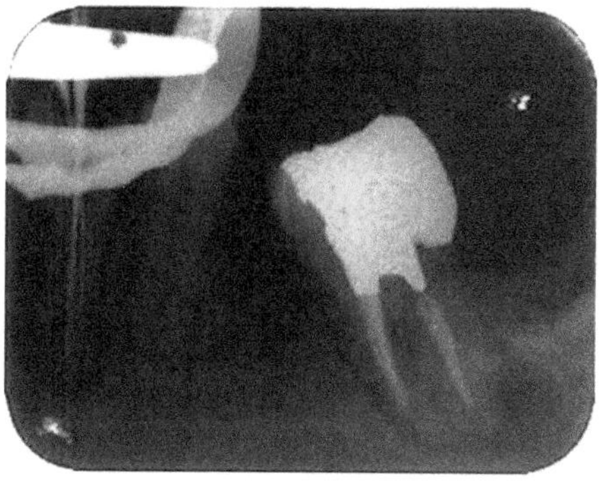

FIGURE 2: Working length radiograph confirming three root canal orifices.

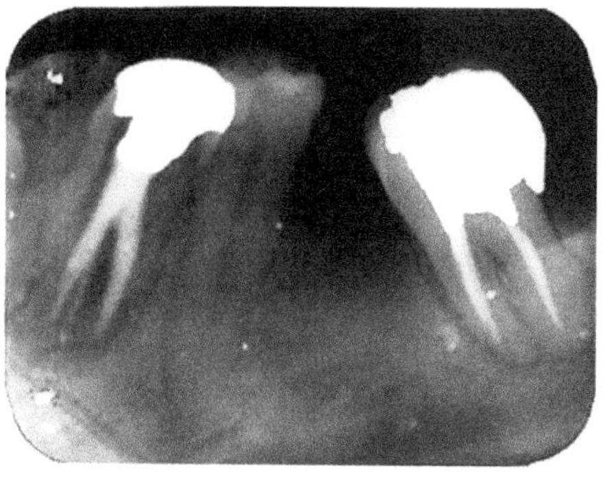

FIGURE 3: Radiograph revealing complete obturation.

2. Case Report

A 42-year-old female with no remarkable medical history was referred to the Endodontics Department of Shahid Beheshti Dental School for root canal treatment of her left first mandibular premolar. The patient had not any complaint about the mentioned tooth and the tooth was asymptomatic. However, an extensive radiolucency associated with periradicular lesion of tooth was detected through routine radiographs (Figure 1). There was no sensitivity to percussion. Vitality testing was negative for the tooth suggesting pulp necrosis. A large defective composite resin coronal restoration was present. Periodontal probing was within the normal limits.

Parallel diagnostic radiograph showed a substantial periradicular lesion, calcification, and division of root canal system at midroot. In this radiograph, an extra canal was obviously diverged distally from the main canal with a sharp angle. 2% Lidocaine plus 1 : 80,000 epinephrine (Darou Pakhsh Co., Tehran, Iran) was used for inferior alveolar nerve block. Rubber dam was applied and access cavity preparation was accomplished. After removing coronal pulpal tissue, only one orifice was observed. Size #2, #3, and #4 Gates Glidden burs (MANI Inc., Japan) were used for initial opening of canal orifice. Through further exploration with a bended #10 and #15 K-files (Maillefer, Switzerland) entrance of divided canals was located. Root canal lengths were estimated with an electronic apex locator (Smarpex, Meta, Korea) and these lengths were confirmed by further radiographs. In this radiograph, trunk of canal seemed to trifurcate at midroot level giving rise to three separate canals and apical foramina (Figure 2). Sodium hypochlorite (5.25%) was used as endodontic irrigant. Apical preparation was performed by using both hand K-files and ProTaper rotary files (DENTSPLY, Switzerland). During preparation, size #15 K-file was used to establish and maintain apical patency. Master apical file was of size #30 for all the root canals. Calcium hydroxide was used as intracanal medicament and access cavity was sealed with temporary filling (Coltosol, Ariadent, Iran). Two weeks later, patient returned for second visit and the tooth was asymptomatic. After application of dental rubber dam, coronal temporary filling was removed. 5.25% sodium hypochlorite was used for removing intracanal calcium hydroxide and root canal irrigation. After drying with paper points, canals were obturated with gutta-percha and AH26 Sealer (DENTSPLY Caulk) via cold lateral compaction technique and access cavity was sealed with temporary filling (Cavit 3M ESPE, St. Paul, MN, USA) (Figure 3). Final radiographic examination showed distal canal diverged from main canal more coronally than mesial canal which divided into two distinct canals at apical one third. At 3-month recall, patient was asymptomatic (Figure 4) and 6-month recall radiograph showed significant healing (Figure 5).

3. Discussion

Knowledge of common root canal morphology and its frequent variations is a prerequisite for successful endodontic treatment. These variations in pulpal anatomy must be considered at the beginning of endodontic treatment [17]. The possibility that there is more than one root canal in lower premolar teeth should always be expected. Accurate straight

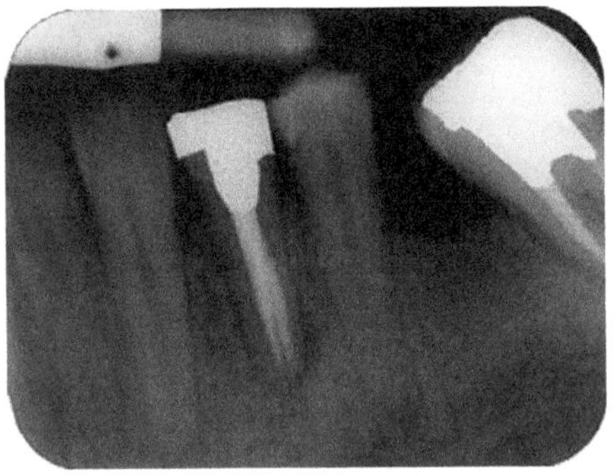

FIGURE 4: A 3-month recall shows dramatic healing.

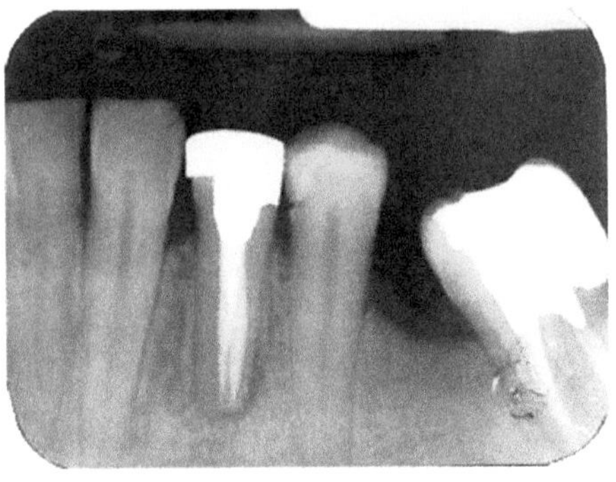

FIGURE 5: A 1-year recall shows complete healing.

and angled preoperative radiographs and clinical clues are essential in exploring the number of roots canals that exist in a tooth. In this case to view individual canals we used 35-degree distal angled radiograph which could separate canals. Presence of untreated canal may be a reason for failure of endodontic therapy [18]. Electronic apex locators are useful adjuncts for determining working length in all cases, particularly complex anatomical variations. Use of both of electronic devices and angled radiographs provides greater accuracy [19]. Missing of anatomic information may be resulted if electronic apex locators are used exclusively. Additional anatomic information about root canals can be obtained by careful observation of positioning and deformation of instruments [20]. It is most important to be on the lookout for additional canals. In this case, a single broad root canal trifurcated into three separate root canals. Enhanced lighting and visibility are important aids for locating root canals. Dental operating microscope provides magnification and illumination which improves the ability to locate and negotiate canals [21]. When working with operating microscope can many times see hypochlorite bubbling in extra canal, marking its presence. On occasion, dyes or transillumination may be helpful in locating additional canal [22].

Although no significant difference was found in periapical healing between one- or two-visit endodontic treatment of necrotic teeth [23], some factors such as the patient's health, anxiety, fatigue, and symptoms, in addition to complexity of treatment, should be considered. Su et al. described that the healing rate of single- and multiple-visit root canal treatment is similar for infected teeth [24]. Multiple-visit and single-visit root canal treatment demonstrated almost equal success but most important aspect for success in treatment is indication of each case and then its subsequent treatment, be it multiple or single visit root canal treatment [25].

Nonsurgical endodontic therapy proved successful in promoting the healing of periapical lesions; irrespective of the size of the lesion every attempt should be made to treat the periapical lesions with non surgical endodontic therapy [26]. Intracanal placement of calcium hydroxide has been proposed because of its antimicrobial properties in necrotic cases that cannot be treated in one visit [27]. It has been reported that treatment with calcium hydroxide resulted in high frequency of periapical healing and some lesions, especially in young patients, were reduced or had completely disappeared only 1 or 3 months after treatment [28]. $Ca(OH)_2$ is proven to assist periapical healing by virtue of its antibacterial properties and also by its biological action facilitating osseous repair [29].

Finally, there is a need for further studies to determine the frequency of anatomic variations in root canal system of Iranian population and referral to an endodontist seems to be mutually beneficial in complex anatomic variations of root canal system.

4. Conclusion

Although frequency of first mandibular premolars with an unusual anatomical configuration is not common, each tooth should be investigated carefully, clinically, and radiographically to detect possible anatomical variations before commencement of endodontic treatment.

References

[1] P. Stashenko, R. Teles, and R. D'Souza, "Periapical inflammatory responses and their modulation," *Critical Reviews in Oral Biology and Medicine*, vol. 9, no. 4, pp. 498–521, 1998.

[2] P. V. Abbott, "The periapical space—a dynamic interface," *Australian Endodontic Journal*, vol. 28, no. 3, pp. 96–107, 2002.

[3] S. J. Card, A. Sigurdsson, D. Orstavik, and M. Trope, "The effectiveness of increased apical enlargement in reducing intracanal bacteria," *Journal of Endodontics*, vol. 28, no. 11, pp. 779–783, 2002.

[4] F. Heard and R. E. Walton, "Scanning electron microscope study comparing four root canal preparation techniques in small curved canals," *International Endodontic Journal*, vol. 30, no. 5, pp. 323–331, 1997.

[5] J. F. Siqueira Jr., C. H. F. Pereira da Suva, M. Das, M. das Cerqueira, H. P. Lopes, and M. de Uzeda, "Effectiveness of four chemical solutions in eliminating *Bacillus subtilis* spores on gutta-percha cones," *Endodontics and Dental Traumatology*, vol. 14, no. 3, pp. 124–126, 1998.

[6] R. E. Walton, "Histologic evaluation of different methods of enlarging the pulp canal space," *Journal of Endodontics*, vol. 2, no. 10, pp. 304–311, 1976.

[7] M.-K. Wu, L. W. M. van der Sluis, and P. R. Wesselink, "The capability of two hand instrumentation techniques to remove the inner layer of dentine in oval canals," *International Endodontic Journal*, vol. 36, no. 3, pp. 218–224, 2003.

[8] P. D. Delivanis, G. D. Mattison, and R. W. Mendel, "The survivability of F43 strain of *Streptococcussanguis* in root canals filled with gutta-percha and procosol cement," *Journal of Endodontics*, vol. 9, no. 10, pp. 407–410, 1983.

[9] B. J. Orban, Ed., *Oral Histology and Embryology*, Mosby, St. Louis, Mo, USA, 4 edition, 1957.

[10] A. Nanci, Ed., *Ten Cate's Oral Histology, Development, Structure and Function*, Mosby, St. Louis, Mo, USA, 7 edition, 2008.

[11] M. Trope, L. Elfenbein, and L. Tronstad, "Mandibular premolars with more than one root canal in different race groups," *Journal of Endodontics*, vol. 12, no. 8, pp. 343–345, 1986.

[12] R. Zillich and J. Dowson, "Root canal morphology of mandibular first and second premolars," *Oral Surgery Oral Medicine and Oral Pathology*, vol. 36, no. 5, pp. 738–744, 1973.

[13] T. Yoshioka, J. C. Villegas, C. Kobayashi, and H. Suda, "Radiographic evaluation of root canal multiplicity in mandibular first premolars," *Journal of Endodontics*, vol. 30, no. 2, pp. 73–74, 2004.

[14] S. Sert and G. S. Bayirli, "Evaluation of the root canal configurations of the mandibular and maxillary permanent teeth by gender in the Turkish population," *Journal of Endodontics*, vol. 30, no. 6, pp. 391–398, 2004.

[15] A. A. Al-Qudah and L. A. Awawdeh, "Root canal morphology of mandibular incisors in a Jordanian population," *International Endodontic Journal*, vol. 39, no. 11, pp. 873–877, 2006.

[16] S. Nallapati, "Three canal mandibular first and second premolars: a treatment approach. A case report," *Journal of Endodontics*, vol. 31, no. 6, pp. 474–476, 2005.

[17] C. Maniglia-Ferreira, F. de Almeida-Gomes, B. C. de Sousa, C. C. Dos Santos Acioli Lins, and R. A. Dos Santos, "A case of unusual anatomy in second mandibular molar with four canals," *European Journal of Dentistry*, vol. 2, no. 3, pp. 217–219, 2008.

[18] F. J. Vertucci, "Root canal morphology and its relationship to endodontic procedures," *Endodontic Topics*, vol. 10, pp. 3–29, 2005.

[19] A. ElAyouti, R. Weiger, and C. Löst, "The ability of root ZX apex locator to reduce the frequency of overestimated radiographic working length," *Journal of Endodontics*, vol. 28, no. 2, pp. 116–119, 2002.

[20] C. E. Jerome and R. J. Hanlon Jr., "Identifying multiplanar root canal curvatures using stainless-steel instruments," *Journal of Endodontics*, vol. 29, no. 5, pp. 356–358, 2003.

[21] M. C. Coelho De Carvalho and M. L. Zuolo, "Orifice locating with a microscope," *Journal of Endodontics*, vol. 26, no. 9, pp. 532–534, 2000.

[22] S. Nallapati and G. Glassman, "Ophthalmic dyes for root canal location," *Endodontic Practice*, vol. 7, pp. 21–26, 2004.

[23] V. A. Penesis, P. I. Fitzgerald, M. I. Fayad, C. S. Wenckus, E. A. BeGole, and B. R. Johnson, "Outcome of one-visit and two-visit endodontic treatment of necrotic teeth with apical periodontitis: a randomized controlled trial with one-year evaluation," *Journal of Endodontics*, vol. 34, no. 3, pp. 251–257, 2008.

[24] Y. Su, C. Wang, and L. Ye, "Healing rate and post-obturation pain of single- versus multiple-visit endodontic treatment for infected root canals: a systematic review," *Journal of Endodontics*, vol. 37, no. 2, pp. 125–132, 2011.

[25] S. Rajesh, M. Nikhil, and D. Samir, "Single visit versus multiple visit root canal therapy, Review," *Jaypee International Journal of Clinical Pediatric Dentistry*, vol. 1, pp. 17–24, 2008.

[26] V. Venugopal, S. Anil Kumar, and K. N. Jyothi, "Successful healing of periapical lesions with non-surgical Endodontic Approach," *Journal of Dental Science and Research*, vol. 2, no. 1, pp. 1–6, 2011.

[27] U. Sjögren, D. Figdor, S. Persson, and G. Sundqvist, "Influence of infection at the time of root filling on the outcome of endodontic treatment of teeth with apical periodontitis," *International Endodontic Journal*, vol. 30, no. 5, pp. 297–306, 1997.

[28] W. H. Binnie and D. F. Mitchell, "Induced calcification in the subdermal tissues of the rat," *Journal of Dental Research*, vol. 52, no. 5, pp. 1087–1091, 1973.

[29] M. Tanomaru Filho, M. R. Leonardo, and L. A. B. da Silva, "Effect of irrigating solution and calcium hydroxide root canal dressing on the repair of apical and periapical tissues of teeth with periapical lesion," *Journal of Endodontics*, vol. 28, no. 4, pp. 295–299, 2002.

47

Oral Rehabilitation of an Osteopetrosis Patient with Osteomyelitis

Tamer Celakil, Merve Dogan, Bilge Gokcen Rohlig, Gulumser Evlioglu, and Haluk Keskin

Department of Prosthodontics, Faculty of Dentistry, Istanbul University, 34093 Istanbul, Turkey

Correspondence should be addressed to Tamer Celakil; tamer.celakil@istanbul.edu.tr

Academic Editor: Leandro N. de Souza

Osteopetrosis is a congenital disorder characterized by increasing osteoclastic function resulting in osteomyelitis in the jaws. Orofacial findings in osteopetrosis patients are unerupted, malformed, or delayed teeth and many dental caries due to vulnerable enamel and dentin and osteomyelitis. Many reports have described that maxilla is an uncommon site of occurrence for osteomyelitis due to cortical bone morphology and collateral circulation. This report aims to discuss clinical features and prosthodontic management of a patient with clinical features of adult form of osteopetrosis and osteomyelitis in both jaws. The patient has reported better masticatory and speech efficiency with removable dentures in maxillary and mandibular jaw and also self-esteem improvement and family interaction.

1. Introduction

Osteopetrosis (OP; Albers-Schönberg disease, marble bone disease, generalized congenital osteosclerosis, ivory bones, and osteosclerosis fragilis generalista) is a hereditary disorder characterized by defective osteoclastic function and impaired bone resorption resulting in dense bone [1–4]. OP is stated in an autosomal recessive form (ARO; Infantile Malignant OP) or autosomal dominant form (ADO; Adult Benign OP) [1, 4]. The estimated prevalence of ARO is approximately 1 in 300000 births, and clinical manifestations are generally hematologic, neurologic, and skeletal abnormalities such as fragile bones, anemia, thrombocytopenia, and impaired vision and hearing [5–8]. Furthermore, clinical manifestations of ADO are primarily skeletal manifestations and the incidence of ADO is 1 in 20000 births [6, 9].

Some studies reported that ADO gene is located in chromosome 1p21 [10]. The pathogenesis of ADO involves diminished osteoclast-mediated skeletal resorption. Bone is not resorbed although the number of osteoclasts is often increased. This defective osteoclastic bone resorption may lead to osteosclerosis [11]. Radiological changes of osteosclerosis, such as "bone within a bone" appearance and transverse radiolucent bands, are typical findings of ADO [5, 12, 13].

Orofacial examination in ADO patients generally results in similar findings such as unerupted, malformed, or delayed teeth and many dental caries due to vulnerable enamel and dentin. Furthermore, osteomyelitis (OM) is the most severe complication and orofacial finding of ADO [11].

OM is an infection of bone, often caused by bacteria, that confines to the medullary cavity [14]. Poor vascular circulation on ADO may lead to OM in jaws after dental extractions [11]. Therefore, infection control before and after dental treatment is of vital importance. Once infection and OM are observed in patients with OP, they can be intractable because of poor-wound healing ability [1, 15]. OM in OP patients generally occurs in mandibular jaw. OM of the maxilla is infrequent due to the cortical bone morphology and collateral circulation [16].

Most of the previous studies have presented surgical procedures of ARO and ADO, fewer reports are available from a prosthetic aspect, and prosthetic management of ADO is unclear [1–4, 6, 7, 17–22]. This clinical report presents the prosthetic rehabilitation of an ADO patient with OM in both jaws. There is no published report on prosthetic management in ADO with OM in both jaws.

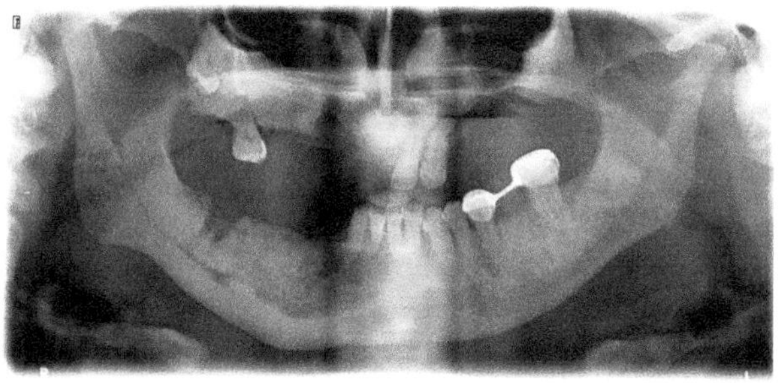

FIGURE 1: Panoramic radiography of the patient before extraction of the left maxillary central and lateral incisor in 2011.

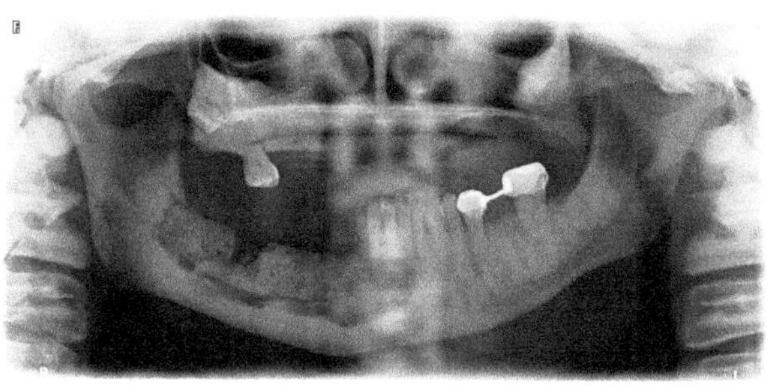

FIGURE 2: Panoramic radiograph showing osteomyelitis in the right mandibula due to extraction of the right mandibular second molar tooth.

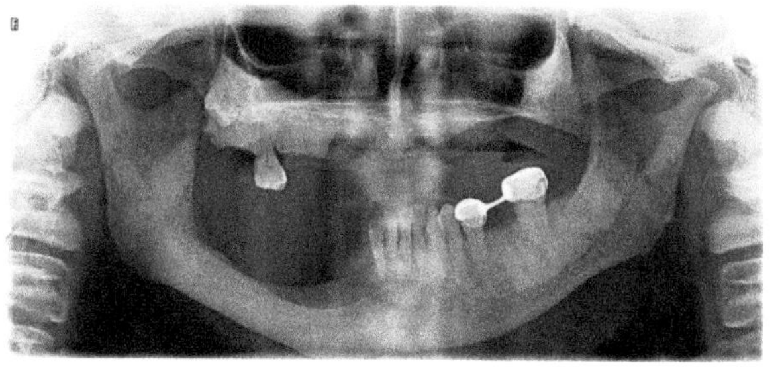

FIGURE 3: Postoperative panoramic radiography after bony sequestra removed in 2013.

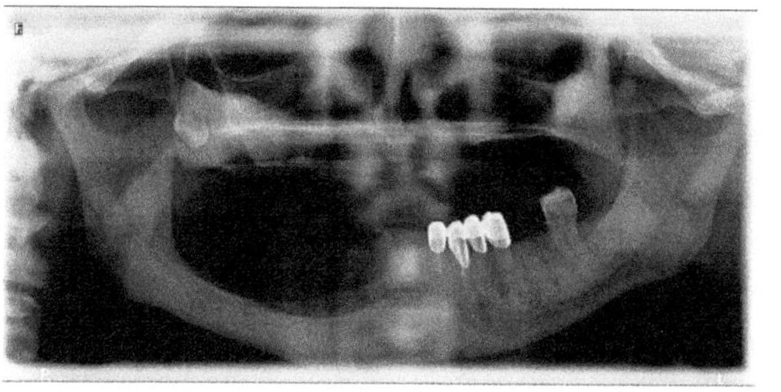

FIGURE 4: Panoramic radiography view of patient before rehabilitation with prostheses in 2014.

2. Case Presentation

A 48-year-old man suffered from ADO without prior family history of the disease and complained of deficiencies in speaking, swallowing, and mastication due to acquired maxillary and mandibular bone defects. He had been first diagnosed with a right femoral fracture in the 2000s. The patient had purulent drainage in the maxilla in 2003 and he informed no treatment performed in this clinical condition. He underwent surgical procedures, including the extraction of the left maxillary central and lateral incisor and right mandibular second molar tooth under local anesthesia in 2011 (Figures 1 and 2) and the sequestrectomy of right mandible under general anesthesia in 2013 (Figure 3). The patient was referred to the Department of Prosthodontics, Faculty of Dentistry, Istanbul University, for dental rehabilitation in 2014 (Figure 4).

At radiographic and oral examination, an unerupted third maxillary molar tooth and extensive bone defects in both jaws without any sign of sequestrum were diagnosed. Extraction of the right maxillary first molar, mandibular central incisors, and right mandibular lateral incisor was planned due to severe periodontal disease. Several treatment options were considered and the patient did not agree to any surgical treatment, so the decision was made to replace missing teeth and separation of nasal cavity from oral cavity with removable dentures in maxillary and mandibular jaw (Figures 5 and 6).

Antibiotics were provided for prophylaxis to prevent the infection of the bone due to extraction of the teeth. Tooth extractions and preparations were performed under local anesthesia, and the irreversible hydrocolloid impression material was used for making the preliminary impression and fabricating acrylic tray. Adhesive was applied to the tray and condensation silicone (Zetaplus System; Zhermack SpA, Badia Polesine, Italy) was loaded into the tray for master impression. Master casts were fabricated and maxillary master cast was mounted to the semiadjustable articulator (Artex CT; Amann Girrbach AG, Koblach, Austria) to locate the condylar (hinge) axis and mandibular master cast was than mounted to the articulator in centric relation. A maxillary obturator and a mandibular resection prosthesis with a fully balanced occlusion were fabricated. A permanent resilient liner was used to increase the comfort of the affected soft and hard tissues in the maxilla (Figure 7). Determination of the occlusal plane and occlusal adjustment was important for obtaining aesthetic and comfortable results.

The patient was satisfied with the aesthetic results and function. The patient has been followed up for 1 year and an oral hygiene program on a 1-month recall schedule was applied (Figure 8). At 1-year follow-up visit, the patient has reported better masticatory and speech efficiency, and also self-esteem improvement and family interaction.

3. Discussion

OP is a hereditary disease characterized by osteosclerosis and OM [22]. OM in OP patients should be treat carefully because OM may lead to some problems such as insufficient function, phonation, and esthetics. This clinical report demonstrates prosthetic treatment of an ADO patient with OM in both jaws.

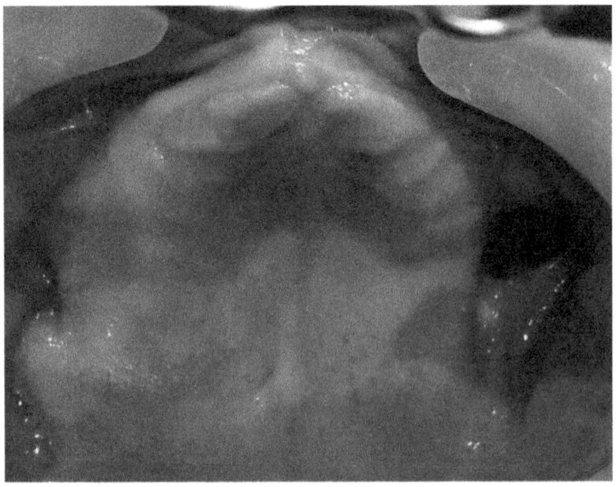

FIGURE 5: Intraoral photograph showing oronasal fistula in maxilla.

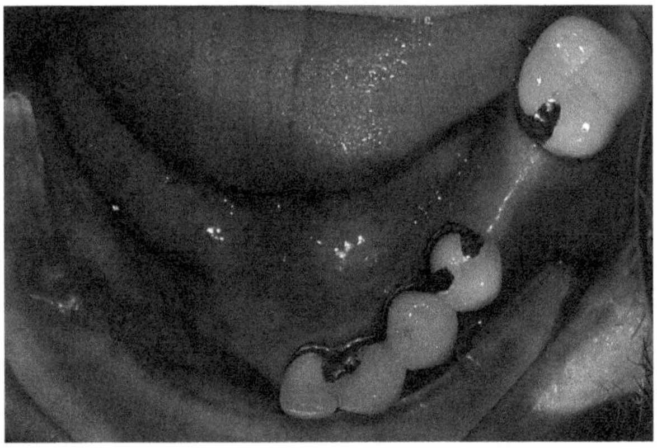

FIGURE 6: Occlusal surface of fixed prostheses and right mandibular defect due to sequestrectomy.

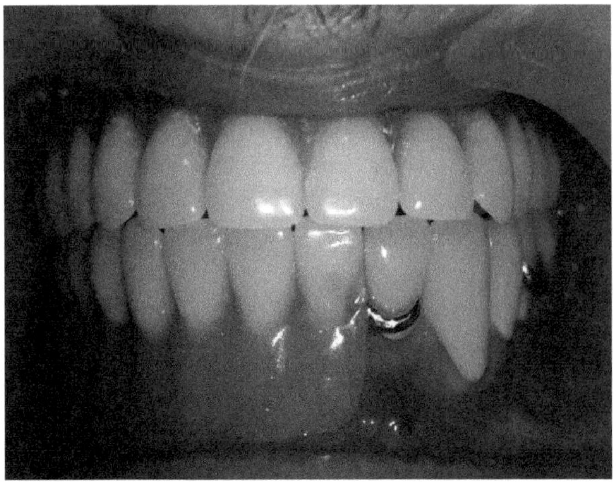

FIGURE 7: Frontal view with definitive prostheses in maxilla and mandibula.

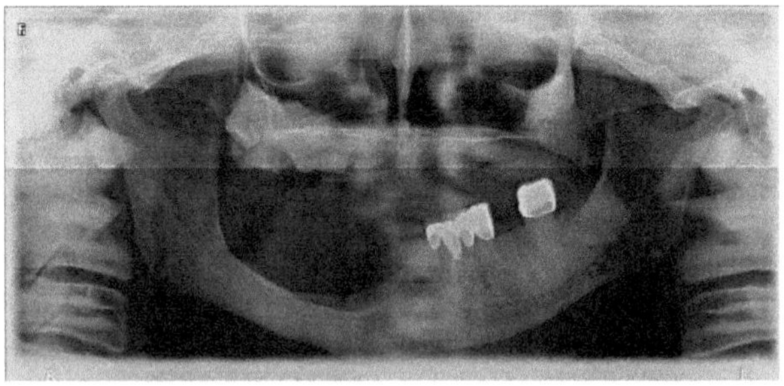

FIGURE 8: Panoramic radiography of patient at 1-year follow-up visit in 2015.

Gene mutations such as mutations in the ClCN7 genes can be responsible for osteosclerosis and these mutations are generally identified by presence of unerupted tooth [22–24]. Radiological examinations and clinical manifestations are generally adequate in ADO and performing a genetic study is unnecessary to confirm the disease [19, 25]. Some researchers state that conventional radiography and conventional computed tomography (CT), cone-beam computed tomography (CBCT), and magnetic resonance imaging (MRI) may evaluate OM in OP patients. Although some studies have reported that CT is more useful to diagnose OM and evaluate maxillofacial infections [14, 26–29], in this situation, the authors preferred to make the decision for the treatment plan on panoramic radiographs, because the patient was referred to our clinic after his control in Department of Oral Diagnosis and Radiology and he was reported to be infection-free. Differential diagnoses of OP are pycnodysostosis, craniometaphyseal dysplasia, endosteal hyperostosis, diaphyseal dysplasia, melorheostosis, osteosclerosis of fluoride poisoning, and osteopathia striata [11, 19]. After diagnostic analysis, the treatment for associated OM includes antibiotherapy and surgical procedures such as surgical removal of necrotic zone and soft tissue therapy [16, 19, 30]. OP patients generally remain asymptomatic and have a normal life expectancy after antibiotherapy [19].

OP associated with OM of the maxilla is a rare situation for reasons already noticed [6, 19]. The few reported patients in literature confirm the rarity of this condition [19]. In contrast, OM of the maxilla and mandibula was seen in this patient. Surgical interventions such as sequestrectomy, tooth extraction, and free bone grafting should be approached with caution due to the compromised blood circulation, and oral rehabilitation with obturator prostheses in the maxilla is the favored method of filling the defect [1, 19, 31, 32]. However, Naval et al. [33] reported the first patient of OP treated with dental implants and described the protocol used to treat OM that developed after failure of one implant. Prosthetic and surgical interventions should be based on clinical judgment, depending on the presenting conditions and patient needs [1].

This clinical report suggests that surgical therapy modalities such as dental extractions in patients with OP may lead to sclerotic bone areas result in OM in the mandibula and oroantral communication in the maxilla.

A patient with OP and OM in both jaws was treated prosthetically and they fulfilled the requirements of the patient. Prosthetic rehabilitation included the separation of nasal cavity from oral cavity with obturator prosthesis in maxilla and the replacement of missing teeth with removable prosthesis in the mandibula. Prosthodontists should be prepared against maxillary defects that may occur depending on the OM in maxillary jaw and knowledgeable about the rules of obturator prosthesis treatment option.

Conflict of Interests

All authors declare that there is no conflict of interests.

References

[1] Y. Ogino, Y. Ayukawa, Y. Tomita, and K. Koyano, "Prosthetic aspects in adult osteopetrosis," *Journal of Prosthetic Dentistry*, vol. 112, no. 4, pp. 736–740, 2014.

[2] H. D. C. de Oliveira, V. A. Pereira Filho, M. F. Real Gabrielli, M. A. Cabrini Gabrielli, and E. H. Vieira, "Marginal resection for treatment of mandibular osteomyelitis associated with osteopetrosis: case report," *Journal of Cranio-Maxillofacial Surgery*, vol. 39, no. 7, pp. 525–529, 2011.

[3] M. Oğütcen-Toller, M. Tek, I. Şener, C. Bereket, S. Inal, and B. Özden, "Intractable bimaxillary osteomyelitis in osteopetrosis: review of the literature and current therapy," *Journal of Oral and Maxillofacial Surgery*, vol. 68, no. 1, pp. 167–175, 2010.

[4] K. Satomura, M. Kon, R. Tokuyama et al., "Osteopetrosis complicated by osteomyelitis of the mandible: a case report including characterization of the osteopetrotic bone," *International Journal of Oral and Maxillofacial Surgery*, vol. 36, no. 1, pp. 86–93, 2007.

[5] J. Tolar, S. L. Teitelbaum, and P. J. Orchard, "Osteopetrosis," *The New England Journal of Medicine*, vol. 351, no. 27, pp. 2839–2849, 2004.

[6] R. G. Long and V. B. Ziccardi, "Osteopetrosis of the maxilla," *Oral Surgery, Oral Medicine, Oral Pathology, Oral Radiology, and Endodontics*, vol. 91, no. 2, pp. 139–140, 2001.

[7] S. Managutti, A. Managutti, and M. Pragasm, "Infantile osteomyelitis secondary to malignant osteopetrosis," *Journal of Maxillofacial and Oral Surgery*, vol. 11, no. 1, pp. 109–114, 2012.

[8] N. Er, O. Kasaboğlu, A. Atabek, K. Öktemer, and M. Akkocaoğlu, "Topical phenytoin treatment in bimaxillary osteomyelitis secondary to infantile osteopetrosis: report of a case," *Journal of Oral and Maxillofacial Surgery*, vol. 64, no. 7, pp. 1160–1164, 2006.

[9] J. Bollerslev and P. E. Andersen Jr., "Radiological, biochemical and hereditary evidence of two types of autosomal dominant osteopetrosis," *Bone*, vol. 9, no. 1, pp. 7–13, 1988.

[10] W. Van Hul, J. Bollerslev, J. Gram et al., "Localization of a gene for autosomal dominant osteopetrosis (Albers-Schönberg disease) to chromosome 1p21," *The American Journal of Human Genetics*, vol. 61, no. 2, pp. 363–369, 1997.

[11] D. K. Lam, G. K. B. Sándor, H. I. Holmes, R. P. Carmichael, and C. M. L. Clokie, "Marble bone disease: a review of osteopetrosis and its oral health implications for dentists," *Journal of the Canadian Dental Association*, vol. 73, no. 9, pp. 839–843, 2007.

[12] F. Shapiro, "Osteopetrosis: current clinical considerations," *Clinical Orthopaedics and Related Research*, vol. 294, pp. 34–44, 1993.

[13] R. Loría-Cortés, E. Quesada-Calvo, and C. Cordero-Chaverri, "Osteopetrosis in children. A report of 26 cases," *The Journal of Pediatrics*, vol. 91, no. 1, pp. 43–47, 1977.

[14] C.-H. An, S.-Y. An, B.-R. Choi et al., "Hard and soft tissue changes of osteomyelitis of the jaws on CT images," *Oral Surgery, Oral Medicine, Oral Pathology and Oral Radiology*, vol. 114, no. 1, pp. 118–126, 2012.

[15] C. C. Johnston Jr., N. Lavy, T. Lord, F. Vellios, A. D. Merritt, and W. P. Deiss Jr., "Osteopetrosis. A clinical, genetic, metabolic, and morphologic study of the dominantly inherited, benign form," *Medicine*, vol. 47, no. 2, pp. 149–167, 1968.

[16] C. P. Barry and C. D. Ryan, "Osteomyelitis of the maxilla secondary to osteopetrosis: report of a case," *Oral Surgery, Oral Medicine, Oral Pathology, Oral Radiology, and Endodontics*, vol. 95, no. 1, pp. 12–15, 2003.

[17] M. Kharazmi, K. Carlson, L. Björnstad, A. Petersson, and G. Warfvinge, "Mandibular osteomyelitis associated with paroxysmal nocturnal hemoglobinuria," *International Journal of Oral and Maxillofacial Surgery*, vol. 40, no. 12, pp. 1441–1444, 2011.

[18] S. M. Khullar, D. Tvedt, K. Chapman, and B. B. Herlofson, "Sixty cases of extreme osteonecrosis and osteomyelitis of the mandible and maxilla in a West African population," *International Journal of Oral and Maxillofacial Surgery*, vol. 41, no. 8, pp. 978–985, 2012.

[19] C. Krithika, R. S. Neelakandan, B. Sivapathasundaram, D. Koteeswaran, P. C. Rajaram, and G. S. Shetkar, "Osteopetrosis-associated osteomyelitis of the jaws: a report of 4 cases," *Oral Surgery, Oral Medicine, Oral Pathology, Oral Radiology and Endodontology*, vol. 108, no. 3, pp. e56–e65, 2009.

[20] P. Goel, N. Pasricha, Sachin, A. Goel, and R. Bedi, "Osteopetrosis-A rare entity with osteomyelitis," *Annals of Maxillofacial Surgery*, vol. 1, no. 2, pp. 155–159, 2011.

[21] V. Jain, G. Pruthi, and K. Mundhe, "Clinical considerations for prosthodontic rehabilitation of intermediate form of osteopetrosis: a report of two cases," *Journal of Oral Biology and Craniofacial Research*, vol. 2, no. 2, pp. 126–130, 2012.

[22] M. H. Helfrich, "Osteoclast diseases and dental abnormalities," *Archives of Oral Biology*, vol. 50, no. 2, pp. 115–122, 2005.

[23] E. Cleiren, O. Bénichou, E. Van Hul et al., "Albers-Schönberg disease (autosomal dominant osteopetrosis, type II) results from mutations in the *ClCN7* chloride channel gene," *Human Molecular Genetics*, vol. 10, no. 25, pp. 2861–2867, 2001.

[24] M. L. Sternberg and J. R. Myer, "Osteopetrosis," *Journal of Emergency Medicine*, vol. 46, no. 6, pp. e183–e184, 2014.

[25] C. M. García, M. A. García, R. G. García, and F. M. Gil, "Osteomyelitis of the mandible in a patient with osteopetrosis," *Journal of Maxillofacial and Oral Surgery*, vol. 12, no. 1, pp. 94–99, 2013.

[26] J. M. Fullmer, W. C. Scarfe, G. M. Kushner, B. Alpert, and A. G. Farman, "Cone beam computed tomographic findings in refractory chronic suppurative osteomyelitis of the mandible," *British Journal of Oral and Maxillofacial Surgery*, vol. 45, no. 5, pp. 364–371, 2007.

[27] D. Schulze, M. Blessmann, P. Pohlenz, K. W. Wagner, and M. Heiland, "Diagnostic criteria for the detection of mandibular osteomyelitis using cone-beam computed tomography," *Dentomaxillofacial Radiology*, vol. 35, no. 4, pp. 232–235, 2006.

[28] T. Kaneda, M. Minami, K. Ozawa et al., "Magnetic resonance imaging of osteomyelitis in the mandible. Comparative study with other radiologic modalities," *Oral Surgery, Oral Medicine, Oral Pathology, Oral Radiology and*, vol. 79, no. 5, pp. 634–640, 1995.

[29] B. F. Schuknecht, F. R. Carls, A. Valavanis, and H. F. Sailer, "Mandibular osteomyelitis: evaluation and staging in 18 patients, using magnetic resonance imaging, computed tomography and conventional radiographs," *Journal of Cranio-Maxillo-Facial Surgery*, vol. 25, no. 1, pp. 24–33, 1997.

[30] R. J. Bakeman, R. A. Abdelsayed, S. H. Sutley, and R. F. Newhouse, "Osteopetrosis: a review of the literature and report of a case complicated by osteomyelitis of the mandible," *Journal of Oral and Maxillofacial Surgery*, vol. 56, no. 10, pp. 1209–1213, 1998.

[31] T. Hanada, S. Furuta, I. Moriyama, Y. Hanamure, T. Miyanohara, and M. Ohyama, "Maxillary osteomyelitis secondary to osteopetrosis," *Rhinology*, vol. 34, no. 4, pp. 242–244, 1996.

[32] D. M. Crockett, R. B. Stanley, and R. Lubka, "Osteomyelitis of the maxilla in a patient with osteopetrosis (Albers-Schönberg disease)," *Otolaryngology—Head and Neck Surgery*, vol. 95, no. 1, pp. 117–121, 1986.

[33] L. Naval, M. S. Molini, G. Herrera, and B. Naval, "Dental implants and osteomyelitis in a patient with osteopetrosis," *Quintessence International*, vol. 45, no. 9, pp. 765–768, 2014.

48

Induction Of Maturogenesis by Partial Pulpotomy: 1 Year Follow-Up

A. Bacaksiz and A. Alaçam

Department of Pediatric Dentistry, Gazi University, 06510 Ankara, Turkey

Correspondence should be addressed to A. Bacaksiz; dtayca@gmail.com

Academic Editors: K.-Y. Fu and E. Nicolas

In cariously exposed immature permanent teeth, the treatment choice is controversial in pediatric dentistry. Radical root canal treatment usually appears to be the solution for these teeth. Even partial pulpotomy is a vital treatment for traumatically exposed immature permanent teeth; extending the borders of indication towards cariously exposed immature permanent teeth with reversible pulpitis may abolish the necessity of pulpectomy. This article describes the partial pulpotomy of a cariously affected immature permanent teeth and the follow-up for 1 year. A healthy 11-year-old male patient was referred to Gazi University Faculty of Dentistry Department of Pediatric Dentistry. The patient had reversible pulpitis symptoms on teeth numbered 45. At radiographic examination, immature apex and deep caries lesion were observed and partial pulpotomy was performed by using calcium hydroxide to maintain vitality of the pulp and allow continued development of root dentin expecting the root will attain full maturity. Clinical and radiographic follow-up demonstrated a vital pulp besides not only closure of the apex (apexogenesis), but also physiologic root development (maturogenesis) after 1 year. Partial pulpotomy is an optional treatment for cariously exposed immature permanent teeth for preserving vitality and physiological root development.

1. Introduction

The treatment of cariously exposed permanent teeth should maintain an arrestment of carious process and vital pulp free of inflammation [1]. The aim of vital pulp therapy is to protect the vitality and function of the coronal or remaining radicular pulp tissue [2]. If cariously exposed teeth not treated, pulpal necrosis or periradicular lesions may occur and patients may complain about pain, swelling, or any discomfort [3]. The treatment of option can be decided due to the maturation of the teeth. In deciduous teeth the aim is maintaining the function thereby, removing the infected coronal pulp or mummifying the radicular pulp tissue are the options. In permanent teeth, the border extends and usually following a pulpectomy, obturation of the root canal system is performed.

Different factors such as trauma or caries can affect immature permanent teeth's root development and maturation. If the damage occurs including the pulp of the immature permanent teeth, the treatment becomes a challenge. It has been stated that pulpectomy is the best treatment choice to prevent and/or heal apical periodontitis [4]. It has been proved that, root canal treatment on vital teeth shows succeeding results [5, 6]. Nevertheless, the survival rate of endodontically treated teeth is not as successful as vital teeth, especially in molars (hazard ratio, 7:1) [7]. Because of that, preserving a vital pulp should be the main goal of treatment options. In cariously exposed immature permanent teeth, besides pulpectomy, vital pulp therapy is an alternative procedure because of the high healing capacity of pulp tissue in young patients [8–10]. By this procedure, while treating the reversible pulpal symptoms, the tissues remain vital and physiologic dentin deposition and root development continues. Thus, further interventional approaches such as root canal treatment may become unnecessary [11].

The overall success of vital pulp therapy mainly depends on which technique is performed, the inflammatory status of the teeth, the type of the agent which is used, the success criteria, and the period of follow-up [12].

As Cvek described in 1978 [13], partial pulpotomy is a form of vital pulp therapy that consists of the surgical amputation of 2 to 3 mm of damaged and inflamed coronal pulp tissue. After removal of the damaged tissue, a dressing agent is placed to stimulate healing and maintain vitality of the remaining pulp [14]. It has showed successful results in the treatment of complicated crown fractures (95%) [15] and in cariously exposed immature posterior, asymptomatic permanent teeth (91–93%) [16, 17].

Calcium hydroxide, has been the material of choice to stimulate dentin formation after a carious exposure of immature permanent teeth for many years [11]. Cvek has reported that partial pulpotomy and pulp capping by using calcium hydroxide in immature permanent teeth had a success rate of 96% [13]. With calcium hydroxide application, a dentine bridge will consist above the healthy pulp tissue. In the absence of a dentin bridge, the remaining pulp becomes unattached which is followed by degeneration, atrophy and shrinkage from the dentine. Therefore, a dentin bridge formation provides a physical barrier from the external factors to protect the pulp.

Not only calcium hydroxide but also mineral trioxide aggregate (MTA) has been suggested as a suitable material to be used in vital pulp therapy [18]. It has good physical characteristics and is biocompatible [19]. It also provides a good seal [20, 21] and has great marginal adaptation [22]. Moreover, it was shown in vitro that MTA did not induce apoptosis of pulp cells but instead induced proliferation of these cells [23].

The term "maturogenesis" has been used for the continued physiologic root development which is not restricted to the apical segment [24]. In this manner, the continued deposition of the root dentin provides a resistant structure against fracture. A case report is presented in which the vitality of the immature teeth maintained after performing an $Ca(OH)_2$ partial pulpotomy allowing the physiological root development.

2. Case Report

An 11-year-old Turkish boy consulted to the Gazi University Faculty of Dentistry Department of Pediatric dentistry clinic (Ankara, Turkey) with sensitivity to cold and sweets. No spontaneous pain was reported by the patient. The medical history was noncontributory. In the clinical examination gross occlusodistal caries was observed on his mandibular right second premolar (number 45) without signs of extraoral or intraoral swelling or sinus tract formation (Figure 1). The lower second premolar tested negative to percussion and palpation tests and the mobility was within the normal limits. Pulp vitality tests using electric pulp test showed a normal positive response without lingering sensation. Additionally, the adjacent teeth responded positive and within the normal limits to the electric pulp test. Radiographic examination revealed a close relation between caries and the pulp horns and undeveloped root with a wide-open apex and no evidence of periradicular pathology (Figure 2).

As a result of clinical and radiographic assessments, the pulpal status of the lower right second premolar was determined as vital with reversible pulpitis due to caries. The treatment plan included the removal of the carious lesion and clinical evaluation of the pulp exposure. Vital pulp therapy including partial pulpotomy with calcium hydroxide was planned and an informed consent was obtained from patient's father.

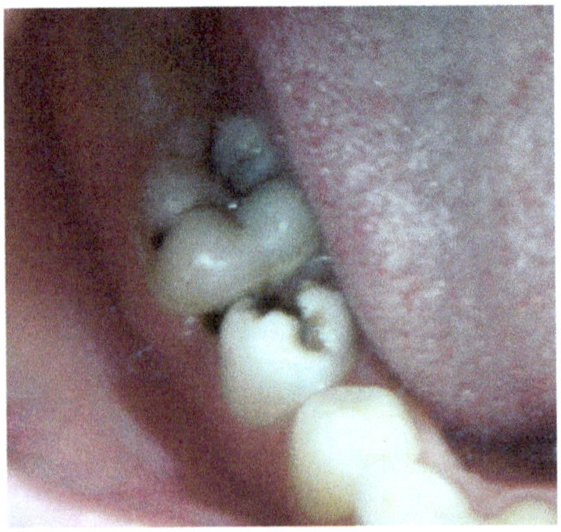

Figure 1

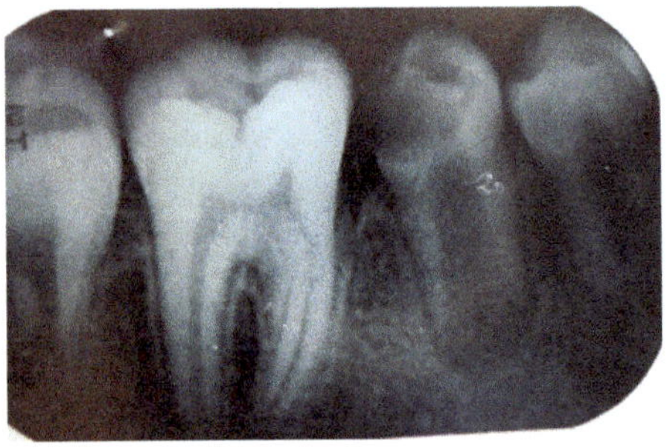

Figure 2

After local anesthesia, the tooth was cleaned with pumice and isolated with a rubber dam. Caries removal was performed with a sterile high-speed 801-016 ML diamond round bur with copious irrigation which was continued with steel round bur and exposure of pulp horns with moderate bleeding was observed. The amputation of the 2-3 mm damaged pulp was executed. The cavity was rinsed with saline and a sterile cotton pellet moistened with saline was used to apply moderate pressure to the exposed pulp for 5 min. After the homeostasis was achieved, calcium hydroxide was gently placed on the exposed pulp. A glass ionomer cement (Kavitan Pro, Spofa Dental, Czech Republic) was used as base material and the tooth was restored with amalgam (Figure 3).

The patient was scheduled for 1 month follow-up in order to assess root developmentvitality and examine any signs or symptoms. The parents were informed to call the dental clinic if the patient reported any pain or discomfort.

At the 1-month follow-up, the clinical examination showed an intact restoration and absence of any abnormal signs or symptoms. The patient reported no pain or discomfort. The tooth tested positive to the electrical pulp test and radiographic examination showed continued development of root and maturation of the root (Figure 4).

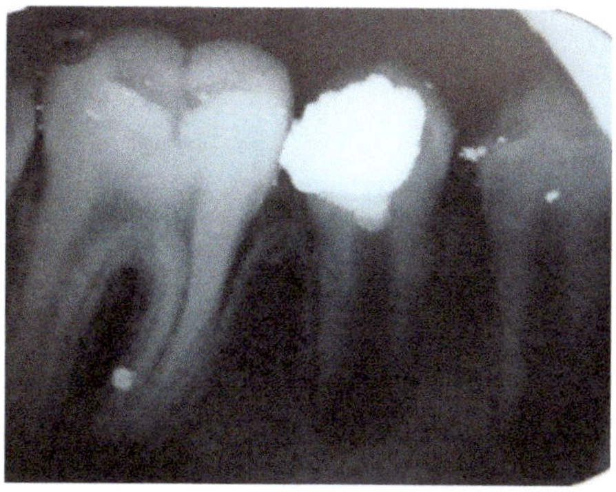

Figure 3

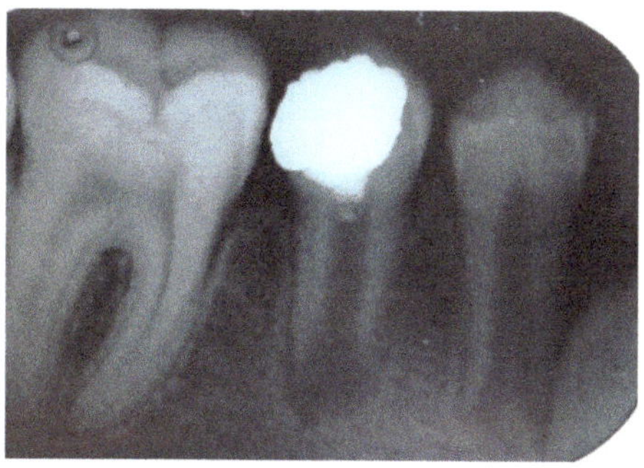

Figure 4

At 3 and 6 months, no abnormal findings were observed, and the clinical examination revealed no changes from the previous visit. The pulp continued to respond positive to the electrical pulp test. Root maturation was observed as a significant progression when compared with the preoperative radiographs (Figures 5 and 6).

The patient was reexamined 12 months after treatment began, and reported as asymptomatic. The pulp tests repeated and the tooth responded normally to the tests. A periapical radiographical assessment showed continued root development and apical closure (Figure 7). Root maturation (maturogenesis) appeared normal with no evidence of internal root resorption or pulp calcification.

3. Discussion

Recently, vital pulp therapy and regeneration of infected pulps have become an alternative treatment procedure for immature permanent teeth [25, 26]. The aim of vital pulp therapy is to protect the reversibly damaged pulp from further injuries and promote the reformation while sustaining vitality [25]. Hence, as dentin deposition continues, a more resistant and mature root will produce against fractures [27]. Zilberman et al. [28] reported that 14 of 15 deeply carious immature permanent teeth showed a vital pulp response at 12–99 months following partial pulpotomy. Mass and Zilberman [17] found successful results up to 91.4% after a minimum of 12 months, performing partial pulpotomy in the treatment of cariously exposed immature permanent molars.

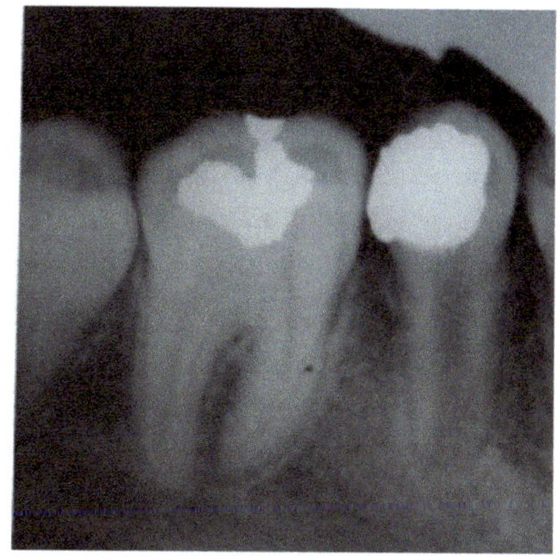

Figure 5

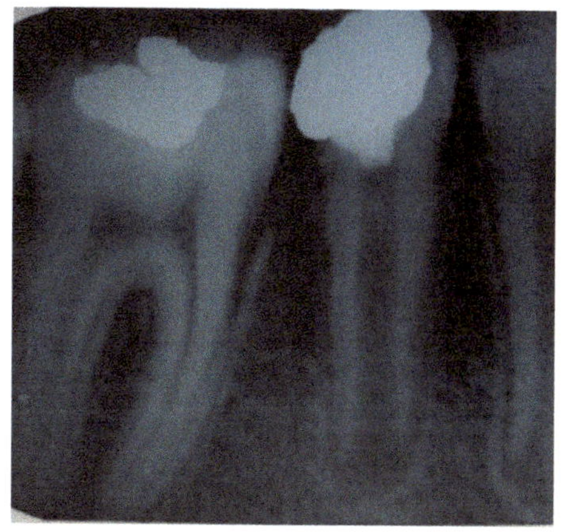

Figure 6

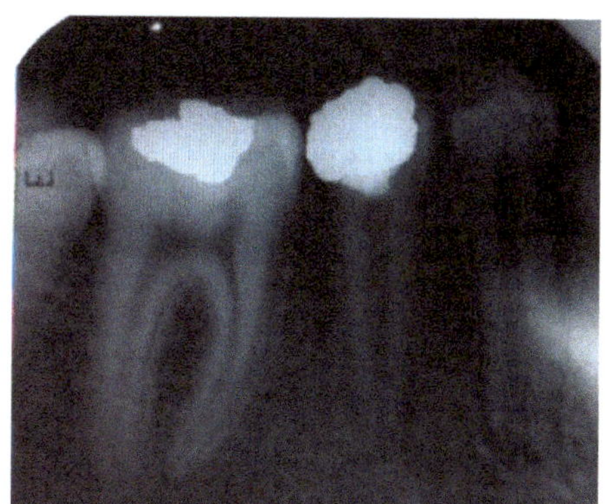

Figure 7

While deciding the treatment options of an exposed teeth, the main consideration should be the degree of infection and inflammation in the pulp, instead of the size or duration of pulp exposure [8]. In contradiction to traumatic exposures, carious can lead to evident modifications in the pulp-dentine structure. These modifications are relevant to the degree of the disease and the maturity of the pulp [29]. Therefore, the important concern should be the selection of the case and treatment planning to acquire better results [30].

Although many new agents were introduced to the market, $Ca(OH)_2$ is still a well-accepted material to stimulate dentin formation after a carious exposure of immature permanent teeth [11]. In the literature, many studies reported that partial pulpotomy of cariously exposed immature permanent teeth with calcium hydroxide have sustained a success rate of 93 [16, 17, 28]. It is still the most accessible material and dentists can perform easily in clinics. Çalişkan [2] reported twenty-six permanent vital molars with carious pulp exposures and radiographic periapical involvement were treated using a full coronal pulpotomy, with calcium hydroxide placed directly on the radicular pulp tissue once bleeding had stopped. Of these, twenty-four teeth showed resolution of radiographic periapical involvement and dentine bridge formation after 16–72 months. The presence of radiographic periapical change accompanying reversible pulpitis can be as a sequel to reversible pulpal inflammation, rather than as a direct response to an infected pulp.

Clinical and radiographical evaluations at 1, 3, 6, and 12 months showed pulpal vitality maintenance. Current vitality tests are still based on neurological inducement, and this is still a contradictory in immature teeth [12]. The radiographical assessment of periapical pathology in immature teeth is also questionable due to the normal radiolucency of the developing root.

In spite of the fact that histological success cannot be evaluated, clinical success can be assessed by the absence of any clinical or radiographic signs of failure and the substantiation of the development of the root dentin and apex closure. Thus, the patient should be recalled and reexamined periodically against any failure even if absence of visible symptoms.

The optimal choice of treatment is, to maintain vitality of an exposed pulp rather than replacing it with a root filling material. However, the technique, the type of the agent which is used, the inflammatory status of the teeth is variable and a challenge to the dentists.

In the light of the literature and this case, for cariously exposed immature permanent teeth, partial pulpotomy is an optional treatment for preserving vitality and physiological root development. In this manner, as well as a vital pulp, not only closure of the apex (apexogenesis) but also physiologic root development (maturogenesis) occurs.

References

[1] J. Ward, "Vital pulp therapy in cariously exposed permanent teeth and its limitations," *Australian endodontic journal : the journal of the Australian Society of Endodontology Inc*, vol. 28, no. 1, pp. 29–37, 2002.

[2] M. K. Çalişkan, "Pulpotomy of carious vital teeth with periapical involvement," *International endodontic journal*, vol. 28, no. 3, pp. 172–176, 1995.

[3] I. V. Nosrat and C. A. Nosrat, "Reparative hard tissue formation following calcium hydroxide application after partial pulpotomy in cariously exposed pulps of permanent teeth," *International Endodontic Journal*, vol. 31, no. 3, pp. 221–226, 1998.

[4] A. Gesi, M. Hakeberg, J. Warfvinge, and G. Bergenholtz, "Incidence of periapical lesions and clinical symptoms after pulpectomy - A clinical and radiographic evaluation of 1- versus 2-session treatment," *Oral Surgery, Oral Medicine, Oral Pathology, Oral Radiology and Endodontology*, vol. 101, no. 3, pp. 379–388, 2006.

[5] K. Kojima, K. Inamoto, K. Nagamatsu et al., "Success rate of endodontic treatment of teeth with vital and nonvital pulps. a meta-analysis," *Oral Surgery, Oral Medicine, Oral Pathology, Oral Radiology, and Endodontics*, vol. 97, no. 1, pp. 95–99, 2004.

[6] Y.-L. Ng, V. Mann, S. Rahbaran, J. Lewsey, and K. Gulabivala, "Outcome of primary root canal treatment: Systematic review of the literature - Part 2. Influence of clinical factors," *International Endodontic Journal*, vol. 41, no. 1, pp. 6–31, 2008.

[7] D. J. Caplan, J. Cai, G. Yin, and B. A. White, "Root canal filled versus non-root canal filled teeth: A retrospective comparison of survival times," *Journal of Public Health Dentistry*, vol. 65, no. 2, pp. 90–96, 2005.

[8] C. D. Fong and M. J. Davis, "Partial pulpotomy for immature permanent teeth, its present and fixture," *Pediatric Dentistry*, vol. 24, no. 1, pp. 29–32, 2002.

[9] P. Aguilar and P. Linsuwanont, "Vital pulp therapy in vital permanent teeth with cariously exposed pulp: A systematic review," *Journal of Endodontics*, vol. 37, no. 5, pp. 581–587, 2011.

[10] E. Mass, U. Zilberman, and A. B. Fuks, "Partial pulpotomy: another treatment option for cariously exposed permanent molars," *ASDC journal of dentistry for children*, vol. 62, no. 5, pp. 342–345, 1995.

[11] R. Weisleder and C. R. Benitez, "Maturogenesis: Is it a new concept?" *Journal of Endodontics*, vol. 29, no. 11, pp. 776–778, 2003.

[12] P. J. Waterhouse, J. H. Nunn, J. M. Whitworth, and J. V. Soames, "Primary molar pulp therapy - Histological evaluation of failure," *International Journal of Paediatric Dentistry*, vol. 10, no. 4, pp. 313–321, 2000.

[13] M. Cvek, "A clinical report on partial pulpotomy and capping with calcium hydroxide in permanent incisors with complicated crown fracture," *Journal of Endodontics*, vol. 4, no. 8, pp. 232–237, 1978.

[14] J. H. Camp, E. J. Barrett, and F. Pulver, "Pediatric endodontics: endodontic treatment for the primary and young permanent dentition.," in *Pathway of the Pulp*, S. B. R. Cohen, Ed., pp. 823–833, Mosby, St. Loius, Mo, USA, 8th edition, 2002.

[15] A. B. Fuks, E. Bimstein, and A. Bruchim, "Radiographic and histologic evaluation of the effect of two concentrations of formocresol on pulpotomized primary and young permanent teeth in monkeys," *Pediatric dentistry*, vol. 5, no. 1, pp. 9–13, 1983.

[16] I. Mejàre and M. Cvek, "Partial pulpotomy in young permanent teeth with deep carious lesions," *Endodontics & dental traumatology*, vol. 9, no. 6, pp. 238–242, 1993.

[17] E. Mass and U. Zilberman, "Clinical and radiographic evaluation of partial pulpotomy in carious exposure of permanent molars," *Pediatric dentistry*, vol. 15, no. 4, pp. 257–259, 1993.

[18] M. Torabinejad and N. Chivian, "Clinical applications of mineral trioxide aggregate," *Journal of Endodontics*, vol. 25, no. 3, pp. 197–205, 1999.

[19] J. Camilleri, F. E. Montesin, S. Papaioannou, F. McDonald, and T. R. Pitt Ford, "Biocompatibility of two commercial forms of mineral trioxide aggregate," *International Endodontic Journal*, vol. 37, no. 10, pp. 699–704, 2004.

[20] K. M. Barrieshi-Nusair and H. M. Hammad, "Intracoronal sealing comparison of mineral trioxide aggregate and glass ionomer," *Quintessence International*, vol. 36, no. 7-8, pp. 539–545, 2005.

[21] M. Tselnik, J. Craig Baumgartner, and J. Gordon Marshall, "Bacterial leakage with mineral trioxide aggregate or a resin-modified glass ionomer used as a coronal barrier," *Journal of Endodontics*, vol. 30, no. 11, pp. 782–784, 2004.

[22] M. Torabinejad, P. W. Smith, J. D. Kettering, and T. R. Pitt Ford, "Comparative investigation of marginal adaptation of mineral trioxide aggregate and other commonly used root-end filling materials," *Journal of Endodontics*, vol. 21, no. 6, pp. 295–299, 1995.

[23] M. Fridland and R. Rosado, "MTA solubility: A long term study," *Journal of Endodontics*, vol. 31, no. 5, pp. 376–379, 2005.

[24] D. R. Anthony and E. S. Senia, "The use of calcium hydroxide as a temporary paste fill," *Texas dental journal*, vol. 99, no. 10, pp. 6–10, 1981.

[25] D. Tziafas, A. J. Smith, and H. Lesot, "Designing new treatment strategies in vital pulp therapy," *Journal of Dentistry*, vol. 28, no. 2, pp. 77–92, 2000.

[26] F. Banchs and M. Trope, "Revascularization of immature permanent teeth with apical periodontitis: New treatment protocol?" *Journal of Endodontics*, vol. 30, no. 4, pp. 196–200, 2004.

[27] R. T. Webber, "Apexogenesis versus apexification," *Dental Clinics of North America*, vol. 28, no. 4, pp. 669–697, 1984.

[28] U. Zilberman, E. Mass, and H. Sarnat, "Partial pulpotomy in carious permanent molars," *American journal of dentistry*, vol. 2, no. 4, pp. 147–150, 1989.

[29] D. Ricketts, "Management of the deep carious lesion and the vital pulp dentine complex," *British Dental Journal*, vol. 191, no. 11, pp. 606–610, 2001.

[30] R. Patel and N. Cohenca, "Maturogenesis of a cariously exposed immature permanent tooth using MTA for direct pulp capping: A case report," *Dental Traumatology*, vol. 22, no. 6, pp. 328–333, 2006.

Permissions

All chapters in this book were first published in CRID, by Hindawi Publishing Corporation; hereby published with permission under the Creative Commons Attribution License or equivalent. Every chapter published in this book has been scrutinized by our experts. Their significance has been extensively debated. The topics covered herein carry significant findings which will fuel the growth of the discipline. They may even be implemented as practical applications or may be referred to as a beginning point for another development.

The contributors of this book come from diverse backgrounds, making this book a truly international effort. This book will bring forth new frontiers with its revolutionizing research information and detailed analysis of the nascent developments around the world.

We would like to thank all the contributing authors for lending their expertise to make the book truly unique. They have played a crucial role in the development of this book. Without their invaluable contributions this book wouldn't have been possible. They have made vital efforts to compile up to date information on the varied aspects of this subject to make this book a valuable addition to the collection of many professionals and students.

This book was conceptualized with the vision of imparting up-to-date information and advanced data in this field. To ensure the same, a matchless editorial board was set up. Every individual on the board went through rigorous rounds of assessment to prove their worth. After which they invested a large part of their time researching and compiling the most relevant data for our readers.

The editorial board has been involved in producing this book since its inception. They have spent rigorous hours researching and exploring the diverse topics which have resulted in the successful publishing of this book. They have passed on their knowledge of decades through this book. To expedite this challenging task, the publisher supported the team at every step. A small team of assistant editors was also appointed to further simplify the editing procedure and attain best results for the readers.

Apart from the editorial board, the designing team has also invested a significant amount of their time in understanding the subject and creating the most relevant covers. They scrutinized every image to scout for the most suitable representation of the subject and create an appropriate cover for the book.

The publishing team has been an ardent support to the editorial, designing and production team. Their endless efforts to recruit the best for this project, has resulted in the accomplishment of this book. They are a veteran in the field of academics and their pool of knowledge is as vast as their experience in printing. Their expertise and guidance has proved useful at every step. Their uncompromising quality standards have made this book an exceptional effort. Their encouragement from time to time has been an inspiration for everyone.

The publisher and the editorial board hope that this book will prove to be a valuable piece of knowledge for researchers, students, practitioners and scholars across the globe.

List of Contributors

Emre Yaprak
Department of Periodontology, Faculty of Dentistry, Kocaeli University, Kocaeli, Turkey

Meryem Gülce Subaşı
Department of Prosthodontics, Faculty of Dentistry, Aydın University, İzzettin Çalışlar Cad., No. 31/A, Bahçelievler, İstanbul, Turkey

Mustafa Avunduk
Department of Pathology, Meram Faculty of Medicine, Necmettin Erbakan University, Konya, Turkey

Filiz Aykent
Department of Prosthodontics, Faculty of Dentistry, Selcuk University, Konya, Turkey

Lorena Gallego
Department of Oral and Maxillofacial Surgery, Cabueñes Hospital, 33394 Gijón, Spain

Tania R. Santamarta and Luis García-Consuegra
Department of Oral and Maxillofacial Surgery, Central University Hospital, 33306 Oviedo, Spain

Verónica Blanco
Department of Pathology, Central University Hospital, 33306 Oviedo, Spain

Tommaso Cutilli
Italy Health Sciences Department, Maxillofacial Surgery Unit, University of L'Aquila, 67100, Italy

Luis Junquera
Department of Oral and Maxillofacial Surgery, Central University Hospital, 33306 Oviedo, Spain
Oral andMaxillofacial Surgery, Dental School,University ofOviedo, Catedŕatico José Serrano Street, 33009 Oviedo, Spain

Neha Jain
Department of Prosthodontics, Manav Rachna Dental College, Faridabad 121004, India

Dinesh Naitam and Ashish Dewangan
Department of Prosthodontics, Rungta College of Dental Sciences and Research, Kohka-Kurud Road, Kurud, Bhilai 490024, India

ArtiWadkar
Department of Prosthodontics, Nair Hospital Dental College, Mumbai 400008, India

Anuradha Nemane
Department of Prosthodontics, YMT Dental College, Navi Mumbai 410210, India

Shiva Katoch
Department of Prosthodontics, D.A.V. Dental College, Solan 173212, India

M. P. V. Prabhat, Chintamaneni Raja Lakshmi, N. SaiMadhavi, Sujana Mulk Bhavana and Gummadapu Sarat
Department of Oral Medicine and Radiology, Drs. Sudha and Nageswara Rao Siddhartha Institute of Dental Sciences, Gannavaram Mandal, Krishna District, Andhra Pradesh 521286, India

Kodali Ramamohan
Department of Oral and Maxillofacial Surgery, Drs. Sudha and Nageswara Rao Siddhartha Institute of Dental Sciences, Gannavaram Mandal, Krishna District, Andhra Pradesh 521286, India

Chiyadu Padmini
Department of Pedodontics and Preventive Dentistry, Malla Reddy Institute of Dental Sciences, Suraram, Zediametla, Hyderabad 500055, Andhra Pradesh, India

K. Yellamma Bai
Department of Pedodontics and Preventive Dentistry, Malla Reddy College of Dental Sciences forWomen, India

Vinil Chaitanya
Department of Oral Medicine and Radiology, Malla Reddy Institute of Dental Sciences, Suraram, Zediametla, Hyderabad 500055, Andhra Pradesh, India

M. Shilpa Reddy
Department of Conservative Dentistry and Endodontics, Malla Reddy Institute of Dental Sciences, Suraram, Zediametla, Hyderabad 500055, Andhra Pradesh, India

Marcus Stoetzer, Martin Ruecker and Nils Claudius Gellrich
Department of Oral and Maxillofacial Surgery, Hanover Medical School, Carl Neuberg-Straße 1, 30625 Hanover, Germany

Constantin von See
Department of Oral and Maxillofacial Surgery, Hanover Medical School, Carl-Neuberg-Straße 1, 30625 Hanover, Germany
Munster Military Medical Center, Munster, Germany

Christoph Kuehlhorn
Munster Military Medical Center, Munster, Germany

Dirk Ziebolz
Department of Preventive Dentistry, Periodontology and Cariology, University of Goettingen Medical Centre, Goettingen, Germany

Appasaheb Naragond
Department of Orthodontics and Dentofacial Orthopedics, P.M.N.M Dental College and Hospital, Bagalkot, Karnataka, India

Smitha Kenganal
Department of Conservative Dentistry and Endodontics, P.M.N.M Dental College and Hospital, Bagalkot, Karnataka, India

K. Rajasigamani
Department of Orthodontics and Dentofacial Orthopedics, RajahMuthiah Dental College and Hospital, Chidambaram, Tamil Nadu, India

N. Sathish Kumar
Sri Manakula Vinayagar Medical College and Hospital, Kalitheerthalkuppam, Puducherry, Tamil Nadu, India

Marília Ferreira Correia
Department of Pediatric Dentistry, Araraquara Dental School, State University of Sao Paulo, Araraquara, SP, R Humaitá 1680, 14801-903 Araraquara, SP, Brazil

Marianne Nicole Nogueira and Telma Blanca Bedran
Department of Diagnosis and Surgery, Araraquara Dental School, State University of Sao Paulo, Araraquara, SP, R Humaitá 1680, 14801-903 Araraquara, SP, Brazil

DeniseMadalena Palomari Spolidorio
Department of Physiology and Pathology, Araraquara Dental School, State University of Sao Paulo, Araraquara, SP, R Humaitá 1680, 14801-903 Araraquara, SP, Brazil

Adrianne Freire de Paula, Manoel Brito-Júnior, Alex Carvalho Quintino and Carla Cristina Camilo
Department of Dentistry, State University of Montes Claros, Avenue Rui Braga s/n, 39401-089, Montes Claros, MG, Brazil

AntônioMiranda Cruz-Filho and Manoel Damião Sousa-Neto
Department of Restorative Dentistry, Faculty of Dentistry, University of São Paulo, Avenue Bandeirantes 3900, 14040-900, Ribeirão Preto, SP, Brazil

Kavitarani Rudagi
Department of Conservative Dentistry and Endodontics, Sharad Pawar Dental College, Sawangi (Meghe), Maharashtra, Wardha, India

B. M. Rudagi
Department of Oral and Maxillofacial Surgery, Sharad Pawar Dental College, Sawangi (Meghe), Wardha, India

Sandeep Metgud and RahulWagle
Department of Conservative Dentistry and Endodontics, Rural Dental College, Pravara Institute of Medical Sciences, Loni, India

Niloufar Khodaeian
Dental Implant Research Center and Department of Prosthodontics, School of Dentistry, Isfahan University of Medical Sciences, Isfahan, Iran

Mahmoud Sabouhi
Torabinejad Dental Research Center, Department of Prosthodontics, School of Dentistry, Isfahan University of Medical Sciences, Isfahan 81746-73461, Iran

Ebrahim Ataei
Department of Restorative Dentistry, School of Dentistry, Shahid Sadoughi University of Medical Sciences, Yazd, Iran

Veena A. Patil and Manthan H. Desai
Department of Periodontology, HKES's S.Nijalingappa Institute of Dental Sciences and Research, Sedam Road, Gulbarga, Karnataka 585105, India

Veerendra S. Patil and Hanisha Reddy Kaveti
Department of Endodontics, HKES's S.Nijalingappa Institute of Dental Sciences and Research, Sedam Road, Gulbarga, Karnataka 585105, India

Kiran Kumar Ganji
Department of Periodontics, Sharad Pawar Dental College & Hospital, Sawangi MegheWardha, Maharashtra 442004, India

Prasanna M. Danappanavar
Department of Oral and Maxillofacial Pathology, MNR Dental College & Hospital, Sangareddy, Medak, Andhra Pradesh 502294, India

Inger Kjær
Department of Orthodontics, Institute of Odontology, Faculty of Health Sciences, University of Copenhagen, 20 Norre Alle, 2200 Copenhagen, Denmark

Carsten Strøm
Private Dental Practice, Lyngbyvej 133, 2100 Copenhagen, Denmark

NilsWorsaae
Department of Oral and Maxillofacial Surgery, Copenhagen University Hospital, Rigshospitalet, 2100 Copenhagen, Denmark

Ashutosh Agrawal and AditiMurari
Department of Oral Pathology and Microbiology, Institute of Dental Sciences, Uttar Pradesh, Bareilly 243006, India

Sunil Vutukuri
Department of Oral Pathology and Microbiology, Padmashree Dr. D. Y. Patil Dental College and Hospital, Nerul, Maharashtra, Navi Mumbai 400706, India

Arun Singh
Department of Oral Pathology and Microbiology, Kothiwal Dental College and Research Centre, Uttar Pradesh, Moradabad 244001, India

Esko Peltonen
Department of Oral Pathology and Oral Radiology, Institute of Dentistry, University of Turku, Lemmink¨aisenkatu 2, 20520 Turku, Finland

Jaana Rautava
Department of Oral Pathology and Oral Radiology, Institute of Dentistry, University of Turku, Lemminkäisenkatu 2, 20520 Turku, Finland
Cell Biology Program, Research Institute, Hospital for Sick Children, University of Toronto, Room 7142, 555 University Avenue, Toronto, ON, Canada M5G 1X8

Tero Soukka and Petri Nurmenniemi
Department ofOral andMaxillofacial Surgery, Institute of Dentistry,University of Turku, Lemminkäisenkatu 2, 20520 Turku, Finland

Markku Kallajoki
Department of Pathology, University of Turku, Kiinanmyllynkatu 4-8, 20520 Turku, Finland

Stina Syrjänen
Department of Oral Pathology and Oral Radiology, Institute of Dentistry, University of Turku, Lemmink¨aisenkatu 2, 20520 Turku, Finland
Department of Pathology, University of Turku, Kiinanmyllynkatu 4-8, 20520 Turku, Finland

A. P.Münevveroglu and B. B. Akgöl
Department of Pedodontics, Faculty of Dentistry, Istanbul Medipol University, Fatih, 34093 Istanbul, Turkey

Krishna Kripal, Senthil Rajan and Ipsita Jayanti
Department of Periodontology, Rajarajeswari Dental College & Hospital, Bangalore, Karnataka 560060, India

Beena Ropak
Department of Oral and Maxillofacial Surgery, Rajarajeswari Dental College & Hospital, Bangalore, Karnataka 560060, India

Aluana Dal Vechio
Department of Stomatology, School of Dentistry, University of São Paulo, 05508-900 São Paulo, SP, Brazil

Edgar Nakajima and Luciane Hiramatsu Azevedo
Laboratory for Laser in Dentistry (LELO), School of Dentistry, University of São Paulo, 05508-900 São Paulo, SP, Brazil

Décio Pinto Jr. and Dante A. Migliari
Department of Stomatology, School of Dentistry, University of São Paulo, Avenida Professor Lineu Prestes 2227, Cidade Universitária, 05508-900 São Paulo, SP, Brazil

Deepak Pandiar, Shaini Basheer, P.M. Shameena, S. Sudha and Lakshmi J. Dhana
Department of Oral and Maxillofacial Pathology, Government Dental College, Kozhikode, Kerala 673008, India

Kiran Kumar Ganji
Department of Periodontics, Sharad Pawar Dental College, Datta Meghe Institute of Medical Sciences (Deemed University), Nagpur, India

ArunKumar Bhimashankar Chakki
Department of Oral and Maxillofacial Pathology, Guru Gobind Singh College of Dental Sciences, Devi Ahilya University, Burhanpur, Indore, India

Sharanbasappa Chandrashekar Nagaral
Department of Prosthodontics, Al-badar Dental College and Hospital, Near PDA Engineering College, Rajiv Gandhi University of Health Sciences, Gulbarga, Bangalore, India

Esha Verma
Department of Periodontics, College of Dental Sciences & Hospital, Devi Ahilya University, Rau, Indore, India

Emin Murat Canger
Department of Oral and Maxillofacial Radiology, Faculty of Dentistry, Erciyes University, Melikgazi, 38039 Kayseri, Turkey

Peruze Çelenk
Department of Oral and Maxillofacial Radiology, Faculty of Dentistry, Ondokuz Mayis University, 55139 Samsun, Turkey

Enci Devrim
Department of Periodontology, Faculty of Dentistry, Ondokuz Mayis University, 55139 Samsun, Turkey

Aysun AvGar
Department of Pediatric Dentistry, Faculty of Dentistry, Ondokuz Mayis University, 55139 Samsun, Turkey

S. Venkata Suman, Raviraj Jayam, B. Vijay Kumar, Suresh Dirasantchu and Sameeulla Sk
Department of Oral Medicine and Radiology, CKS Theja Dental College, Hospital and Research Centre, Tirupati, Andhra Pradesh 517501, India

K. Venkata Suneel Kumar
Department of Oral Medicine and Radiology, Narayana Dental College and Hospital, Nellore, Andhra Pradesh 524001, India

Mehmet Fatih Fentürk
Department of Oral and Maxillofacial Surgery, Faculty of Dentistry, University of Süleyman Demirel, East Campus, 32260 C¸ ünür Isparta, Turkey

Recep Kestane and Ahmet Keskin
Department of Oral and Maxillofacial Surgery, Faculty of Dentistry, University of Ankara, Ankara, Turkey

Elif Naz Yakar
Department of Dentomaxillofacial Radiology, Faculty of Dentistry, University of Ankara, Ankara, Turkey

Hossein Aghili and Mahdjoube Goldani Moghadam
Department of Orthodontics, Faculty of Dentistry, Shahid Sadoughi University of Medical Sciences, Yazd 89195/165, Iran

Amin Rahpeyma
Oral and Maxillofacial Surgery, Oral and Maxillofacial Diseases Research Center, Faculty of Dentistry, Mashhad University of Medical Sciences, Vakilabad Boulevard, Mashhad, Iran

Seyed Hosein Hoseini Zarch
Oral and Maxillofacial Radiology, Dental Research Center, Faculty of Dentistry, Mashhad University of Medical Sciences, Vakilabad Boulevard, Mashhad, Iran

Saeedeh Khajehahmadi
Oral and Maxillofacial Pathology, Dental Research Center, Faculty of Dentistry, Mashhad University of Medical Sciences, Vakilabad Boulevard, P.O. Box 91735-984, Mashhad, Iran

Faysal Ugurlu, Coskun YJldJz, B. C. Sener and Atilla Sertgoz
Department of Oral and Maxillofacial Surgery, Dentistry Faculty, Marmara University, 34365 Istanbul, Turkey

Sunil Pendor, Vidya Baliga, A. Prasad V. Dhadse, Kiran Kumar Ganji and Kaustubh Thakare
Department of Periodontics, Sharad Pawar Dental College and Hospital, Sawangi (M),Wardha, Maharashtra 442004, India

Muthukumaraswamy
Department of Periodontics, Tamilnadu Government Dental College and Hospital, Chennai, Tamilnadu 600003, India

Biji Balan
Department of Conservative Dentistry and Endodontics, Kannur Dental College, Anjarakandy, Kannur, Kerala 670612, India

Chengappa Madanda Uthaiah
Department of Prosthodontics, Kannur Dental College, Anjarakandy, Kannur, Kerala 670612, India

Sreejesh Narayanan
DistrictHQHospital, Kannur, Kerala 670017, India

Priyadarshini Mookalamada Monnappa
Kannur Medical College, Anjarakandy, Kannur, Kerala 670612, India

Krishna Priya Vellore, Brahmananda Dutta, Sri Ram and Arun Parsa
Department of Pedodontics and Preventive Dentistry,MNR Dental College and Hospital, Andhra Pradesh, Sangareddy 502001, India

Srinivas Gadipelly and Vijay Bhaskar Reddy
Department of Oral and Maxillofacial Surgery, MNR Dental College and Hospital, Andhra Pradesh, Sangareddy 502001, India

Michael Leizerovitz and Olga Leizerovitz
UCLA School of Dentistry, 10833 Le Conte Avenue, Los Angeles, CA 90095-1668, USA

Kumar T. S.Mahesh and Peeyush Shivhare
Department of Oral Medicine and Radiology, Rajarajeswari Dental College and Hospital, Ramohalli Cross, Kumbalagodu, Mysore Road, Bangalore 560060, Karnataka, India

Indira Annamalai Ponnuswamy and Maria Priscilla David
Department ofOralMedicine and Radiology, M. R. Ambedkar Dental College and Hospital, 1/36 Cline Road, Cooke Town, Bangalore 560005, Karnataka, India

Mahalakshmi Ikkanur Puttaranganayak and Pooja Sinha
Department of Oral Medicine and Radiology, Sri Rajiv Gandhi College of Dental Science and Hospital, Chola Nagar, R. T. Nagar, Bangalore 560032, Karnataka, India

Divya Gopinath
Department of Oral Pathology & Microbiology, Government of Dental College, Calicut, Kerala 673008, India

V. T. Beena, G. Sugirtharaj, K. Vidhyadharan, K. Salmanul Faris and Sajai J. Kumar
Department of Oral & Maxillofacial Pathology, Government of Dental College, Trivandrum Kerala 695011, India

V. Nagalaxmi, Mithare Sangmesh, Kotya Naik Maloth, Srikanth Kodangal, Vani Chappidi and Stuti Goyal
Sri Sai College of Dental Surgery, H. No. 5-5-47/1, MustafaNagar, Khammam 507 001, Vikarabad, Andhra Pradesh, India

Kunio Yoshizawa, AkinoriMoroi and Koichiro Ueki
Department ofOral andMaxillofacial Surgery, Division of Medicine, Interdisciplinary Graduate School of Medical and Engineering, University of Yamanashi, 1110 Shimokato, Chuo, Yamanashi 409-3898, Japan

Shuichi Kawashiri
Department of Oral and Maxillofacial Surgery, Kanazawa University Graduate School of Medical Science, 13-1 Takaramachi, Kanazawa, Ishikawa 920-8641, Japan

D. P. Vinuth
Department of Oral Pathology and Microbiology, Hitkarini Dental College and Hospital, Jabalpur 482005, India

Poonam Agarwal
Department of Oral Medicine Diagnosis and Radiology, Hitkarini Dental College and Hospital, Jabalpur 482005, India

Gunjan Dube
Department of Oral and Maxillofacial Surgery, Hitkarini Dental College and Hospital, Jabalpur 482005, India

S. Abhilash
Department of Conservative Dentistry, Hitkarini Dental College and Hospital, Jabalpur, Madhya Pradesh 482005, India

Pallavi Dube
Dube Surgical & Dental Hospital, Jabalpur, Madhya Pradesh 482005, India

Hisashi Ozaki, Hirohiko Tachibana, Shigeo Ishikawa, Kazuyuki Yusa, Kenichirou Kitabatake and Mitsuyoshi Iino
Department of Dentistry, Oral and Maxillofacial-Plastic and Reconstructive Surgery, Faculty of Medicine, Yamagata University, 2-2-2 Iida-Nishi, Yamagata 990-9585, Japan

Vincenzo Ariano, ManueleMancini, Roberta Condò, Loredana Cerroni and Guido Pasquantonio
Department of Dental Materials, University of Rome "Tor Vergata", Viale Oxford 81, 00133 Rome, Italy

Andrea Cardi
Private Practice, Rome, Italy

Yashwant Ingale
Department of Dentistry, Yashwantrao Chavan Memorial Hospital, Pimpri, Pune 410018, India

Akhil A. Shankar
Department of Oral Pathology and Microbiology, YMT Dental College, Kharghar, Navi Mumbai, India

Samapika Routray
Department of Oral Pathology and Microbiology, Institute of Dental Sciences, SOA University, Bhubaneswar, Odisha 751003, India

Manoj Agrawal
Oral andMaxillofacial Surgeon, Talera Hospital, Pimpri, Pune 410018, India

Ajit Kadam
Department of Oral Pathology and Microbiology, Seema Dental College, Rishikesh, Uttarakhand, India

Tushar Patil
Department of Pathology, Yashwantrao Chavan Memorial Hospital, Pimpri, Pune 410018, India

Snigdha Pattanaik and SumitaMishra
Department of Orthodontics and Dentofacial Orthopaedics, Institute of Dental Sciences, Siksha 'O' Anusandhan University, Bhubaneswar, Odisha 751003, India

Bora Korkut, Funda Yanikoglu and Dilek Tagtekin
Department of Restorative Dentistry, Faculty of Dentistry, Marmara University, 34746 Istanbul, Turkey

Kenji Yamagata, Hiroki Nagai, Osamu Baba, Fumihiko Uchida, Naomi Kanno,Shogo Hasegawa, Toru Yanagawa and Hiroki Bukawa
Department of Oral and Maxillofacial Surgery, Institute of Clinical Medicine, Faculty of Medicine, University of Tsukuba, 1-1-1 Tennodai, Tsukuba, Ibaraki 305-8575, Japan

Cristina Dupim Presoto, Janaina Freitas Bortolatto, Priscila Petrucelli Freire de Carvalho, Tamara Carolina Trevisan and Osmir Batista de Oliveira Junior
Department of Restorative Dentistry, Araraquara Dental School, Universidade Estadual Paulista (UNESP), 1680 Humaitá Street, 14801-903 Araraquara, SP, Brazil

Michael Christopher Floros
Departments of Physics & Astronomy and Chemistry, Trent Centre for Biomaterials Research, Trent University, Peterborough, ON, Canada K9J 7B8

Soghra Yassaei and Mahdjoube Goldani Moghadam
Department of Orthodontics, Faculty of Dentistry, Shahid Sadoughi University of Medical Sciences, Yazd 89195/165, Iran

S. M. Ali Tabatabaei
Private Practice, Yazd 89195/165, Iran

Emma Brown
Oral Medicine Department, Bristol Dental Hospital, Lower Maudlin Street, Bristol BS1 2LY, UK

Konrad Staines
Oral Medicine Department, University of Bristol Dental School, Lower Maudlin Street, Bristol BS1 2LY, UK

Hamid RezaMozaffari and Fetemeh Rezaei
Department of Oral Medicine, School of Dentistry, Kermanshah University of Medical Sciences, Kermanshah, Iran

Roohollah Sharifi
Department of Endodontics, School of Dentistry, Kermanshah University of Medical Sciences, Kermanshah, Iran

S. GhasemMirbahari
Department of Pathology, School of Medicine, Kermanshah University of Medical Sciences, Kermanshah, Iran

Hengameh Ashraf, Payam Paymanpour and Maryam Mojtahed Bidabadi
Department of Endodontics, Shahid Beheshti University of Medical Science, Tehran, Iran

Reihaneh Hajrezai
Department of Orthodontics, Dental Branch, Islamic Azad University, Tehran, Iran

Tamer Celakil,Merve Dogan, Bilge Gokcen Rohlig, Gulumser Evlioglu and Haluk Keskin
Department of Prosthodontics, Faculty of Dentistry, Istanbul University, 34093 Istanbul, Turkey

A. Bacaksiz and A. Alaçam
Department of Pediatric Dentistry, Gazi University, 06510 Ankara, Turkey

Index